Endoscopic Endonasal Skull Base Surgery

Editor

DANIEL M. PREVEDELLO

NEUROSURGERY
CLINICS OF NORTH AMERICA

www.neurosurgery.theclinics.com

Consulting Editors
RUSSELL LONSER
ISAAC YANG

July 2015 • Volume 26 • Number 3

ELSEVIER

1600 John F. Kennedy Boulevard ● Suite 1800 ● Philadelphia, Pennsylvania, 19103-2899

http://www.theclinics.com

NEUROSURGERY CLINICS OF NORTH AMERICA Volume 26, Number 3
July 2015 ISSN 1042-3680, ISBN-13: 978-0-323-39107-8

Editor: Jennifer Flynn-Briggs
Developmental Editor: Colleen Viola

Neurosurgery Clinics of North America (ISSN 1042-3680) is published quarterly by Elsevier Inc., 360 Park Avenue South, New York, NY 10010-1710. Months of issue are January, April, July, and October. Business and Editorial Offices: 1600 John F. Kennedy Blvd., Suite 1800, Philadelphia, PA 19103-2899. Customer Service Office: 11830 Westline Industrial Drive, St. Louis, MO 63146. Periodicals postage paid at New York, NY, and additional mailing offices. Subscription prices are $380.00 per year (US individuals), $572.00 per year (US institutions), $415.00 per year (Canadian individuals), $711.00 per year (Canadian institutions), $525.00 per year (international individuals), $711.00 per year (international institutions), $185.00 per year (US students), and $255.00 per year (international and Canadian students). International air speed delivery is included in all *Clinics* subscription prices. All prices are subject to change without notice. **POSTMASTER:** Send address changes to *Neurosurgery Clinics of North America*, Elsevier Periodicals Customer Service, 11830 Westline Industrial Drive, St. Louis, MO 63146. **Customer Service: 1-800-654-2452 (US and Canada). From outside the US and Canada, call: 1-314-453-7041. Fax: 1-314-453-5170. E-mail: JournalsCustomerService-usa@elsevier.com (for print support) and journalsonlinesupport-usa@elsevier.com (for online support).**

Reprints. For copies of 100 or more, of articles in this publication, please contact the Commercial Reprints Department, Elsevier Inc., 360 Park Avenue South, New York, NY 10010-1710. Tel. 212-633-3874; Fax: 212-633-3820; E-mail: reprints@elsevier.com.

Neurosurgery Clinics of North America is covered in *MEDLINE/PubMed (Index Medicus), EMBASE/Excerpta Medica, and Current Contents/Clinical Medicine (CC/CM).*

Contributors

CONSULTING EDITORS

RUSSELL LONSER, MD
Professor and Chair, Department of
Neurological Surgery, The Ohio State
University Wexner Medical Center, Columbus,
Ohio

ISAAC YANG, MD
Attending Neurosurgeon, Assistant Professor
Department of Neurosurgery, Director of
Medical Student Education, David Geffen
School of Medicine at UCLA, Jonsson
Comprehensive Cancer Center, University
of California Los Angeles, Los Angeles,
California

EDITOR

DANIEL M. PREVEDELLO, MD
Departments of Neurological Surgery and
Otolaryngology – Head and Neck Surgery,
Wexner Medical Center, The Ohio State
University, Columbus, Ohio

AUTHORS

YAZEED ALGHONAIM, MD
Department of Otolaryngology-Head and
Neck Surgery, Mount Sinai Hospital,
University of Toronto, Toronto, Ontario,
Canada

MUHAMAD A. AMINE, MD, MS
Department of Otolaryngology, Weill Cornell
Medical College, New York–Presbyterian
Hospital, New York, New York

VIJAY ANAND, MD
Department of Otolaryngology, Weill Cornell
Medical College, New York–Presbyterian
Hospital, New York, New York

JÖRG BALDAUF, MD
Department of Neurosurgery, Ernst Moritz
Arndt University, Greifswald, Germany

LEONARDO BALSALOBRE, MD
Neurosurgical Department, São Paulo Skull
Base Center; ENT Department, São Paulo ENT
Center, Professor Edmundo Vasconcelos
Hospital, São Paulo, Brazil

GARNI BARKHOUDARIAN, MD
The Brain Tumor Center and Pituitary Disorders
Program, Providence Saint John's Health
Center, John Wayne Cancer Institute, Santa
Monica, California

PAOLO BATTAGLIA, MD
Unit of Otorhinolaryngology, Department of
Biotechnology and Life Sciences (DBSV),
Ospedale di Circolo e Fondazione Macchi,
University of Insubria; Head and Neck Surgery
& Forensic Dissection Research center
(HNS&FDRc), DBSV, University of Insubria,
Varese, Italy

ANDRÉ BEER-FURLAN, MD
Neurosurgical Department, São Paulo Skull
Base Center; DFV Neuro Neurosurgical Group,
São Paulo, Brazil

DAMIEN BRESSON, MD
Department of Neurosurgery, Hôpital
LARIBOISIERE, Assistance Publique –
Hôpitaux de Paris, Université Paris Diderot,
Paris, France

RAEWYN CAMPBELL, MD
Department of Otolaryngology–Head and Neck
Surgery, Wexner Medical Center, The Ohio
State University, Columbus, Ohio

PAOLO CAPPABIANCA, MD
Division of Neurosurgery, Department of
Neurosciences, Reproductive and
Odontostomatological Sciences, Federico II
University of Naples, Naples, Italy

RICARDO L. CARRAU, MD
Departments of Neurological Surgery and
Otolaryngology – Head and Neck Surgery,
Wexner Medical Center, The Ohio State
University, Columbus, Ohio

PAOLO CASTELNUOVO, MD
Unit of Otorhinolaryngology, Department of
Biotechnology and Life Sciences (DBSV),
Ospedale di Circolo e Fondazione Macchi,
University of Insubria; Head and Neck Surgery
& Forensic Dissection Research center
(HNS&FDRc), DBSV, University of Insubria,
Varese, Italy

LUIGI MARIA CAVALLO, MD, PhD
Division of Neurosurgery, Department of
Neurosciences, Reproductive and
Odontostomatological Sciences, Federico II
University of Naples, Naples, Italy

CARMELA CHIARAMONTE, MD
Division of Neurosurgery, Department of
Neurosciences, Reproductive and
Odontostomatological Sciences, Federico II
University of Naples, Naples, Italy

IACOPO DALLAN, MD
Head and Neck Surgery & Forensic
Dissection Research center (HNS&FDRc),
DBSV, University of Insubria, Varese,
Italy; First Otorhinolaryngologic Unit,
Azienda Ospedaliero-Universitaria Pisana,
Pisa, Italy

MICHELANGELO DE ANGELIS, MD
Division of Neurosurgery, Department of
Neurosciences, Reproductive and
Odontostomatological Sciences, Federico II
University of Naples, Naples, Italy

ORESTE DE DIVITIIS, MD
Division of Neurosurgery, Department of
Neurosciences, Reproductive and

Odontostomatological Sciences, Federico II
University of Naples, Naples, Italy

LEO F.S. DITZEL FILHO, MD
Department of Neurological Surgery, Wexner
Medical Center, The Ohio State University,
Columbus, Ohio

RICARDO L. DOLCI, MD
Department of Otolaryngology – Head and
Neck Surgery, Wexner Medical Center, The
Ohio State University, Columbus, Ohio

JEAN ANDERSON ELOY, MD, FACS
Professor and Vice Chairman, Department of
Otolaryngology - Head and Neck Surgery;
Director, Rhinology and Sinus Surgery;
Co-Director, Endoscopic Skull Base Surgery
Program, Neurological Institute of New Jersey,
Rutgers New Jersey Medical School, Newark,
New Jersey

JAMES EVANS, MD
Professor, Department of Otolaryngology –
Head and Neck Surgery; Professor,
Department of Neurological Surgery, Thomas
Jefferson University, Philadelphia,
Pennsylvania

ALEXANDER FARAG, MD
Department of Otolaryngology – Head and
Neck Surgery, Thomas Jefferson University,
Philadelphia, Pennsylvania

GIORGIO FRANK, MD
Department of Neurosurgery, Center of
Pituitary Tumors and Endoscopic Skull Base
Surgery, IRCCS Scienze Neurologiche,
Bologna, Italy

SÉBASTIEN FROELICH, MD
Department of Neurosurgery, Hôpital
LARIBOISIERE, Assistance Publique –
Hôpitaux de Paris, Université Paris Diderot,
Paris, France

FRED GENTILI, MD
Division of Neurosurgery, Toronto Western
Hospital, University of Toronto, Toronto,
Ontario, Canada

BERNARD GEORGE, MD
Department of Neurosurgery, Hôpital
LARIBOISIERE, Assistance Publique –
Hôpitaux de Paris, Université Paris Diderot,
Paris, France

LIOR GONEN, MD
Division of Neurosurgery, Toronto Western Hospital, University of Toronto, Toronto, Ontario, Canada

CHESTER F. GRIFFITHS, MD
The Brain Tumor Center and Pituitary Disorders Program, Providence Saint John's Health Center, John Wayne Cancer Institute, Santa Monica, California; Department of Otolaryngology, Pacific Eye and Ear Specialists, Los Angeles, California

ELLINA HATTAR, BA
Department of Neurological Surgery, Neurological Institute of New Jersey, Rutgers New Jersey Medical School, Newark, New Jersey

PHILIPPE HERMAN, MD
ENT Department, Hôpital LARIBOISIERE, Assistance Publique – Hôpitaux de Paris, Université Paris Diderot, Paris, France

WERNER HOSEMANN, MD
Department of Otorhinolaryngology, Ernst Moritz Arndt University, Greifswald, Germany

ALI O. JAMSHIDI, MD
Department of Neurological Surgery, Wexner Medical Center, The Ohio State University, Columbus, Ohio

DANIEL F. KELLY, MD
The Brain Tumor Center and Pituitary Disorders Program, Providence Saint John's Health Center, John Wayne Cancer Institute, Santa Monica, California

EDWARD E. KERR, MD
Department of Neurological Surgery, Wexner Medical Center, The Ohio State University, Columbus, Ohio

GEORGE KLIRONOMOS, MD, PhD
Division of Neurosurgery, Toronto Western Hospital, University of Toronto, Toronto, Ontario, Canada

JAMES K. LIU, MD, FACS, FAANS
Director, Center for Skull Base and Pituitary Surgery; Co-Director, Endoscopic Skull Base Surgery Program; Associate Professor,

Departments of Neurological Surgery and Otolaryngology-Head and Neck Surgery, Neurological Institute of New Jersey, Rutgers New Jersey Medical School, Newark, New Jersey

BJORN LOBO, MD
The Brain Tumor Center and Pituitary Disorders Program, Providence Saint John's Health Center, John Wayne Cancer Institute, Santa Monica, California

DAVIDE LOCATELLI, MD
Head and Neck Surgery & Forensic Dissection Research center (HNS&FDRc), DBSV, University of Insubria, Varese, Italy; Unit of Neurosurgery, Civic Hospital, Legnano, Italy

CARMELO MASCARI, MD
Department of Neurosurgery, Center of Pituitary Tumors and Endoscopic Skull Base Surgery, IRCCS Scienze Neurologiche, Bologna, Italy

DIEGO MAZZATENTA, MD
Department of Neurosurgery, Center of Pituitary Tumors and Endoscopic Skull Base Surgery, IRCCS Scienze Neurologiche, Bologna, Italy

ERIC MONTEIRO, MD
Department of Otolaryngology-Head and Neck Surgery, Mount Sinai Hospital, University of Toronto, Toronto, Ontario, Canada

BRADLEY A. OTTO, MD
Departments of Neurological Surgery and Otolaryngology – Head and Neck Surgery, Wexner Medical Center, The Ohio State University, Columbus, Ohio

ERNESTO PASQUINI, MD
ENT Department, Azienda USL, Bologna, Italy

DANIEL M. PREVEDELLO, MD
Departments of Neurological Surgery and Otolaryngology – Head and Neck Surgery, Wexner Medical Center, The Ohio State University, Columbus, Ohio

SHAAN M. RAZA, MD
Department of Neurosurgery, The University of Texas MD Anderson Cancer Center, Houston, Texas

MARC ROSEN, MD
Professor, Department of Otolaryngology –
Head and Neck Surgery; Professor,
Department of Neurological Surgery, Thomas
Jefferson University, Philadelphia,
Pennsylvania

HENRY W.S. SCHROEDER, MD
Department of Neurosurgery, Ernst Moritz
Arndt University, Greifswald, Germany

THEODORE H. SCHWARTZ, MD
Departments of Neurosurgery, Otolaryngology,
and Neuroscience, Weill Cornell Medical
College, New York–Presbyterian Hospital,
New York, New York

DOMENICO SOLARI, MD, PhD
Division of Neurosurgery, Department of
Neurosciences, Reproductive and
Odontostomatological Sciences, Federico II
University of Naples, Naples, Italy

ALDO C. STAMM, MD, PhD
Neurosurgical Department, São Paulo Skull
Base Center; ENT Department, São Paulo ENT
Center, Professor Edmundo Vasconcelos
Hospital, São Paulo, Brazil

MARIO TURRI-ZANONI, MD
Unit of Otorhinolaryngology, Department of
Biotechnology and Life Sciences (DBSV),
Ospedale di Circolo e Fondazione Macchi,
University of Insubria; Head and Neck Surgery
& Forensic Dissection Research center

(HNS&FDRc), DBSV, University of Insubria,
Varese, Italy

ADELAIDE VALLUZZI, MD
Department of Neurosurgery, Center of
Pituitary Tumors and Endoscopic Skull Base
Surgery, IRCCS Scienze Neurologiche,
Bologna, Italy

EDUARDO A.S. VELLUTINI, MD, PhD
Neurosurgical Department, São Paulo Skull
Base Center; DFV Neuro Neurosurgical Group,
São Paulo, Brazil

ALLAN VESCAN, MD
Department of Otolaryngology-Head and Neck
Surgery, Mount Sinai Hospital, University of
Toronto, Toronto, Ontario, Canada

GELAREH ZADEH, MD, PhD
Division of Neurosurgery, Toronto Western
Hospital, University of Toronto, Toronto,
Ontario, Canada

XIN ZHANG, MD
The Brain Tumor Center and Pituitary Disorders
Program, Providence Saint John's Health
Center, John Wayne Cancer Institute, Santa
Monica, California

MATTEO ZOLI, MD
Department of Neurosurgery, Center of
Pituitary Tumors and Endoscopic Skull Base
Surgery, IRCCS Scienze Neurologiche,
Bologna, Italy

Contents

The management of giant and large pituitary adenomas with wide intracranial extension or infrasellar involvement of nasal and paranasal cavities is a big challenge for neurosurgeons and the best surgical approach indications are still controversial. Endoscopic extended endonasal approaches have been proposed as a new surgical technique for the treatment of such selected pituitary adenomas. Surgical series coming from many centers all around the world are flourishing and results, in terms of outcomes and complications, seem encouraging. This technique could be considered a valid alternative to the transcranial route for the management of giant and large pituitary adenomas.

 Videos of the endoscopic views of a spontaneous cribriform plate defect with associated meningoencephalocele and an iatrogenic frontal sinus CSF leak accompany this article

This article presents an overview of endoscopic endonasal repair of cerebrospinal fluid (CSF) rhinorrhea. In recent years, endoscopic repair has become the standard of care for managing this condition, because it gradually replaces the traditional open transcranial approach. Discussion includes the etiologic classification of CSF rhinorrhea, management paradigm for each category, diagnosis algorithm, comprehensive description of the surgical technique, and an updated review of the literature regarding the safety and efficacy of this procedure. In addition, the authors present their experience, including 2 surgical videos demonstrating endoscopic repair of CSF rhinorrhea in two distinct clinical scenarios.

Tuberculum sellae meningiomas are challenging lesions; their critical location and often insidious growth rate enables significant distortion of the superjacent optic apparatus before the patient notices any visual impairment. This article describes the technical nuances, selection criteria, and complication avoidance strategies for the endonasal resection of tuberculum sellae meningiomas. A stepwise description of the surgical technique is presented; indications, adjuvant technologies, pitfalls and the relevant anatomy are also reviewed. Tuberculum sellae meningiomas may be safely and effectively resected through the endonasal route; invasion of the optic canals does not represent a limitation.

nuances, and complication management of the endonasal resection of skull base chondrosarcomas.

Based on the anatomic relationship between sinonasal complex and orbit, endoscopic transnasal procedures could be a smart solution for approaching the medial orbital region. These techniques should be considered a valid option for optic nerve or orbital wall decompression in cases of Graves ophthalmopathy and posttraumatic optic neuropathy as well as for addressing extraconal or intraconal lesions placed medially to the optic nerve course. This article describes the anatomic principles, indications, technical nuances, and limitations of the endoscopic endonasal approaches for the management of selected orbital pathologic abnormalities.

The surgical management of trigeminal schwannomas (TNs) entails the use of a variety of cranial base approaches for their effective surgical management. Although an extended middle fossa or posterior petrosal approach may be more appropriate for disease with primarily posterior fossa involvement, the expanded endoscopic approaches are suited for tumors with predominately middle fossa and/or extracranial involvement along the V2 and V3 divisions and limited posterior fossa extension. The endoscopic endonasal resection of TNs within the middle fossa, pterygopalatine fossa, and infratemporal fossa is reviewed in this article with a brief discussion of reported outcomes.

NEUROSURGERY CLINICS OF NORTH AMERICA

THE CLINICS ARE AVAILABLE ONLINE!
Access your subscription at:
www.theclinics.com

NEUROSURGERY CLINICS OF NORTH AMERICA

Preface

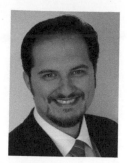

Daniel M. Prevedello, MD
Editor

Immediately following its introduction, expanded endonasal approaches to intracranial lesions faced substantial criticism due to their high risk of postoperative cerebrospinal fluid (CSF) leak and the perceived risk of intracranial infection with sinonasal flora. Progressive development of the technique, led by multiple pioneering centers around the world, reduced these pertinent concerns. We are approaching the 10th anniversary of the pedicled nasoseptal flap, which was quickly adopted worldwide and dramatically reduced postoperative CSF leak rates, making the technique reliable and reproducible. Furthermore, the apprehension regarding high rates of postoperative infection proved to be unfounded. Consequently, endoscopic endonasal approaches (EEAs) to address intracranial diseases became a viable alternative to traditional approaches.

Technical feasibility should not be the only motivation to continue doing EEA skull-base surgery. Often a ventral approach to the skull base allows for direct access to pathologic abnormality, minimizing or eliminating the need for manipulation of neurovascular structures compared with open approaches. In many instances, EEAs transform skull-base tumors into "convexity tumors," as they share the same surgical strategy. For example, in the case of a midline skull-base meningioma, the tumor origin is reached early in the surgery, and its blood supply is interrupted before the tumor is exposed. Most or even all involved dura can be removed. The nearly avascular tumor may be centrally debulked to facilitate its extracapsular resection, which is done using standard principles of bimanual dissection and microsurgical technique.

Over the last decade, as more centers are performing EEAs, we are discovering that the initial impressions of EEA's pioneers were correct: that EEAs can offer comparable resection rates while offering, in appropriately selected cases, the potential to minimize morbidity when compared with traditional approaches. Conversely, it is clear that EEAs cannot replace traditional skull-base approaches in every instance; therefore, surgeons should strive to be facile with both open and endonasal techniques to provide the safest, most efficient means to address specific clinical situations.

I thank all my colleagues who contributed articles to this work not only for their efforts hereby presented but also for all their previous contributions to establish and refine EEA for the benefit of our patients.

Daniel M. Prevedello, MD
Departments of Neurological Surgery, and
Otolaryngology
and Head & Neck Surgery
Wexner Medical Center
The Ohio State University
Columbus, OH 43210, USA

E-mail address:
Daniel.Prevedello@osumc.edu

Neurosurg Clin N Am 26 (2015) xiii
http://dx.doi.org/10.1016/j.nec.2015.05.001
1042-3680/15/$ – see front matter © 2015 Published by Elsevier Inc.

Endoscopic Endonasal Extended Approaches for the Management of Large Pituitary Adenomas

 CrossMark

Paolo Cappabianca, MD, Luigi Maria Cavallo, MD, PhD,
Oreste de Divitiis, MD, Michelangelo de Angelis, MD,
Carmela Chiaramonte, MD, Domenico Solari, MD, PhD*

KEYWORDS

- Transsphenoidal surgery • Extended approach • Pituitary adenoma • Giant adenoma
- Endoscopic endonasal surgery

KEY POINTS

- The endoscopic endonasal approach is a valuable treatment of large and giant adenomas.
- The extended approach gives the opportunity to access pituitary lesions via a double corridor (ie, intracapsular and extracapsular).
- The reconstruction of the osteodural defect is mandatory for extended approach.

INTRODUCTION

Among all the intracranial tumors, pituitary adenomas represent the third most common lesion, with a prevalence of 16.9% in autopsy studies.[1] The management of these lesions can become particularly challenging especially in those classified as large or giant and with wide intracranial extension or prevalent inferior involvement down into the nasal and paranasal cavities.[2,3] Adenoma can be defined as "giant" if the maximum diameter is bigger than 4 cm, but there is no consensus about the definition of large pituitary adenomas.[3–8] The conventional transcranial approach has been traditionally the first choice for the removal of large intracranial adenomas, because of limited visualization beyond the sella provided by microscopic transsphenoidal approaches.[9] The improved visualization gained with the introduction of the endoscope, adopted over the past two decades for the treatment of pituitary adenomas and other sellar lesions, has opened the possibility of removing lesions that grow considerably beyond the sella, thus greatly increasing the number of tumors being approached via the transsphenoidal route.[2,3] Although in many neurosurgical centers worldwide endoscopic approaches are now routinely used in clinical practice,[10–16] there are still some controversies concerning the safety and effectiveness of approaching large and giant pituitary adenomas via an endoscopic endonasal approach.

INDICATIONS

Pituitary adenomas are a heterogeneous group of lesions. According to the biologic, endocrinologic, and pathologic viewpoint, the main goal of surgery for the removal of giant or large lesions should be, regardless of the hormonal status, relief of mass effect, preservation or restoration of normal neurologic function, and decompression of the pituitary gland to improve or preserve residual hormonal

Division of Neurosurgery, Department of Neurosciences, Reproductive and Odontostomatological Sciences, Federico II University of Naples, Naples, Italy
* Corresponding author. Division of Neurosurgery, Department of Neurosciences, Reproductive and Odontostomatological Sciences, Università degli Studi di Napoli Federico II, Via Pansini 5, Naples 80131, Italy.
E-mail address: domenico.solari@unina.it

Neurosurg Clin N Am 26 (2015) 323–331
http://dx.doi.org/10.1016/j.nec.2015.03.007
1042-3680/15/$ – see front matter © 2015 Elsevier Inc. All rights reserved.

function. The extended endonasal transsphenoidal approach has become well established in a conspicuous number of centers, and it is adopted with expanding indications for a variety of midline skull-base lesions.[2,17–34]

The transtuberculum/transplanum approach has been introduced during the last decade to address selected midline suprasellar lesions, such as craniopharyngiomas, Rathke cleft cysts, or tuberculum sellae meningiomas.[35] Currently, several authors[10–16] report on pituitary adenomas series treated with such an extended approach, thus expanding the indications for endonasal resection of these lesions, especially for those tumors with a prevalent intracranial extension.[11] Nowadays, it is possible to use extended endonasal approaches for dumbbell-shaped adenomas, pure suprasellar adenomas or adenomas whose suprasellar component fails to descend within the sella after sellar debulking, adenomas extended over the tuberculum or planum sphenoidale, giant symmetric or asymmetric adenomas, or adenomas invading the cavernous sinuses (**Figs. 1–3**). However, we should conceive an "extended approach" not only targeted to suprasellar or parasellar regions: an infrasellar variation of the technique with a wider removal of nasal structures allows the surgeon to obtain an easier removal of those lesions with a prevalent extracranial extension, such as adenomas invading the whole sphenoid sinus cavity, with erosion of the clivus or extension to the pterygoid fossa or the nasal cavities (**Table 1**).

At our institution the endoscopic endonasal route, with either standard or extended variations, is adopted as first choice in almost all the cases of pituitary adenomas, regardless of the most relevant features (ie, size and shape).[36] However, it is worth reminding that the transcranial route is reserved for those tumors showing a significant lateral intracranial extension that results from the visibility and maneuverability of the endoscopic endonasal route; in this regard, we respect the policy suggested by Kassam and colleagues[37,38] of adopting a transcranial approach in case of vascular encroachment or to avoid crossing the plane of cranial nerves.

Although the surgeon should always attempt the maximum-allowed tumor surgical removal, it is important to keep in mind the wide variety of different treatment options (medical, surgical, radiotherapy, and radiosurgery) that are currently effective in terms of long-term results. The surgeon should focus the goal of surgery to the patient's needs, selecting the best option for the actual condition of the patient among all the available options.[36]

SURGICAL TECHNIQUE
Preoperative Planning

The preoperative planning for a binostril endoscopic endonasal extended approach involves

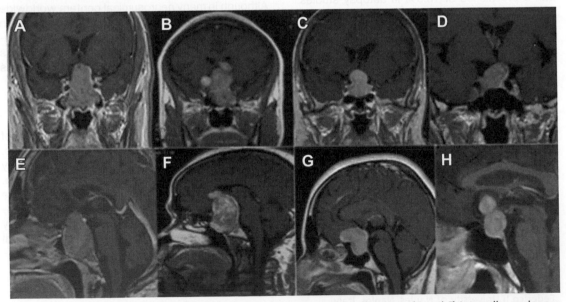

Fig. 1. MRI showing the different growth pathways of giant pituitary adenomas. (*A* and *E*) Intrasellar and suprasellar pituitary adenoma with erosion of the sellar floor and extension into the sphenoidal sinus with invasion of its lateral recesses. (*B* and *F*) Asymmetric giant pituitary adenoma with intracranial extension up to the third ventricle. (*C* and *G*) Intrasellar and suprasellar pituitary adenoma with extension into the anterior cranial fossa. (*D* and *H*) Sand-glass–shaped pituitary adenoma.

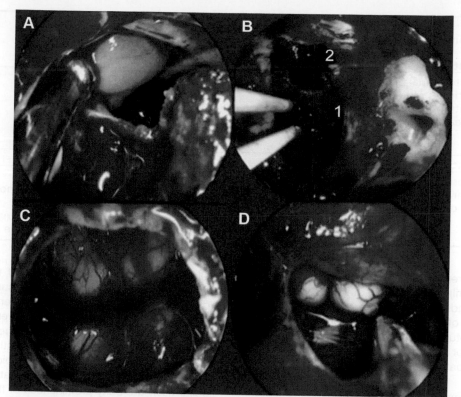

Fig. 2. (*A*) Intraoperative imaging showing the surgical removal of the suprasellar portion of a large adenoma. (*B*) Surgical cavity after adenoma removal. It is possible to see the double intracapsular and extracapsular corridor (1, intracapsular corridor; 2, extracapsular corridor). (*C* and *D*) Close-up view of suprasellar and retrosellar space after the extracapsular removal of the suprasellar portion of two different large adenomas.

several experts working as a team. The neuroradiologist, the endocrinologist, the ophthalmologist, the ear-nose-throat surgeon, and the anesthesiologist work with the neurosurgeon to define the

right indication for each case and weigh in on each aspect of the multidisciplinary management for pituitary adenoma surgery.

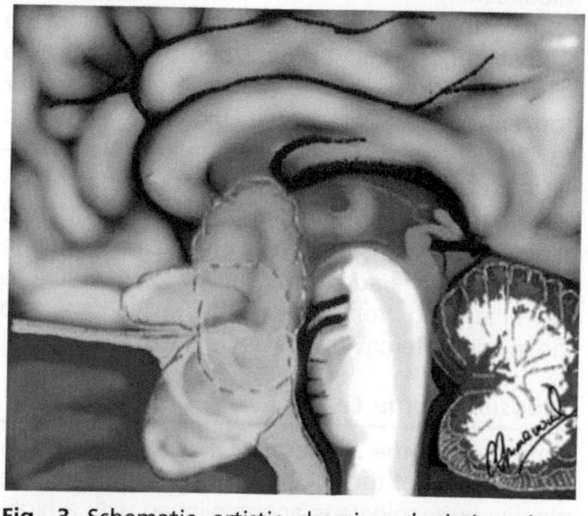

Patient Positioning

Extended transsphenoidal approaches may require the use of a three-point Mayfield-Kees headrest to allow the use of the neuronavigation system. The patient is supine and, depending on the surgical target area, the head is extended about 10° to 20° to achieve a more anterior trajectory (as for planum sphenoidale or olfactory groove approach) or is slightly flexed in case of downward extension of the adenoma. The position should avoid the impinging of the patient's thorax with either the endoscope and/or the surgical instruments.

Nasal Disinfection and Decongestion

Using a small Killian-type nasal speculum, cotton pledgets soaked in 3.5% polyvidone-iodine solution are placed for approximately 5 minutes along the floor of the nasal cavities and in between the nasal septum and the middle turbinate. The cotton pledgets soaked with polyvidone-iodine solution

Fig. 3. Schematic artistic drawing depicting three different patterns of growth of large and giant pituitary adenomas. (*Courtesy of* Carmela Chiaramonte, MD, Napoli, Italy.)

Table 1
Indications for extended approach for pituitary adenomas according to tumor features

Prevalent intracranial extension	
Often intentional extracapsular dissection is required	Dumbbell-shaped adenomas
	Pure suprasellar adenomas
Often intraoperative cerebrospinal fluid leak is present	Adenomas extended over the tuberculum or planum sphenoidale
	Giant symmetric adenomas
	Giant asymmetric adenomas
Prevalent extracranial extension	
Extracapsular resection is rarely necessary	Adenomas with cavernous sinuses invasion
Intraoperative cerebrospinal fluid leak rarely occurs	Giant adenomas involving the whole sphenoid cavity including the lateral recesses
	Giant adenomas involving sphenoid sinus, nasal and paranasal cavities, and/or other skull-base areas

are then removed and eight cotton pledgets (four per nostril) soaked in a decongestant solution (2 mL of adrenaline, 5 mL of 20% diluted lidocaine, and 4 mL of saline solution) are placed between the nasal septum and the middle turbinate. They are left in place for approximately 15 minutes, during which time the patient is prepared with sterile draping.

Nasal Step

The endoscope is introduced into the right nostril to identify the inferior turbinate laterally and the nasal septum medially, with the head of the middle turbinate slightly behind and superiorly. The gently lateral dislocation of the middle turbinate protected with a cottonoid allows enlargement of the working space and creation of an adequate surgical pathway; often the middle turbinate of the left nostril is removed. The endoscope is then moved further to identify the choana and the sphenoethmoid recess with the sphenoid ostium. The mucosa that covers the anterior wall of the sphenoid sinus is dissected, preserving the septal branch of the sphenopalatine artery, which is important in case there is a need to harvest the nasoseptal flap.[39] The nasal septum is then detached with the microdrill from the sphenoid bone and the anterior wall of the sphenoid sinus is exposed.

Sphenoid Step

The anterior sphenoidotomy is performed using a microdrill or bone punches, paying particular attention in the inferolateral direction, where the sphenopalatine artery or its major branches lie. Thereafter the corridor is enlarged with removal of the superior and/or the supreme turbinates and the opening of the posterior othmoid cells. The wide opening of the anterior wall of the sphenoid sinus is a key point during surgery, because it

allows the proper maneuverability of the instruments and avoids having debris obscure the lens during in-and-out endoscope movements.

The identification of septa and their removal permits identification and exposure of the anatomic features inside the sphenoid cavity with the sellar floor at the center, the planum sphenoidale above it, and the clival indentation below; lateral to the sellar floor, the bony prominences of the intracavernous carotid artery (ICA) and the optic canals can be seen with respective optocarotid recess between them bilaterally. In those cases when the identification of all these landmarks is not possible because of minimal pneumatization, the ICA protuberance, the planum sphenoidale, and the clival indentation allow some orientation to define the position of the sella; in patients with a presellar or a conchal sphenoid sinus, the use of an image guidance system helps in preventing misdirection.

From this point a second surgeon holds the endoscope, so that the first can work with two instruments through one or both nostrils, as per conventional microsurgery. Once the sphenoid cavity is exposed and all the landmarks are recognized, according to the anatomic conditions of the sellar floor (intact, eroded, or thinned), it is opened in different ways as required by the volume and the extension of the adenoma, usually from an ICA to the other and from tuberculum sellae down to the inferior intercavernous sinus.

Exposure of the Lesion

Approach to the suprasellar area

The removal of the tuberculum sellae and of the planum sphenoidale is accomplished with a high-speed drill, whereas a thin footplate Kerrison rongeur helps to refine and flatten the bone edges. The opening can be extended in anterior direction up to

1.5 to 2 cm, minding not to extend beyond the anterior wall of the sphenoid sinus. Laterally, the protuberances of the optic nerves define the limits: at the level of the tuberculum sellae these latter are distant about 14 mm, whereas they diverge anteriorly after piercing the optic canal; thus the opening of the planum has the shape of a trapezium, with the smaller base posteriorly. On dural opening, the adenoma removal starts from the inferior and the lateral aspects to avoid the premature descent of the redundant diaphragm; this event indeed could obscure the vision of the lateral or posterior portion of the lesion, thus reducing the chance of a radical removal. The suprasellar aspect of the lesion is then debulked and its capsule is separated from the distended pituitary gland. However, giant pituitary adenomas often spread to the subarachnoid space, so it is dissected from the surrounding neurovascular structures, using microscissors and sharp dissection from arachnoid, as in a conventional microsurgical approach. This extended variation gives the advantage of a double surgical corridor for the management of the suprasellar portion of the lesion: the first, intracapsular, allows the debulking of the adenoma; the second, extracapsular, permits the dissection of the capsule from the surrounding neurovascular structures (see **Fig. 2**).[11]

At the end, the use of angled endoscopes (30° or 45°) allows the visualization of blind corners, permitting recognition of eventual tumor remnants. This is of utmost importance, especially in the case of giant adenomas with prevalent intracranial extension, because of the high risk of intralesional hemorrhage of the residual tumor, which often results in severe complications, seldom to death.

Approach to the cavernous sinus

In case of adenomas extending into the cavernous sinus, two different surgical corridors can be used to gain access to different areas of the cavernous sinus, as related to the position of the ICA: one permits access to a compartment medial to the ICA, whereas the other allows access to a cavernous sinus compartment lateral to it. The first approach is indicated for pituitary adenomas projecting through the medial wall of the cavernous sinus. The tumor itself enlarges the C-shaped parasellar segment of the internal carotid artery, thus making easier suctioning and curettage through this corridor. The approach to the lateral compartment of the cavernous sinus is indicated in case of tumors involving the entire cavernous sinus (ie, grade 4 Knosp adenomas).[40] Such tumors, occupying mainly the lateral compartment of the cavernous sinus, usually displace the ICA medially and push the cranial nerves laterally. The exposure of these lesions can be gained by enlarging the

corridor, flattening the pterygoid process and the bone enclosed between the vidian canal and the foramen rotundum, at the level of the anterior wall of the sphenoid sinus.[41] These maneuvers allow the exposure of the pterygoid fossa, thus making possible the removal of adenomas invading this area and along their growth path inside the cavernous sinus.[41] Delicate maneuvers of curettage and suction usually allow the removal of the parasellar portion of the lesion, in the same fashion as for the intrasellar portion, because usually the oculomotor nerves are pushed in a lateral direction by the adenoma.

Approach to the nasal and paranasal cavities

When extended into the nasal or paranasal cavities, giant adenomas have to be approached via a lower trajectory. The surgical approach has to be tailored to the extension of the lesion, so that some nasal and or paranasal structures have to be removed to improve the width of the surgical field and the maneuverability of surgical instruments.

If the adenoma extends downward, eroding the clivus and down to the rhinophariynx, it is important to remove the prow and the floor of the sphenoid sinus; if the whole sphenoid sinus is invaded, it is necessary to remove the posterior portion of the nasal septum, whereas to approach a lesion invading the lateral recess of the sinus the medial pterygoid process needs to be flattened to access this area.

Reconstruction

In case of giant adenomas with a prevalent downward extension, the reconstruction does not require peculiar strategies, especially when the suprasellar cistern (this latter has to be protected) has not been violated. However, when the suprasellar cistern has been opened, the reconstruction of the osteodural breach with a multilayer technique is required.[42,43] When performing the reconstruction after removal of giant adenomas with predominant intracranial extension, the same technique already described for craniopharingiomas or tuberculum sellae meningiomas is used; the pedicled nasoseptal flap and the lumbar drainage can be used to ensure a better result.[39,42,44] Recently, we adopted the "sandwich technique": the surgical cavity is filled with fat sutured to the inner layer of a three-layer foil of fascia lata or dural substitute; the first layer is positioned intradurally, the second between the dura and the bone, and the third outside to cover the bone. A vascular flap of septal mucosa[39,45] is used to cover the skull base defect and a moderate inflated Foley balloon catheter is then placed in the sphenoid sinus to support the reconstruction.[42,46–48]

Table 2
Complications and corresponding management strategies

Complications	Management
Cerebrospinal Fluid leak	Reoperation for reconstruction
Infections	Antibiotics
Intracranial hemorrhage	Reoperation for evacuation
Chiasm, optic and oculomotor nerves injury	Corticosteroid therapy
ICA injury	Intraoperative sphenoidal packing, angiography, stent positioning, or embolization
Tensive pneumocephalus	Computed tomography scan, bed rest, hydration therapy
Bleeding from the mucosal branches of the sphenopalatine artery	Nasal packing or reoperation with coagulation of the sphenopalatine artery
Sinusitis and mucocele	Aerosol therapy, reoperation when symptomatic
Anterior pituitary deficiency	Hormonal replacement
Diabetes insipidus (transient or permanent)	Medical therapy (vasopressine)

OUTCOMES AND COMPLICATIONS

According to the pertinent literature, the extended endoscopic endonasal approach for the removal of giant and large pituitary adenomas has shown encouraging outcomes in terms of extent of removal, postoperative visual function, and complication rates. Analyzing the main series,[10–16] the most intriguing data are represented by the improvement of visual function reported in 82% of cases. However, cerebrospinal fluid leakage still represents the most frequent and feared complication of this approach, although its rate is decreasing.[38] Data concerning results and complications of the recent surgical series are summarized in **Tables 2–4**.

Table 3
Outcomes of main series of extended endoscopic endonasal approaches for pituitary adenomas

Author, Year	Number of Patients	Extent of Removal			Preoperative Visual Defect (Number of Patients)	Visual Function		
		GTR	STR	PR		Improved	Unchanged	Worsened
De Paiva Neto et al,[16] 2010	51	41.2%	58.8%	0%	38	81.6%	0%	0%
Nakao & Itakura,[15] 2011	43	47%	53%	0%	43	97.7%	2.3%	0%
Zhao et al,[14] 2010	126	61.9%	34.1%	3.9%	104	93.3%	2.8%	3.8%
Di Maio et al,[13] 2011	20	60%	30%	5%	14	85.7%	7.1%	7.1%
Koutourousiou et al,[12] 2013	54	20.4%	46.3%	33.3%	45[a]	80%	13.3%	4.4%
Gondim et al,[11] 2014	50	38%	18%	44%	50	76%	22%	2%
Juraschka et al,[10] 2014	66[b]	24.2%	16.7%	58.9%	33	61.8%	38.2%	0%

Abbreviations: GTR, gross total removal; PR, partial removal; STR, subtotal removal.
[a] In one patient who presented with visual impairment, postoperative visual examination was not available.
[b] Preoperative and postoperative MRI were available in 66 patients.
Data from Refs.[10–16]

Table 4
Complications of main series of extended endoscopic endonasal approaches for pituitary adenomas

Author, Year	Number of Patients	CSF Leak	Sinusitis	SIADH	Epistaxis	Meningitis	Hydrocephalus	Hematoma	Transient CN Palsy	Permanent DI	Pulmonary Embolism	Apoplexy of Residual Tumor	Respiratory Failure	TIA Hemiparesis	New Pituitary Deficit	Rupture of ICA	Nasal Septum Perforation
De Paiva Neto et al,[16] 2010	51	1.9%	5.8%	0%	0%	0%	0%	3.9%	0%	9.8%	3.9%	0%	0%	1.9%	13.7%	0%	0%
Nakao & Itakura,[15] 2011	43	0%	0%	0%	0%	0%	0%	0%	0%	0%	0%	0%	0%	0%	4.6%	0%	0%
Zhao et al,[14] 2010	126	5.5%	0%	0%	0%	0%	0%	0%	3.9%	0.79%	0%	0%	0%	0%	3.9%	1.58%	1.58%
Di Maio et al,[13] 2011	20	5%	0%	0%	0%	0%	0%	0%	0%	0%	0%	0%	0%	0%	15%	0%	0%
Koutourousiou et al,[12] 2013	54	16.6%	0%	3.7%	0%	5.5%	0%	0%	11.1%	9.2%	5.5%	3.7%	3.7%	1.8%	16.6%	0%	0%
Gondim et al,[11] 2014	50	8%	0%	0%	6%	2%	0%	0%	0%	10%	0%	0%	0%	0%	36%	0%	0%
Juraschka et al,[10] 2014	73	9.6%	13.7%	4.1%	2.7%	2.7%	2.7%	0%	0%	0%	0%	0%	0%	0%	7.4%	0%	0%

Abbreviations: CN, cranil nerve; CSF, cerebrospinal fluid; DI, diabetes insipidus; SIADH, syndrome of inappropriate antidiuretic hormone secretion; TIA, transient ischemic attack.
Data from Refs.[10–16]

SUMMARY

Surgical decompression of cerebrovascular structures, especially the optic apparatus, and control of disease progression are the main goals of surgery, particularly when approaching giant pituitary adenomas with frank intracranial extension. Although a complete removal of the tumor without recurrence is desirable, a subtotal resection accomplishing the aforementioned goals sometimes can be well accepted. Along with the widespread use of endoscopic transsphenoidal surgery for pituitary adenomas, its progress and refinements have permitted expansion of its indications. The resection of large and giant pituitary adenomas performed via an endoscopic endonasal approach provides reasonable resection rates, favorable clinical outcomes, and acceptably low complication rates. The indications for this route must be carefully evaluated and tailored to each case, according to lesion inner features. Sometimes it is reasonable to accept a near-total resection. Subtotal resection with decompression of the optic apparatus can be an acceptable result, especially for those patients with severe comorbidities or in elderly patients, where progression of residual tumor is not as relevant as in younger patients.

Cerebrospinal fluid leak rate continues to decrease with the use of vascularized nasoseptal flap and the refinement of the reconstruction techniques. The complications and removal rate of extended endonasal transsphenoidal approach for large and giant pituitary adenomas seem to be similar to those reported for transcranial approaches. For these reasons, the extended endoscopic approach can be considered a valid option in the management of large and giant pituitary adenomas.

REFERENCES

1. Ezzat S, Asa SL, Couldwell WT, et al. The prevalence of pituitary adenomas: a systematic review. Cancer 2004;101(3):613–9.
2. Cappabianca P, Cavallo LM, Esposito F, et al. Extended endoscopic endonasal approach to the midline skull base: the evolving role of transsphenoidal surgery. Adv Tech Stand Neurosurg 2008;33:151–99.
3. Cusimano MD, Kan P, Nassiri F, et al. Outcomes of surgically treated giant pituitary tumours. Can J Neurol Sci 2012;39(4):446–57.
4. Garibi J, Pomposo I, Villar G, et al. Giant pituitary adenomas: clinical characteristics and surgical results. Br J Neurosurg 2002,10(2):100–0.
5. Goel A, Nadkarni T, Muzumdar D, et al. Giant pituitary tumors: a study based on surgical treatment of 118 cases. Surg Neurol 2004;61(5):436–45 [discussion: 445–6].
6. Jane JA Jr, Laws ER Jr. The surgical management of pituitary adenomas in a series of 3,093 patients. J Am Coll Surg 2001;193(6):651–9.
7. Laws ER, Jane JA Jr. Neurosurgical approach to treating pituitary adenomas. Growth Horm IGF Res 2005;15(Suppl A):S36–41.
8. Mohr G, Hardy J, Comtois R, et al. Surgical management of giant pituitary adenomas. Can J Neurol Sci 1990;17(1):62–6.
9. Sinha S, Sharma BS. Giant pituitary adenomas–an enigma revisited. Microsurgical treatment strategies and outcome in a series of 250 patients. Br J Neurosurg 2010;24(1):31–9.
10. Juraschka K, Khan OH, Godoy BL, et al. Endoscopic endonasal transsphenoidal approach to large and giant pituitary adenomas: institutional experience and predictors of extent of resection. J Neurosurg 2014;121(1):75–83.
11. Di Maio S, Cavallo LM, Esposito F, et al. Extended endoscopic endonasal approach for selected pituitary adenomas: early experience. J Neurosurg 2011;114(2):345–53.
12. Koutourousiou M, Gardner PA, Fernandez-Miranda JC, et al. Endoscopic endonasal surgery for giant pituitary adenomas: advantages and limitations. J Neurosurg 2013;118(3):621–31.
13. Gondim JA, Almeida JP, Albuquerque LA, et al. Giant pituitary adenomas: surgical outcomes of 50 cases operated on by the endonasal endoscopic approach. World Neurosurg 2014;82(1–2):e281–90.
14. Zhao B, Wei YK, Li GL, et al. Extended transsphenoidal approach for pituitary adenomas invading the anterior cranial base, cavernous sinus, and clivus: a single-center experience with 126 consecutive cases. J Neurosurg 2010;112(1):108–17.
15. Nakao N, Itakura T. Surgical outcome of the endoscopic endonasal approach for non-functioning giant pituitary adenoma. J Clin Neurosci 2011;18(1):71–5.
16. de Paiva Neto MA, Vandergrift A, Fatemi N, et al. Endonasal transsphenoidal surgery and multimodality treatment for giant pituitary adenomas. Clin Endocrinol (Oxf) 2010;72(4):512–9.
17. Ceylan S, Koc K, Anik I. Endoscopic endonasal transsphenoidal approach for pituitary adenomas invading the cavernous sinus. J Neurosurg 2010; 112(1):99–107.
18. Couldwell WT, Weiss MH, Rabb C, et al. Variations on the standard transsphenoidal approach to the sellar region, with emphasis on the extended approaches and parasellar approaches: surgical experience in 105 cases. Neurosurgery 2004;55(3):539–50.
19. de Divitiis E, Cappabianca P, Cavallo LM. Endoscopic transsphenoidal approach: adaptability of the procedure to different sellar lesions. Neurosurgery 2002; 51(3):699–705 [discussion: 705–7].

20. Dusick JR, Esposito F, Kelly DF, et al. The extended direct endonasal transsphenoidal approach for non-adenomatous suprasellar tumors. J Neurosurg 2005;102(5):832–41.

21. Frank G, Pasquini E, Farneti G, et al. The endoscopic versus the traditional approach in pituitary surgery. Neuroendocrinology 2006;83(3–4):240–8.

22. Hashimoto N, Handa H, Yamagami T. Transsphenoidal extracapsular approach to pituitary tumors. J Neurosurg 1986;64(1):16–20.

23. Jho HD, Carrau RL. Endoscopy assisted transsphenoidal surgery for pituitary adenoma. Technical note. Acta Neurochir (Wien) 1996;138(12):1416–25.

24. Kaptain GJ, Vincent DA, Sheehan JP, et al. Transsphenoidal approaches for the extracapsular resection of midline suprasellar and anterior cranial base lesions. Neurosurgery 2001;49(1):94–101.

25. Kassam A, Snyderman CH, Mintz A, et al. Expanded endonasal approach: the rostrocaudal axis. Part I. Crista galli to the sella turcica. Neurosurg Focus 2005;19(1):E3.

26. Kato T, Sawamura Y, Abe H, et al. Transsphenoidal-transtuberculum sellae approach for supradiaphragmatic tumours: technical note. Acta Neurochir (Wien) 1998;140(7):715–9.

27. Kim J, Choe I, Bak K, et al. Transsphenoidal supradiaphragmatic intradural approach: technical note. Minim Invasive Neurosurg 2000;43(1):33–7.

28. Kitano M, Taneda M. Extended transsphenoidal surgery for suprasellar craniopharyngiomas: infrachiasmatic radical resection combined with or without a suprachiasmatic trans-lamina terminalis approach. Surg Neurol 2009;71(3):290–8 [discussion: 298].

29. Kouri JG, Chen MY, Watson JC, et al. Resection of suprasellar tumors by using a modified transsphenoidal approach. Report of four cases. J Neurosurg 2000;92(6):1028–35.

30. Laufer I, Anand VK, Schwartz TH. Endoscopic, endonasal extended transsphenoidal, transplanum transtuberculum approach for resection of suprasellar lesions. J Neurosurg 2007;106(3):400–6.

31. Liu JK, Das K, Weiss MH, et al. The history and evolution of transsphenoidal surgery. J Neurosurg 2001;95(6):1083–96.

32. Schwartz TH, Fraser JF, Brown S, et al. Endoscopic cranial base surgery: classification of operative approaches. Neurosurgery 2008;62(5):991–1002 [discussion: 1002–5].

33. Schwartz TH, Anand VK. The endoscopic endonasal transsphenoidal approach to the suprasellar cistern. Clin Neurosurg 2007;54:226–35.

34. Tabaee A, Anand VK, Barron Y, et al. Endoscopic pituitary surgery: a systematic review and meta-analysis. J Neurosurg 2009;111(3):545–54.

35. de Divitiis E, Cavallo LM, Cappabianca P, et al. Extended endoscopic endonasal transsphenoidal approach for the removal of suprasellar tumors: Part 2. Neurosurgery 2007;60(1):46–58 [discussion: 58–9].

36. Cappabianca P, Cavallo LM, Solari D, et al. Size does not matter. The intrigue of giant adenomas: a true surgical challenge. Acta Neurochir (Wien) 2014;156(12):2217–20.

37. Kassam AB, Vescan AD, Carrau RL, et al. Expanded endonasal approach: vidian canal as a landmark to the petrous internal carotid artery. J Neurosurg 2008;108(1):177–83.

38. Kassam AB, Prevedello DM, Carrau RL, et al. Endoscopic endonasal skull base surgery: analysis of complications in the authors' initial 800 patients. J Neurosurg 2011;114(6):1544–68.

39. Hadad G, Bassagasteguy L, Carrau RL, et al. A novel reconstructive technique after endoscopic expanded endonasal approaches: vascular pedicle nasoseptal flap. Laryngoscope 2006;116(10):1882–6.

40. Knosp E, Steiner E, Kitz K, et al. Pituitary adenomas with invasion of the cavernous sinus space: a magnetic resonance imaging classification compared with surgical findings. Neurosurgery 1993;33(4):610–7 [discussion: 617–8].

41. Frank G, Pasquini E. Approach to the cavernous sinus. In: de Divitiis E, Cappabianca P, editors. Endoscopic endonasal transsphenisal surgery. Vienna (Austria): Springer - Verlag; 2003. p. 159–75.

42. Cavallo LM, Messina A, Esposito F, et al. Skull base reconstruction in the extended endoscopic transsphenoidal approach for suprasellar lesions. J Neurosurg 2007;107(4):713–20.

43. Leng P, Ding CR, Zhang HN, et al. Reconstruct large osteochondral defects of the knee with hIGF-1 gene enhanced mosaicplasty. Knee 2012;19(6):804–11.

44. Kassam AB, Thomas A, Carrau RL, et al. Endoscopic reconstruction of the cranial base using a pedicled nasoseptal flap. Neurosurgery 2008;63(1 Suppl 1):ONS44–52 [discussion: ONS52–3].

45. Rivera-Serrano CM, Snyderman CH, Gardner P, et al. Nasoseptal "rescue" flap: a novel modification of the nasoseptal flap technique for pituitary surgery. Laryngoscope 2011;121(5):990–3.

46. Eloy JA, Kuperan AB, Choudhry OJ, et al. Efficacy of the pedicled nasoseptal flap without cerebrospinal fluid (CSF) diversion for repair of skull base defects: incidence of postoperative CSF leaks. Int Forum Allergy Rhinol 2012;2(5):397–401.

47. van Aken MO, Feelders RA, de Marie S, et al. Cerebrospinal fluid leakage during transsphenoidal surgery: postoperative external lumbar drainage reduces the risk for meningitis. Pituitary 2004;7(2):89–93.

48. Hu F, Gu Y, Zhang X, et al. Combined use of a gasket seal closure and a vascularized pedicle nasoseptal flap multilayered reconstruction technique for high-flow cerebrospinal fluid leaks after endonasal endoscopic skull base surgery. World Neurosurg 2015;83:181–7.

Endoscopic Endonasal Repair of Spontaneous and Traumatic Cerebrospinal Fluid Rhinorrhea
A Review and Local Experience

Lior Gonen, MD[a], Eric Monteiro, MD[b],
George Klironomos, MD, PhD[a], Yazeed Alghonaim, MD[b],
Allan Vescan, MD[b], Gelareh Zadeh, MD, PhD[a],
Fred Gentili, MD[a,*]

KEYWORDS

- Paranasal sinuses • Cerebrospinal fluid • Endoscopic endonasal approach • Rhinorrhea

KEY POINTS

- Surgical repair is the mainstay of management in cases of persisting cerebrospinal fluid (CSF) rhinorrhea.
- The principal indication is prevention of the possible complications that include ascending meningitis, intracranial abscess, and pneumocephalus.
- Endoscopic endonasal repair is an effective and well-tolerated procedure for the vast majority of CSF rhinorrhea cases, with primary closure rates of greater than 90% in large series and systematic reviews.
- Compared with the traditional open approaches, endoscopic endonasal repair carries similar results with fewer complications.

 Videos of the endoscopic views of a spontaneous cribriform plate defect with associated meningoencephalocele and an iatrogenic frontal sinus CSF leak accompany this article at www.neurosurgery.theclinics.com/

INTRODUCTION
General

Cerebrospinal fluid (CSF) rhinorrhea is caused by an abnormal communication between the subarachnoid space and the nasal cavity. This condition most commonly occurs secondary to a predisposing event, such as accidental or iatrogenic trauma. Nevertheless, CSF rhinorrhea may also occur spontaneously, a condition associated with benign intracranial hypertension (BIH). Surgical repair of CSF rhinorrhea is recommended to prevent the potential serious sequelae that include ascending meningitis, intracranial abscess, and pneumocephalus.

The most common anatomic sites leading to CSF rhinorrhea are located in the anterior skull

Funding Sources: None.
Conflict of Interest: None.
[a] Division of Neurosurgery, Toronto Western Hospital, University of Toronto, 399 Bathurst Street, Toronto, Ontario M5T 2S8, Canada; [b] Department of Otolaryngology-Head and Neck Surgery, Mount Sinai Hospital, University of Toronto, 600 University Avenue, Toronto, Ontario M5G 1X5, Canada
* Corresponding author.
E-mail address: Fred.Gentili@uhn.ca

Neurosurg Clin N Am 26 (2015) 333–348
http://dx.doi.org/10.1016/j.nec.2015.03.003
1042-3680/15/$ – see front matter © 2015 Elsevier Inc. All rights reserved.

base (ASB), namely the ethmoid roof, the olfactory groove, the roof of the sphenoid sinus, and the posterior wall of the frontal sinus. Historically, these defects have been repaired via an external approach, including a frontal craniotomy, and pericranial flap closure. However, the development of endoscopic endonasal skull base approaches in the last 2 decades provides an alternative to the traditional open approaches and has gradually gained popularity.

Following a thorough review of the existing literature, this article discusses the pathophysiology, diagnosis, and management of spontaneous and traumatic CSF rhinorrhea and provides a comprehensive description of the endoscopic endonasal approach (EEA) for repairing ASB CSF leaks.

Anatomic Considerations

CSF rhinorrhea refers to CSF leakage into the nasal cavity. Most commonly, CSF enters the nasal cavity through defects in the ASB. Understanding the anatomy of the related components of the cranial base, nasal cavity, and paranasal sinuses is essential for successful management of this condition. This section focuses on the anatomic interface between the intracranial and sinonasal cavities, outlining the areas that are prone to injury.

The ASB is formed by the ethmoid, sphenoid, and frontal bones and is separated from the middle cranial base by the sphenoid ridge, joined medially by the chiasmic sulcus. Two parts form the medial part of the ASB: the crista galli and the cribriform plate of the ethmoid bone anteriorly, and posteriorly, the planum and the body of the sphenoid bone.[1] The nasal cavity is bounded superiorly by the anterior cranial fossa above and is divided sagittally into 2 compartments by the nasal septum.[2] The paranasal sinuses are 4 pairs of pneumatic cavities: namely, the frontal, ethmoid, sphenoid, and maxillary sinuses. Each paranasal sinus is named after the bone in which it is located, and they all communicate directly with the nasal cavity. Excluding the maxillary sinuses, all the paranasal sinuses are superiorly bounded by the cranium.[3]

The frontal sinuses are housed in the frontal bone between the inner and outer tables. The inner table forms the posterior wall of the sinus, separating it from the anterior cranial fossa. Anatomically, it is much thinner than the outer table, and thus prone to injury.[3] The frontal recess constitutes the frontal sinus outflow tract.[4]

The ethmoid sinuses are formed by 5 components: the crista galli, cribriform plate, perpendicular plate, and paired lateral ethmoidal labyrinths, which contain the ethmoid air cells. The ethmoid cells are divided by the basal lamella of the middle turbinate into anterior and posterior divisions, which drain into the middle meatus and the sphenoethmoidal recess, respectively.[5] The roof of the ethmoid labyrinth, which separates the ethmoidal cells from the anterior cranial fossa, is formed by the relatively thick orbital plate of the frontal bone, called the fovea ethmoidalis. The fovea ethmoidalis attaches medially to the thinner lateral lamella of the cribriform plate (LLCP), completing the roof of the ethmoid air cells. Therefore, the ethmoid roof contains a transition from a thick bony part laterally to the thinner LLCP medially. The olfactory fossa is the region of depression of the horizontal cribriform plate below the level of the fovea ethmoidalis, and between the lateral lamellas. The vertical attachment of the middle turbinate divides the ASB into the cribriform plate medially and the fovea ethmoidalis laterally. Consequently, the anterior part of the nasal cavity's roof between the vertical attachment of the middle turbinate and the nasal septum is located directly under the horizontal cribriform plate (**Fig. 1**).[3]

The sphenoid sinus originates in the sphenoid bone at the junction of the anterior and middle cranial fossa and separates the pituitary gland from the nasal cavity. The sphenoid bone has a central portion called the body, which contains the sphenoid sinus. Three pairs of extensions spread out of the sphenoid body to form the complete sphenoid bone: 2 lesser wings that spread outward from the superolateral part of the body, 2 greater wings that spread upward from the lower part, and 2 pterygoid processes that are directed downward.[2] During embryogenesis, the sphenoid bone is formed from the ossification and fusion of 5 cartilaginous areas that subsequently fuse into a single bone. As first described in 1888 by Sternberg, incomplete fusion of the greater wing with the central cartilaginous precursors can result in a persistent lateral craniopharyngeal canal, called Sternberg canal.[6]

Following a systematic literature review of endoscopic approaches for repairing CSF leaks, Psaltis and colleagues[7] reported that the central part of the ASB is the most susceptible region to injury. Specifically, the ethmoid roof and cribriform region were found to be affected in more than half of the cases, independent of cause. This observation might be explained by several previously reported anatomic findings: first, the LLCP was found to be the thinnest, and therefore, the most vulnerable structure of the entire skull base.[5,8] Second, it has been reported that the horizontal cribriform plate is a thin and fragile bone that is covered only by an arachnoid layer, and hence, missing the protection of a true dural investment.

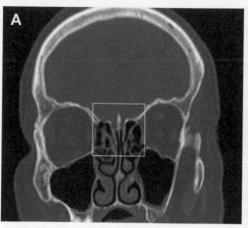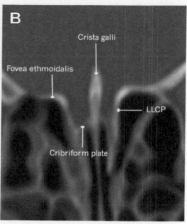

Fig. 1. Normal coronal HRCT images demonstrating medial ASB structures including cribriform plate, LLCP, and the fovea ethmoidalis. (*B*) An enlargement of the region marked within the box in (*A*).

Moreover, it is located in the midline of the anterior fossa, and CSF may preferentially gravitate to this area.[9] Finally, there is a firm adherence of the dura mater to the cribriform plate, ethmoidal roof, and the roof and lateral wall of sphenoid sinus. As a result, any pathologic process located in these structures can easily result in CSF rhinorrhea.[10]

Psaltis and colleagues[7] also identified the sphenoid sinus to be the second most common site of injury, affecting 30% of cases. Shetty and colleagues[11] demonstrated that an overpneumatized sphenoid sinus, especially in the lateral recess, is a common site of CSF rhinorrhea. A proposed explanation includes extensive lateral pneumatization, leading to weakening of the bony sphenoid roof. According to another theory, persistence of Sternberg canal may act as a susceptible site for CSF fistula within the lateral sphenoid sinus.[12]

DIAGNOSIS AND PREOPERATIVE CONSIDERATIONS

Establishing the diagnosis of CSF rhinorrhea in cases with suggestive clinical scenarios (ie, clear nasal discharge, recurrent meningitis) is crucial for prompt and successful management of this condition. The following 3 steps, completed in a stepwise fashion, are essential to establishing the diagnosis:

1. Cause-based classification: to develop a clinical suspicion by obtaining an accurate history
2. Confirmation of CSF leak: to verify the presence of CSF in the nasal discharge
3. Localization of the leak site: to preoperatively identify the site of the leak.

Cause-based Classification

Discussions about CSF rhinorrhea usually use a cause-based classification system. This breakdown is important because the specific cause may significantly alter the course of the disease and its management. Specifically, each cause requires a different management paradigm because of differences in rates of spontaneous closure, risk of ascending meningitis, size and location of the bony defect, and the long-term success rates of surgical repair.

The most commonly used cause-based classification of CSF rhinorrhea is the one presented by Schlosser and Bolger,[13] who described 5 categories: accidental trauma, surgical trauma, tumor-related, congenital, and spontaneous rhinorrhea. Tumor-related leaks are usually operatively addressed following primary tumor resection. Likewise, congenital encephaloceles and CSF rhinorrhea are rarely encountered and constitute a separate entity. These 2 categories are beyond the scope of this review, and consequently, this discussion is devoted to spontaneous and traumatic rhinorrhea. **Table 1** summarizes the different features of these categories.

Accidental traumatic cerebrospinal fluid leaks

Accidental traumatic CSF leaks, which were found to complicate up to 30% of nonpenetrating head injuries, present in either an acute or a delayed fashion. Most begin in the first 48 hours following the injury; however, up to 70% present within the first week. It is extremely uncommon for CSF leaks to present later than 3 months in this etiologic category.[14–17]

Despite slight variations between different studies, the most common sites of accidental traumatic CSF leaks are the cribriform plate and frontal sinus.[7] There are several important considerations when selecting a management strategy for these patients. On one hand, the vast majority of these cases resolve spontaneously or with conservative

Table 1
Comparison between different categories of cerebrospinal fluid rhinorrhea

Features	Accidental Trauma	Surgical Trauma	Spontaneous
Most common site locations	Cribriform plate and frontal sinus	Sphenoid sinus and ethmoid roof	Cribriform plate, ethmoid roof, and lateral recess of sphenoid sinus
Approximate nonsurgical resolution rates	Up to 85%	20% with lumbar drainage	Not relevant
Approximate overall risk of ascending meningitis (in unrepaired fistulae)	30%	20%	10%
Management paradigm	ASB defect: 3 d of conservative treatment 3 d of lumbar drainage Surgical repair for persistent cases Temporal bone defect: ≤7 d of conservative treatment ≤7 d of lumbar drainage Surgical repair for persistent cases	Immediate postoperative leak: Consider short trial (of ≤7 d) conservative treatment, with or without lumbar drainage All other cases and persistent cases: Surgical repair	Surgical repair (consider postoperative CSF pressure measurement to identify the need for subsequent VPS)

treatment, such as bed rest and external CSF diversion (40% resolution after 3 days and 85% after 7 days).[13,14,16–20] On the other hand, the incidence of ascending meningitis in accidental post-traumatic leaks is relatively high, with an approximate 30% risk overall in unrepaired fistulae and a weekly risk of 7.5% during the first month after the injury. Importantly, CSF rhinorrhea secondary to temporal bone trauma is more likely to resolve with conservative management, compared with ASB defects.[17,19,21–23]

Accordingly, Prosser and colleagues[14] suggested a graduated management paradigm for accidental traumatic leaks. The first stage should be a trial of conservative treatment, followed by a second stage in which CSF diversion is used in persistent cases. Surgical repair should be reserved for cases that do not resolve after these 2 stages. Considering the different probability for nonsurgical resolution, each of these stages should be pursued over a different time period, depending on the site of the defect. The threshold for surgical repair of ASB leaks is lower, and 3 days for each stage is sufficient. Conversely, with temporal bone leaks, a week for each stage seems more appropriate, given the lower rate of meningitis and the higher rate of spontaneous closure.

Surgical traumatic cerebrospinal fluid leaks
Surgical traumatic CSF leaks most frequently occur secondary to either functional endoscopic sinus surgery (FESS) or neurosurgical procedures. Overall, the most common sites of surgical traumatic CSF leaks are the ethmoid roof and the sphenoid sinus.[7]

Expectedly, the most common site of traumatic CSF leaks following neurosurgical procedures is the sphenoid sinus, Which is due to the increased use of EEA for various skull base pathologic conditions, predominantly pituitary adenomas. Kassam and colleagues[24] reported that CSF leaks represented the most common postoperative complication in 800 cases using EEA approaches, with an overall rate of 15.9%. Of these, 23.6% were treated with short-term CSF drainage through a lumbar drain. The remaining 76.4% required endoscopic endonasal reconstruction. Only one of these failed, requiring a transcranial repair. Recent reports show that postoperative leak rates have declined significantly, occurring in less than 3% of cases in experienced centers, likely due to improved closure techniques and increased surgeon experience.[25,26] Several factors are associated with a higher risk of CSF leaks following EEAs. These factors include expanded EEAs, certain pathologic conditions (ie, craniopharyngioma), postoperative adjuvant therapies, idiopathic intracranial hypertension, and transplanum approaches with exposure of the third ventricle.[24,27–29] Similarly, although the incidence of postoperative CSF leaks following resection of even large pituitary adenomas is less than 10%, EEAs for ventral skull base meningiomas are associated with a considerably higher incidence (more than 30% for olfactory groove and more than 20% for tuberculum sellae meningiomas).[30,31] CSF leaks following FESS are most commonly associated with injury to the ethmoid roof or the LLCP.[13] The overall risk of ascending meningitis in unrepaired cases of surgical traumatic leaks is approximately 20%.[21]

In addition to the different features already discussed, surgical leaks are distinct from accidental ones because they tend to be much larger and associated with a higher volume of flow.[13] Furthermore, the later the CSF leak presents following the surgery, the lower the likelihood of achieving durable repair with nonsurgical measures. Accordingly, the management paradigm suggested by Prosser and colleagues[14] for surgical traumatic leaks differs from accidental leaks, encouraging a more aggressive approach. The management of select, recently operated, iatrogenic leaks may include short-term conservative measures limited to no longer than 1 week. All other cases, as well as all cases failing conservative measures, require surgical repair.

Spontaneous cerebrospinal fluid leaks

Spontaneous CSF leaks are classified by a lack of any identifiable cause and represent a diagnostic and therapeutic challenge. Despite being commonly referred to as idiopathic, there is growing evidence suggesting a strong association between spontaneous leaks and BIH. Schlosser and his group[32–36] published several studies providing evidence of a link between spontaneous CSF leaks and BIH. Both disorders share common clinical and radiographic features, including a high prevalence in women, patients with obesity, and individuals with radiographic evidence of empty sellae. Furthermore, mildly elevated intracranial pressure (ICP) was frequently encountered when evaluating patients with spontaneous leaks by lumbar puncture. Finally, more than 70% of patients with spontaneous CSF satisfy the modified Dandy criteria that are commonly used for diagnosing BIH.[33] The association between spontaneous CSF leaks and high-pressure hydrocephalus contributes to the high risk for recurrence in these patients, despite attempts at surgical repair.[37]

Spontaneous leaks most commonly originate from cribriform plate defects. The lateral sphenoid recess is also a relatively common location, especially in patients with an extensively pneumatized lateral sphenoid sinus.[7,32] Another important observation regarding spontaneous leaks is the frequent presence of multiple leak sites, occurring in approximately 35% of the cases. The overall risk of ascending meningitis in cases of unrepaired spontaneous leaks is approximately 10%.[21]

When analyzed by subtype, spontaneous CSF leaks have the highest recurrence rate after surgical repair.[10,32] Difficulty in achieving durable repair of spontaneous leaks is attributed to several reasons: occult elevated ICP, multiple skull base defects, and a high rate of meningoencephalocele formation.[38]

Appropriate management of spontaneous leaks includes surgical repair. Nevertheless, there is an ongoing debate about the management of these cases, specifically regarding the use of transient lumbar drainage or a ventriculoperitoneal shunt (VPS). One hypothesis is that surgical repair may further increase the CSF pressure postoperatively, resulting in an increased risk of leak recurrence. Carrau and colleagues[37] reported that 6 of 18 patients with spontaneous CSF leaks were found to have high-pressure CSF when evaluated postoperatively. All 6 subsequently underwent ventriculoperitoneal shunting, with no recurrences observed at long-term follow-up. Accordingly, the investigators suggest that CSF pressure be routinely measured postoperatively through a lumbar puncture in patients with spontaneous leaks. This approach has yet to gain wide acceptance, because of the possible complications associated with postoperative lumbar drainage, and the contradictory reports in the literature.[7,39]

Confirmation of Cerebrospinal Fluid Leak

Definitive confirmation of active CSF rhinorrhea in suspected cases is done noninvasively by analysis of the nasal discharge for the presence of CSF biomarkers. In light of this, every effort should be made to obtain nasal secretions and perform chemical analysis before other diagnostic methods, especially invasive ones. Moreover, Zapalac and colleagues[40] encourage repeated collection of rhinorrhea for CSF biomarker analysis before pursuing invasive diagnostic methods.

Since it was introduced in 1979, β2-transferrin is the most commonly used CSF biomarker, with high sensitivity and specificity (approaching 97% and 99%, respectively). Another protein that is used for this purpose is β-trace protein. Although the latter carries similar advantages as the former, including even higher sensitivity and specificity (both approaching 100%), it is not widely used, mainly because its utility is limited in cases of bacterial meningitis or reduced glomerular filtration.[20,41–43]

Radionuclide cisternography, which is a nonlocalizing invasive modality involving lumbar puncture and radiation exposure, is rarely used for confirmation of CSF rhinorrhea and should be reserved for highly suggestive cases in which confirmation could not be obtained with CSF biomarkers.[40]

Localization of the Leak Site

Following definitive confirmation of CSF rhinorrhea, accurate localization of the leak site is the next imperative step for establishing the diagnosis.

Coronal, sagittal, and axial high-resolution thin-cut (1-mm) computed tomography scan (HRCT) with bone algorithm is considered by most groups to be the best modality for depicting any bony defects, as exemplified in **Fig. 2**.[10,13,44] MRI may also be a valuable localization modality, primarily T2-weighted sequences. Although the sensitivity of each of these modalities for detecting the leak site approaches 90%, combining both increases the sensitivity to almost 97%.[7,45,46]

Nowadays, computed tomography (CT) cisternography is rarely used because of its invasiveness and low sensitivity (40%) in detecting inactive leaks.[40] If additional localization is required, some investigators advocate for specific MRI techniques for CSF leak detection, which uses a fast spin-echo sequence with fat suppression and image reversal. This modality has a reported sensitivity and specificity of 92% and 100%, respectively.[20,47,48] However, the combination of a suggestive clinical history, confirmation by positive β2-transferrin, and approximate localization with HRCT and routine MRI is usually sufficient to establish the diagnosis.[44]

ENDOSCOPIC ENDONASAL REPAIR OF CEREBROSPINAL FLUID RHINORRHEA
Perioperative Adjunctive Modalities

Lumbar drain

The use of lumbar drainage following surgical repair of CSF leak remains controversial. Some groups oppose routine use of lumbar drainage in these cases, for 2 main reasons: first, the fear of drainage-related complications (mainly pneumocephalus), and second, because there is no solid evidence that it improves closure rates.[38] In this regard, according to recent systematic review of the literature, the benefit of lumbar drains in CSF leak repair could not be supported by the available data.[7] Nevertheless, most investigators report using it selectively, and 67% of otolaryngologists that were recently surveyed use lumbar drains routinely as part of their management of CSF fistulae.[49] Commonly cited indications for perioperative lumbar drainage include all the high-risk factors for repair failure: large defects, coexistent meningoencepahloceles, associated high ICP, body mass index greater than 30, radiographic empty sella syndrome, and previous CSF fistula repair.[50,51]

In the authors' institution, they use lumbar drainage selectively. As described by other groups, the drain is placed in the supine position before or immediately after the operation, and it is opened at a low rate of approximately 5 mL/h. The drain is usually removed 24 to 48 hours after the operation.[38] During this period, any neurologic deterioration prompts an immediate closure of the drain, followed by urgent CT scan to exclude expanding pneumocephalus.

Intrathecal fluorescein

Fluorescein is a green fluorescent dye that alters the color of CSF when introduced intrathecally,

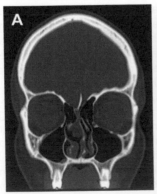
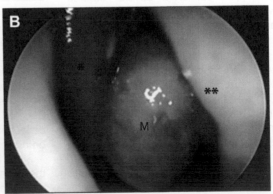

Fig. 2. (A) HRCT coronal image clearly demonstrating meningoencephalocele herniating through a right cribriform plate defect. (B) Endoscopic view of the same meningoencephalocele (M), located between the middle turbinate laterally (*asterisk*) and the nasal septum medially (*double asterisks*).

thus making it more easily visible, especially in a surgical field. Intrathecal injection of fluorescein is a useful adjuvant method in endoscopic endonasal repair of CSF leak. By enhancing the visualization of CSF, fluorescein facilitates the identification of the leak, especially in cases of multiple leak sites, and helps to verify a watertight closure of the repair at the end of the procedure. Intrathecal administration of fluorescein was reported to be neurotoxic, with potential complications including transient paraparesis, numbness, opisthotonus, and cranial nerve deficits.[52] Despite these major safety concerns, its use remains common practice.[53–55] Keerl and colleagues[56] reported an acceptable safety profile of intrathecal fluorescein at low doses in a large series of 420 administrations. The most significant complications were seen in 2 patients who experienced grand mal seizures on the day of the intrathecal injection. In another recent case series, Seth and colleagues[54] demonstrated that intrathecal fluorescein has a sensitivity of 73.8% and a specificity of 100% in detecting the intraoperative CSF leak site, along with a false-negative rate of 26.2%.

Placantonakis and colleagues[53] established an administration protocol that includes intravenous administration of 10 mg of dexamethasone and 50 mg of diphenhydramine after intubation, performing a lumbar puncture and withdrawal of 10 mL of CSF, mixing this with 0.25 mL of 10% fluorescein solution, and slow intrathecal injection of the solution for about an hour before its visualization. In the authors' institution, they use a similar protocol, with a few modifications: the lumbar drain is placed preoperatively while the patient is awake, so any possible side effects, such as epileptic seizures, can be recognized. The patient is then kept in the recovery area for at least 2 hours in a slight Trendelenburg position to allow for the fluorescein to enter the cranial cavity and mix with the intracranial CSF.

Image-guidance system

Despite considered by many to be an invaluable adjunctive tool in endoscopic endonasal skull base surgeries, the role of image-guidance systems using multiple planar CT or MRI information has not, to date, been widely studied. Tabaee and colleagues[57] retrospectively analyzed the possible correlation between successful endoscopic endonasal repair of CSF rhinorrhea and use of computer-assisted surgery. Although the study failed to establish clear correlation, the investigators concluded that the use of computer assistance may improve the confidence of the surgeon and is a valuable adjunct in this procedure. In the authors' institution, image-guidance systems

are used routinely in every endoscopic endonasal skull base surgeries.

Surgical Technique

The objectives of surgical repair of CSF leaks include reconstruction of the tissue barriers separating the cranial cavity from the sinonasal tract, while preserving neurovascular as well as sinonasal function. Despite slight variations, most groups uniformly advocate the following basic principles of endoscopic repair of CSF rhinorrhea to achieve the above objectives (**Box 1**).[10,13,38,44,58]

Positioning and Preoperative Preparation

In most institutions, endoscopic endonasal skull base surgeries are carried out by an interdisciplinary team, including a neurosurgeon and a skull base rhinologist. After inducing general anesthesia, the patient is positioned supine with the head placed in a rigid 3-point fixation. The head is slightly rotated toward the surgeon by approximately 10°, whereas the degree of flexion or extension depends on the location of the fistula. The head is fixated in a neutral position when approaching the sphenoid sinus, and slightly hyperextended for more anterior locations. The operating table is set in a 20° reverse Trendelenburg position to further enhance ASB visualization. The authors mainly use 0° angle 4-mm rigid endoscopes, occasionally switching to 30° or 45° endoscopes if an angled view is required.

After inducing general anesthesia, the patient is positioned supine with the head placed in a rigid 3-point fixation in a neutral position, or slightly rotated toward the surgeon by approximately 10°. The operating table is set in a 20° reverse Trendelenburg position to further enhance ASB visualization. The authors mainly use 0° angle 4-mm rigid endoscopes, occasionally switching to 30° or 45° endoscopes if an angled view is required.

To assure a clear field during the procedure, topical decongestant is applied to the nasal cavity (1/1000 topical epinephrine or oxymetazoline), and the nasal septum, middle turbinate, and lateral nasal wall are infiltrated with lidocaine 1% and epinephrine 1/200,000.

Location-based Exposure

Depending on the site of the leak, various endoscopic corridors and degrees of sinus dissection are required to achieve adequate exposure. The initial endoscopic approach, whether direct transnasal (paraseptal), transsphenoidal, transethmoidal, transpterygoidal, or any combination of these, is dictated by the preoperative HRCT localization. The extent of the exposure can be

> **Box 1**
> **Essential surgical steps and principles in endoscopic endonasal repair of cerebrospinal fluidrhinorrhea**
>
> 1. Position and preparation
>   - Consider lumbar drain and intrathecal fluorescein administration
>   - Patient positioned supine, head rotated to the right by 10°, operating table in a 20° reverse Trendelenburg position
>   - Image-guidance registration
>   - Nasal decongestion
> 2. Location-based approach
>   - Initial approach is guided by the preoperative defect localization (see **Table 2**)
>   - Exposing a wide corridor is favorable to enhance defect accessibility
>   - Consider septal flap harvest according to the expected size of skull base defect (free graft vs NSF)
>   - Include opening of adjacent sinuses to prevent iatrogenic sinus obstruction
>   - Expansion of the exposure might be required according to intraoperative findings
> 3. Leak site identification
>   - Guided mainly by preoperative localization
>   - Image guidance should be used routinely
>   - Provocative iatrogenic ICP elevation might help identifying leak site
>   - Use of intrathecal fluorescein might also be helpful and should be considered in selective cases
> 4. Leak site preparation
>   - Herniated meningoencephalocele is amputated and reduced to the skull base level
>   - Meticulous removal of surrounding mucosa around the defect is mandatory
>   - To stimulate osteogenesis, consider abrading the surrounding exposed bone margins
> 5. Skull base reconstruction
>   - Individualized and tailored method of reconstruction is required for different CSF leaks
>   - General reconstruction principles
>   ○ Simple defects (≤4 mm, low-flow, easily accessible and prepared) ⇒ free soft tissue overlay graft
>   ○ Complex defects (>4 mm, high-flow, suspected underlying elevated CSF pressure) ⇒ combined underlay graft and overlay vascularized flap

expanded as necessary according to intraoperative findings. Importantly, in some cases opening of additional intact sinuses, which are adjacent to the sinus that contains the leak site, is also performed. The rationale includes preventing iatrogenic sinus obstruction because of postoperative scarring, with subsequent risk of mucocele development, and for creating adequate space for maneuvering surgical instrumentation.

The endoscopic approaches for the 3 common skull base leak sites are described later in discussion and summarized in **Table 2**.

Cribriform plate and anterior ethmoid roof defects

Cribriform plate and anterior ethmoid roof defects can be exposed via either direct transnasal approach medial to the turbinates (without violating ethmoidal integrity) or a transethmoidal approach. Generally, a wider exposure including maxillary antrostomy along with complete anterior and posterior ethmoidectomy is more likely to provide adequate exposure. Opening of the natural drainage pathways of the frontal and sphenoid sinuses (ie, frontal sinusotomy and sphenoidotomy) as well as the need for middle turbinectomy should be considered intraoperatively on the basis of 2 factors: requirement for additional exposure and ensuring sinus patency (see **Fig. 2**).

Sphenoid sinus defects

Sphenoid sinus defects should be further divided into central versus lateral recess defects. *Central defects* can be adequately exposed via both

Table 2
Location-based approach in endoscopic endonasal repair of cerebrospinal fluid rhinorrhea

Cribriform Plate and Anterior Ethmoid Roof Defects	Sphenoid Sinus Defects	Frontal Sinus Defects

Direct transnasal approach without violating ethmoidal integrity, or transethmoidal approach
Additional exposure could be achieved with middle turbinectomy, sphenoidotomy, and frontal sinusotomy
	Central sphenoid defect:
	  Direct transnasal or transethmoidal approaches with a wide sphenoidotomy
	Lateral sphenoid recess defect:
	  Direct transnasal or transethmoidal approaches with a wide sphenoidotomy for little or medium degree of lateral pneumatization of the sphenoid sinus, respectively
	Transpterygoidal approach for extensive lateral pneumatization
		Frontal recess:
		  Direct transnasal approach (with removal of the agger nasi cell and widening the frontal recess)
		Posterior wall defects:
		  Direct transnasal approach, unless the defect can only be partially visible (in the presence of a well-pneumatized agger nasi cell)
		In this case, further extension with enlargement of frontal ostium and frontal sinusotomy is required

Note: Superior and lateral aspects of the frontal sinus usually require an open approach.

approaches described for cribriform plate defects, namely direct transnasal and transethmoidal. Regardless of the chosen approach, a wide sphenoidotomy is performed. When using the transnasal approach, the sphenoid sinus is accessed unilaterally or bilaterally through the sphenoid ostium in the superior meatus and sphenoidotomy is accomplished in the same manner as for sellar surgery. The transethmoidal approach includes anterior and posterior ethmoidectomy and creation of a large transethmoidal sphenoidotomy. *Lateral sphenoid recess defects* represent a surgical challenge because of limited accessibility.[59] Recently, Tabaee and colleagues[6] redescribed 3 valid options to approach these defects, in accordance with the extent of lateral sphenoid pneumatization: transnasal, transethmoidal, and the most extensive transpterygoidal approach. In cases with little sphenoid pneumatization, the transnasal approach with wide sphenoidotomy, achieved by creating a common sinus cavity connecting sphenoid ostia and removing the sphenoid rostrum, is probably sufficient. Transethmoidal sphenoidotomy is appropriate for cases in which additional lateral exposure is required to address larger degrees of lateral pneumatization. Finally, in cases of extensive lateral pneumatization, the transpterygoidal approach may be favorable.

This approach initiates with a transethmoidal wide sphenoidotomy as described above, followed by maxillary antrostomy to provide wide exposure of the posterior wall of the maxillary sinus. The bony posterior wall is then exposed by reflecting a medially based flap of mucosa off the bone. Afterward, the palatine bone is dissected and defined;

its anterior perpendicular process is removed, and the sphenopalatine artery is mobilized. At that stage, the posterior wall of the maxillary sinus adjoining the palatine bone is drilled to allow entry to the pterygopalatine fossa. The neurovasculature structures of the fossa, including the internal maxillary artery, maxillary branch of the trigeminal nerve, the vidian nerve, and the sphenopalatine ganglion, are reflected laterally. The anterior wall of the sphenoid sinus and the anterior aspect of the pterygoid process are removed to expose the lateral sphenoid sinus extension.

Frontal sinus defects

Frontal sinus defects constitute a separate entity in regard to endoscopic repair. Until recently, the surgical dogma has dictated that frontal sinus CSF leaks should be repaired by open intracranial or an external transfrontal approach, such as cranialization or osteoplastic flap with obliteration. However, surgical options have changed with the introduction of the 45° and 70° angled telescope and development of suitable instruments, making endoscopic repair of frontal sinus leaks possible.[60,61] Despite this evolution, leak sites located at an extreme superior or lateral location within the sinus are beyond the reach of current instruments and should be approached by open techniques.[62] Generally, frontal sinus CSF leaks are anatomically located either within the frontal recess or within the posterior wall of the proper sinus. Shi and colleagues[63] recently described endoscopic approaches for specific leak site locations within the frontal sinus. First, defects located within the frontal recess or at the posterior wall of the frontal sinus that are less than 1 cm in diameter can be adequately exposed via a direct transnasal endoscopic approach, with removal of the agger nasi cell and widening of the frontal recess. Second, defects located in the posterior wall of the frontal sinus that are only partially visible in the presence of a well-pneumatized agger nasi cell can be adequately exposed via a direct transnasal endoscopic approach, with enlargement of the frontal ostium and frontal sinusotomy (**Fig. 3**). Superior and lateral aspects of the frontal sinus usually require an open approach. Finally, reports describing endoscopic repair of traumatic frontal sinus CSF leaks via a frontal trephine, and not endonasally, show promising results.[64]

Leak Site Identification

Accurate leak site identification remains the cornerstone of successful repair. It is crucial that the entire defect is identified and accessible. Designing the surgical approach based on accurate preoperative radiographic leak site location, together with using an intraoperative image-guidance system, promotes straightforward identification.

Nevertheless, accurate intraoperative localization of leak sites can be challenging. Two additional intraoperative methods may assist in identifying the leak site. First, the use of intrathecal fluorescein might be helpful. Second, transiently elevating ICP by initiating a Valsalva maneuver will increase CSF extrusion from the defect. In the authors' institution, they use image-guidance routinely, and intraoperative fluorescein selectively.

Leak Site Preparation

Following identification of the leak site, the recipient bed is prepared for reconstruction. This stage involves removing all the surrounding mucosa circumferentially around the defect. Dissecting the mucosa is crucial for allowing a firm adherence of the flap or graft to the recipient bony skull base. Any overlap between the skull base mucosa and the overlay mucosal graft may lead to the development of a mucocele that can gradually expand with time and violate the reconstruction.[65] To stimulate osteogenesis, which is mainly relevant when using bone grafts, the exposed bone around the defect can be abraded using a diamond burr or curette.[66]

If a meningoencephalocele is present, it has to be either resected or reduced to the level of the bone. Herniated brain tissue in the nasal cavity is considered to be nonfunctional and should be amputated. Usually, the herniated tissue is progressively ablated until leaving just a pedicle, which eventually is reduced into the intracranial cavity using bipolar cautery (**Fig. 4**).

Skull Base Reconstruction

The final stage of the repair is reconstructing the skull base in a manner that will provide a durable, watertight seal. Various skull base reconstruction techniques have been described in the literature, and although a decisive algorithm has yet to be established, the basic principles of a successful reconstruction are widely accepted. The main factors that dictate the reconstructive choice are the cause of the leak, size and location of the defect, and the underlying CSF pressure.[13,44,66]

Different closure methods are generally based on free grafts or pedicled flaps. *Free grafts* can be autologous, such as fascia lata, turbinate, or septal mucosa, or a variety of available allografts. Free grafts may be further divided into soft tissue or rigid grafts. Furthermore, there are different strategies for positioning the graft at the site of the defect, including underlay grafting (graft is positioned intracranially and supported against the cranial side of the skull base by the ICP), overlay grafting (graft is positioned outside the skull base and supported by nasal packing), combined underlay and overlay, "gasket-seal" watertight

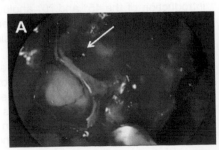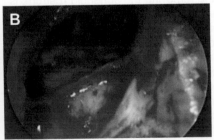

Fig. 3. Endoscopic view of an iatrogenic frontal sinus CSF leak. (*A*) CSF egress from frontal sinus recess (*arrow*) identified after wide exposure that includes uncinectomy and maxillary antrostomy, complete anterior and posterior ethmoidectomy, and a wide sphenoidotomy. (*B*) A wider view of the opened frontal sinus following frontal sinusotomy (This case is presented in Video 2).

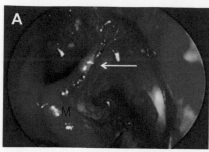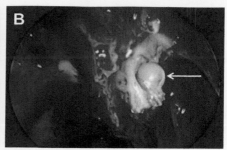

Fig. 4. Endoscopic view of a spontaneous cribriform plate defect with associated meningoencephalocele, before and after site preparation. (*A*) The site before completing the preparation, with a meningoencephalocele (M) still hanged on its pedicle (*arrow*), and the defect is still covered with mucosa. (*B*) The site just before being completely prepared, with only the stump of the pedicle (*arrow*) to be reduced to the skull base level. The defect is surrounded by well-exposed bone only (This case is presented in Video 1).

closure, and the "bath plug" technique.[67,68] *Pedicled flaps*, which are rotated to cover the recipient bed while remaining attached to a vascular pedicle, have evolved significantly in the past decade, extending the limits of endoscopic skull base reconstruction. The nasoseptal flap (NSF), first described by Hadad and colleagues[69] in 2006, is a nasal septal mucoperiosteal and muco-perichondrial flap, based on a terminal branch of the sphenopalatine artery. This flap has certainly become the workhorse of endoscopic skull base reconstruction, used either alone or in multilayered closure strategies.

There are some available studies, comparing different closure materials and techniques, in an attempt to establish an evidence-based algorithm for skull base reconstruction. Before the popularity of the NSF, Hegazy and colleagues[70] performed a meta-analysis reviewing the endoscopic reconstruction of 289 CSF fistulae. The investigators found that high rates of successful repair (more than 90% following the first surgical attempt) are achieved regardless of the technique and materials used. More recently, Harvey and colleagues[50] and Soudry and colleagues[71] performed 2 additional systematic reviews of endoscopic skull base reconstruction. Harvey and colleagues reviewed 609 patients who underwent endoscopic reconstruction of large dural defects, either with a free graft (326) or with a vascularized flap. Soudry and colleagues reviewed 673 patients who underwent endoscopic reconstruction of various defects. According to these reviews, there are 3 clinical situations in which vascularized flaps are significantly superior to free grafting. Harvey and colleagues found that vascularized flaps for reconstructing large skull base defects are associated with a lower failure rate compared with free grafts (failure rates were 15.6% and 6.7% for free graft and vascularized reconstruction, respectively);

Soudry and colleagues demonstrated better reconstructive results with vascularized repair in cases of either high-flow intraoperative CSF leaks (82% and 94% success rates were found with free grafts and vascularized repairs, respectively) or Clival defects. Notwithstanding, 92% success rates were achieved in cases of low flow leaks regardless of the closure technique; it appears that graft choice or closure technique does not seem to influence closure rates for simple, small-size defects.

The above findings support an individualized and tailored method of reconstruction for different CSF leaks.[13,44,65,72] Simple defects (ie, small ≤4 mm, low-flow leaks, and easily accessible sites) are generally reconstructed with a free soft tissue overlay graft (**Fig. 5**). Inserting underlay graft might be technically challenging in these cases and may not be justified. Moreover, an attempt to force a graft into the intracranial cavity might risk an intracranial vessel, causing intracranial hemorrhage. Multilayer overlay closure is frequently used in these cases; for example, abdominal fat graft is applied first, covered with a free septal mucosal graft, and eventually supported by Gelfoam or Surgicel (Johnson and Johnson, New Brunswick, NJ, USA). More complex defects (ie, size >4 mm, high-flow leaks, underlying elevated CSF pressure) are generally reconstructed with a combination of an underlay graft, followed by an overlay vascularized flap, such as the NSF.

POSTOPERATIVE CARE

Patients usually leave the operating room with some form of nasal packing, which can include Foley catheters, Merocel sponges, Vaseline gauze, and various absorbable packing such as Gelfoam and Surgicel. In the authors' institution, they often use a Foley catheter inflated with sterile water to

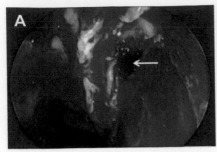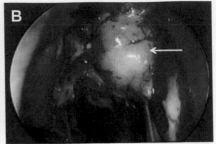

Fig. 5. Endoscopic view of a spontaneous cribriform plate defect with associated meningoencephalocele before and after positioning the reconstruction graft. (*A*) The small skull base defect, circumferentially surrounded by bony margins, is marked by the bipolar cautery sign (*arrow*). (*B*) Overlay reconstruction free septal mucoperiosteal graft (*arrow*) (This case is presented in Video 1).

help support the graft. This catheter is usually removed on the third to fifth postoperative day. Patients are kept on bed rest with bathroom privileges until the nasal packing is removed, and they are instructed to avoid any straining. Patients are also provided with stool softeners and given antibiotics while the packing is in situ. Patients are instructed to slowly resume normal physical activity; however, excessive straining is avoided for 6 weeks.

Nasal saline is prescribed postoperatively, and patients are encouraged in its liberal use. Patients are also instructed to avoid excessive nose blowing and any other activity that may increase ICP. The otolaryngology team assesses patients 2 weeks postoperatively, wherein gentle debridement is performed in areas distant from the skull base reconstruction site, to avoid dislodging the graft. Patients are seen again at 6 weeks when further debridement is performed as required. Subsequent appointments are scheduled according to the individual needs of the patient.

The need for postoperative debridement remains a controversial topic in both skull base surgery and rhinology. Alsaffar and colleagues[73] performed a randomized control trial comparing postoperative debridement to no debridement in patients following FESS for chronic rhinosinusitis. In addition, both groups were given high-volume saline irrigation twice daily. At 4 weeks, there were no differences between the groups in disease-specific outcomes; however, the debridement group did have statistically higher pain scores as assessed by a visual analogue scale. Furthermore, assessment at 6 months continued to show no difference in disease-specific outcomes between the groups. A subsequent systematic review also assessed the role of postoperative debridement following FESS. Short-term benefits in patient symptom scores were seen in 4 of the 6 studies analyzed. However, no long-term statistical differences were seen in objective endoscopic or symptom-based scores.[74]

Future studies are needed to further elucidate the role of postoperative debridement in endoscopic skull base surgery, and until that point, its use should be tailored to the individual patient and clinical situation.

OUTCOME OF ENDOSCOPIC ENDONASAL REPAIR OF CEREBROSPINAL FLUID RHINORRHEA

Four systematic reviews evaluating the outcome of endoscopic endonasal repair of CSF rhinorrhea, with or without a comparison to open approaches, can be found in the literature. The main results of these studies are summarized in **Table 3**.

Of the 4 reviews, the first 2 were published more than a decade ago, supporting the endoscopic approach as a valid alternative to open approach in select patients. Hegazy and colleagues[70] conducted a meta-analysis of all the relevant studies in the literature and found a first repair attempt success rate of 90% in 289 cases of CSF leaks. About half of the persistent leaks were successfully repaired with a second attempt, leading to an overall endoscopic success rate of 97%. Furthermore, the endoscopic approach was associated with low morbidity, with rates of less than 1% for each of the major complications (meningitis, subdural hematoma, and intracranial abscess). In 2001, Senior and colleagues[49] used a questionnaire that was completed by members of the American Rhinologic Society to collect data on 522 cases of endoscopic repair of CSF leaks, reporting a success rate of 90% on first attempt and 98% overall. The complication rate was 2.5%. The results of both reviews emphasize the potential for high closure rates following endoscopic CSF leak repair, with relatively low surgical morbidity.

Recently, 2 additional systematic reviews confirmed the favorable outcomes of endoscopic

Table 3
Summary of main results from systematic reviews: outcome of endoscopic endonasal repair of cerebrospinal fluid leak

Study	Study Design	Sample Size	Successful Repair Rates	Complications Rate
Hegazy et al, 2000	Meta analysis of available studies of endoscopic CSF leak repair	14 studies, 289 cases	First attempt success rate: 90%; overall success rate: 97%	<1% for each major complications
Senior et al, 2001	Retrospective assessment of endoscopic CSF leak repair from various centers	522 cases	First attempt success rate: 90%; overall success rate: 98%	Overall: 2.5%, 1 mortality
Psaltis et al, 2012	Systematic review of studies of endoscopic CSF leak repair	55 studies, 1778 cases	First attempt success rate: 90%; overall success rate: 97%	<0.03%
Komotar et al, 2013	Systematic review comparing endoscopic with open ASB CSF leak repair	71 studies, 1178 cases Endoscopic cohort: 884 Open cohort: 294	Similar first attempt success rate of both endoscopic and open cohorts of approximately 90%	Endoscopic cohort: <2%, significantly lower than in the open cohort

Data from Refs.[7,49,70,75]

CSF leak repair and underlined the decreased morbidity of this approach in comparison with an open approach. Psaltis and colleagues[7] systemically reviewed 55 studies involving 1778 CSF fistulae repaired endoscopically. The overall success rate was 90% following the first attempt and as high as 97% for secondary repairs. In the following year, Komotar and colleagues[75] compared the outcomes of endoscopic and open approaches in more than 1170 cases, finding no significant difference in the rate of successful repair (~90%) between the 2 groups. Nevertheless, complications in the endoscopic cohort were significantly lower compared with the open cohort, including meningitis, abscess/wound infection, and sepsis. Therefore, both of these reviews provide convincing evidence supporting the EEA as a safe and effective option for treating CSF leaks.

THE UNIVERSITY OF TORONTO EXPERIENCE

The authors present 2 surgical videos demonstrating endoscopic repair of CSF leaks in 2 distinct clinical scenarios (Videos 1 and 2).

Video 1 presents the case of a young 23-year-old woman who presented with clear right nasal discharge and 2 episodes of pneumococcal meningitis. CSF rhinorrhea was confirmed by chemical analysis showing β2-transferrin positivity. HRCT scan showed a right frontal mass extending to the nasal cavity through the right cribriform plate, compatible with a meningoencephalocele. The video demonstrates the endoscopic repair via a transethmoidal approach, including maxillary antrostomy, anterior and posterior ethmoidectomy, and a wide sphenoidotomy. Finally, the reconstruction with a free septal mucosal graft is presented.

Video 2 presents a challenging case of an 80-year-old man with a remote history of a right frontotemporal craniotomy for clipping of a paraophthalmic aneurysm. Forty years later, he presented with rhinorrhea and 2 episodes of meningitis, again proven to be CSF rhinorrhea by chemical analysis. HRCT showed an area in the planum sphenoidale of suspected bony erosion underneath the location of the clips. The suspected area was approached endoscopically via a transethmoidal approach, including maxillary antrostomy, anterior and posterior ethmoidectomy, and a wide sphenoidotomy. Surprisingly, exploration of the planum surface was negative. The video presents how the leak was eventually localized to the posterior wall of the right frontal sinus. The intraoperative management of this leak is illustrated.

SUMMARY

CSF rhinorrhea might occur either spontaneously or secondary to accidental trauma or iatrogenic injury. Diagnosis of CSF rhinorrhea is established in a stepwise fashion; it starts with developing a solid clinical suspicion, continues with confirming the presence of CSF in the nasal discharge by chemical analysis, and ends with locating the site of the leak by imaging studies.

Surgical repair remains the mainstay of management in cases of persisting CSF rhinorrhea, for prevention of the possible serious complications that include ascending meningitis, intracranial abscess, and pneumocephalus. Over the past 2 decades, endoscopic endonasal surgeries have grown in popularity for approaching ventral skull base pathologic conditions. Concurrently, CSF rhinorrhea repair has advanced from open transcranial procedures to the far less invasive endoscopic endonasal procedures.

Nowadays, most leak sites leading to CSF rhinorrhea are accessible endoscopically, including the frontal recess. Based on current data, endoscopic endonasal repair is an effective and well-tolerated procedure for the vast majority of CSF rhinorrhea cases, with primary closure rates of greater than 90% in large series. Moreover, compared with the traditional open approaches, this procedure carries similar results with fewer complications.

SUPPLEMENTARY DATA

Supplementary data related to this article can be found online at http://dx.doi.org/10.1016/j.nec. 2015.03.003.

REFERENCES

1. Rhoton AL Jr. The anterior and middle cranial base. Neurosurgery 2002;51(4):S273–302.
2. Rhoton AL Jr. The sellar region. Neurosurgery 2002; 51(4):S335–74.
3. Ogle OE, Weinstock RJ, Friedman E. Surgical anatomy of the nasal cavity and paranasal sinuses. Oral Maxillofac Surg Clin North Am 2012;24(2):155–66.
4. Beale TJ, Madani G, Morley SJ. Imaging of the paranasal sinuses and nasal cavity: normal anatomy and clinically relevant anatomical variants. Semin Ultrasound CT MR 2009;30(1):2–16.
5. Stammberger HR, Kennedy DW. Anatomic terminology group. Paranasal sinuses: anatomic terminology and nomenclature. Ann Otol Rhinol Laryngol Suppl 1995;167:7–16.
6. Tabaee A, Anand VK, Cappabianca P, et al. Endoscopic management of spontaneous meningoencephalocele of the lateral sphenoid sinus. J Neurosurg 2010;112(5):1070–7.
7. Psaltis AJ, Schlosser RJ, Banks CA, et al. A systematic review of the endoscopic repair of cerebrospinal fluid leaks. Otolaryngol Head Neck Surg 2012;147(2):196–203.
8. Kainz J, Stammberger H. The roof of the anterior ethmoid: a locus minoris resistentiae in the skull base. Laryngol Rhinol Otol (Stuttg) 1988;67(4): 142–9.
9. Sakas DE, Beale DJ, Ameen AA, et al. Compound anterior cranial base fractures: classification using computerized tomography scanning as a basis for selection of patients for dural repair. J Neurosurg 1998;88(3):471–7.
10. Locatelli D, Rampa F, Acchiardi I, et al. Endoscopic endonasal approaches for repair of cerebrospinal fluid leaks: nine-year experience. Neurosurgery 2006;58(4 Suppl 2):ONS-246–56 [discussion: ONS-256–7].
11. Shetty PG, Shroff MM, Fatterpekar GM, et al. A retrospective analysis of spontaneous sphenoid sinus fistula: MR and CT findings. AJNR Am J Neuroradiol 2000;21:337–42.
12. Castelnuovo P, Dallan I, Pistochini A, et al. Endonasal endoscopic repair of Sternberg's canal cerebrospinal fluid leaks. Laryngoscope 2007;117(2): 345–9.
13. Schlosser RJ, Bolger WE. Nasal cerebrospinal fluid leaks: critical review and surgical considerations. Laryngoscope 2004;114(2):255–65.
14. Prosser JD, Vender JR, Solares CA. Traumatic cerebrospinal fluid leaks. Otolaryngol Clin North Am 2011;44(4):857–73.
15. Scholsem M, Scholtes F, Collignon F, et al. Surgical management of anterior cranial base fractures with cerebrospinal fluid fistulae: a single-institution experience. Neurosurgery 2008;62(2):463–71.
16. Yilmazlar S, Arslan E, Kocaeli H, et al. Cerebrospinal fluid leakage complicating skull base fractures: analysis of 81 cases. Neurosurg Rev 2006;29(1): 64–71.
17. Friedman JA, Ebersold MJ, Quast LM. Post-traumatic cerebrospinal fluid leakage. World J Surg 2001;25(8):1062–6.
18. Bell RB, Dierks EJ, Homer L, et al. Management of cerebrospinal fluid leak associated with craniomaxillofacial trauma. J Oral Maxillofac Surg 2004;62(6): 676–84.
19. Bernal-Sprekelsen M, Bleda-Vázquez C, Carrau RL. Ascending meningitis secondary to traumatic cerebrospinal fluid leaks. Am J Rhinol 2000;14(4):257–9.
20. Ziu M, Savage JG, Jimenez DF. Diagnosis and treatment of cerebrospinal fluid rhinorrhea following accidental traumatic anterior skull base fractures. Neurosurg Focus 2012;32(6):E3.
21. Daudia A, Biswas D, Jones NS. Risk of meningitis with cerebrospinal fluid rhinorrhea. Ann Otol Rhinol Laryngol 2007;116(12):902–5.
22. Brodie HA. Prophylactic antibiotics for posttraumatic cerebrospinal fluid fistulae: a meta-analysis. Arch Otolaryngol Head Neck Surg 1997;123:749–52.
23. MacGee EE, Cauthen JC, Brackett CE. Meningitis following acute traumatic cerebrospinal fluid fistula. J Neurosurg 1970;33:312–6.

24. Kassam AB, Prevedello DM, Carrau RL, et al. Endoscopic endonasal skull base surgery: analysis of complications in the authors' initial 800 patients. J Neurosurg 2011;114(6):1544–68.

25. McCoul ED, Anand VK, Singh A, et al. Long-term effectiveness of a reconstructive protocol using the nasoseptal flap after endoscopic skull base surgery. World Neurosurg 2014;81(1):136–43.

26. Patel KS, Komotar RJ, Szentirmai O, et al. Case-specific protocol to reduce cerebrospinal fluid leakage after endonasal endoscopic surgery. J Neurosurg 2013;119(3):661–8.

27. Banu MA, Szentirmai O, Mascarenhas L, et al. Pneumocephalus patterns following endonasal endoscopic skull base surgery as predictors of postoperative CSF leaks. J Neurosurg 2014;121(4): 961–75.

28. Dlouhy BJ, Madhavan K, Clinger JD, et al. Elevated body mass index and risk of postoperative CSF leak following transsphenoidal surgery. J Neurosurg 2012;116(6):1311–7.

29. Komotar RJ, Starke RM, Raper DM, et al. Endoscopic skull base surgery: a comprehensive comparison with open transcranial approaches. Br J Neurosurg 2012;26(5):637–48.

30. Juraschka K, Khan OH, Godoy BL, et al. Endoscopic endonasal transsphenoidal approach to large and giant pituitary adenomas: institutional experience and predictors of extent of resection. J Neurosurg 2014;121(1):75–83.

31. Komotar RJ, Starke RM, Raper DM, et al. Endoscopic endonasal versus open transcranial resection of anterior midline skull base meningiomas. World Neurosurg 2012;77(5–6):713–24.

32. Wise SK, Schlosser RJ. Evaluation of spontaneous nasal cerebrospinal fluid leaks. Curr Opin Otolaryngol Head Neck Surg 2007;15(1):28–34.

33. Schlosser RJ, Woodworth BA, Wilensky EM, et al. Spontaneous cerebrospinal fluid leaks: a variant of benign intracranial hypertension. Ann Otol Rhinol Laryngol 2006;115(7):495–500.

34. Schlosser RJ, Wilensky EM, Grady MS, et al. Cerebrospinal fluid pressure monitoring after repair of cerebrospinal fluid leaks. Otolaryngol Head Neck Surg 2004;130(4):443–8.

35. Schlosser RJ, Wilensky EM, Grady MS, et al. Elevated intracranial pressures in spontaneous cerebrospinal fluid leaks. Am J Rhinol 2003;17(4): 191–5.

36. Schlosser RJ, Bolger WE. Spontaneous nasal cerebrospinal fluid leaks and empty sella syndrome: a clinical association. Am J Rhinol 2003; 17(2):91–6.

37. Carrau RL, Snyderman CH, Kassam AB. The management of cerebrospinal fluid leaks in patients at risk for high-pressure hydrocephalus. Laryngoscope 2005;115(2):205–12.

38. Nyquist GG, Anand VK, Mehra S, et al. Endoscopic endonasal repair of anterior skull base nontraumatic cerebrospinal fluid leaks, meningoceles, and encephaloceles. J Neurosurg 2010;113(5): 961–6.

39. Mirza S, Saeed SR, Ramsden RT. Extensive tension pneumocephalus complicating continuous lumbar CSF drainage for the management of CSF rhinorrhoea. ORL J Otorhinolaryngol Relat Spec 2003; 65(4):215–8.

40. Zapalac JS, Marple BF, Schwade ND. Skull base cerebrospinal fluid fistulas: a comprehensive diagnostic algorithm. Otolaryngol Head Neck Surg 2002;126(6):669–76.

41. Warnecke A, Averbeck T, Wurster U, et al. Diagnostic relevance of beta2-transferrin for the detection of cerebrospinal fluid fistulas. Arch Otolaryngol Head Neck Surg 2004;130(10):1178–84.

42. Schnabel C, Di Martino E, Gilsbach JM, et al. Comparison of beta2-transferrin and beta-trace protein for detection of cerebrospinal fluid in nasal and ear fluids. Clin Chem 2004;50(3):661–3.

43. Arrer E, Meco C, Oberascher G, et al. beta-Trace protein as a marker for cerebrospinal fluid rhinorrhea. Clin Chem 2002;48(6 Pt 1):939–41.

44. Sanderson JD, Kountakis SE, McMains KC. Endoscopic management of cerebrospinal fluid leaks. Facial Plast Surg 2009;25(1):29–37.

45. Lloyd KM, DelGaudio JM, Hudgins PA. Imaging of skull base cerebrospinal fluid leaks in adults. Radiology 2008;248(3):725–36.

46. Cui S, Han D, Zhou B, et al. Endoscopic endonasal surgery for recurrent cerebrospinal fluid rhinorrhea. Acta Otolaryngol 2010;130(10):1169–74.

47. Shetty PG, Shroff MM, Sahani DV, et al. Evaluation of high-resolution CT and MR cisternography in the diagnosis of cerebrospinal fluid fistula. AJNR Am J Neuroradiol 1998;19(4):633–9.

48. Sillers MJ, Morgan CE, el Gammal T. Magnetic resonance cisternography and thin coronal computerized tomography in the evaluation of cerebrospinal fluid rhinorrhea. Am J Rhinol 1997;11(5):387–92.

49. Senior BA, Jafri K, Benninger M. Safety and efficacy of endoscopic repair of CSF leaks and encephaloceles: a survey of the members of the American Rhinologic Society. Am J Rhinol 2001;15(1):21–5.

50. Harvey RJ, Parmar P, Sacks R, et al. Endoscopic skull base reconstruction of large dural defects: a systematic review of published evidence. Laryngoscope 2012;122(2):452–9.

51. Wise SK, Harvey RJ, Patel SJ, et al. Endoscopic repair of skull base defects presenting with pneumocephalus. J Otolaryngol Head Neck Surg 2009; 38(4):509–16.

52. Moseley JI, Carton CA, Stern WE. Spectrum of complications in the use of intrathecal fluorescein. J Neurosurg 1978;48(5):765–7.

53. Placantonakis DG, Tabaee A, Anand VK, et al. Safety of low-dose intrathecal fluorescein in endoscopic cranial base surgery. Neurosurgery 2007; 61(3 Suppl):161–6.

54. Seth R, Rajasekaran K, Benninger MS, et al. The utility of intrathecal fluorescein in cerebrospinal fluid leak repair. Otolaryngol Head Neck Surg 2010; 143(5):626–32.

55. Tabaee A, Placantonakis DG, Schwartz TH, et al. Intrathecal fluorescein in endoscopic skull base surgery. Otolaryngol Head Neck Surg 2007;137(2): 316–20.

56. Keerl R, Weber RK, Draf W, et al. Use of sodium fluorescein solution for detection of cerebrospinal fluid fistulas: an analysis of 420 administrations and reported complications in Europe and the United States. Laryngoscope 2004;114(2): 266–72.

57. Tabaee A, Kassenoff TL, Kacker A, et al. The efficacy of computer assisted surgery in the endoscopic management of cerebrospinal fluid rhinorrhea. Otolaryngol Head Neck Surg 2005;133(6):936–43.

58. Tormenti MJ, Paluzzi A, Pinheiro-Nieto C, et al. Endoscopic endonasal repair of spontaneous CSF fistulae. J Neurosurg 2012;32(Suppl):E6.

59. Al-Nashar IS, Carrau RL, Herrera A, et al. Endoscopic transnasal transpterygopalatine fossa approach to the lateral recess of the sphenoid sinus. Laryngoscope 2004;114(3):528–32.

60. Gross WE, Gross CW, Becker D, et al. Modified transnasal endoscopic Lothrop procedure as an alternative to frontal sinus obliteration. Otolaryngol Head Neck Surg 1995;113(4):427–34.

61. Woodworth BA, Schlosser RJ, Palmer JN. Endoscopic repair of frontal sinus cerebrospinal fluid leaks. J Laryngol Otol 2005;119(9):709–13.

62. Jones V, Virgin F, Riley K, et al. Changing paradigms in frontal sinus cerebrospinal fluid leak repair. Int Forum Allergy Rhinol 2012;2(3):227–32.

63. Shi JB, Chen FH, Fu QL, et al. Frontal sinus cerebrospinal fluid leaks: repair in 15 patients using an endoscopic surgical approach. ORL J Otorhinolaryngol Relat Spec 2010;72(1):56–62.

64. Bhavana K, Kumar R, Keshri A, et al. Minimally invasive technique for repairing CSF leaks due to defects of posterior table of frontal sinus. J Neurol Surg B Skull Base 2014;75(3):183–6.

65. Bedrosian JC, Anand VK, Schwartz TH. The endoscopic endonasal approach to repair of iatrogenic and noniatrogenic cerebrospinal fluid leaks and encephaloceles of the anterior cranial fossa. World Neurosurg 2014;82(6S):S86–94.

66. Chin D, Harvey RJ. Endoscopic reconstruction of frontal, cribiform and ethmoid skull base defects. Adv Otorhinolaryngol 2013;74:104–18.

67. Leng LZ, Brown S, Anand VK, et al. "Gasket-seal" watertight closure in minimal-access endoscopic cranial base surgery. Neurosurgery 2008;62(5 Suppl 2):ONSE342–3 [discussion: ONSE343].

68. Wormald PJ, McDonogh M. The bath-plug closure of anterior skull base cerebrospinal fluid leaks. Am J Rhinol 2003;17(5):299–305.

69. Hadad G, Bassagasteguy L, Carrau RL, et al. A novel reconstructive technique after endoscopic expanded endonasal approaches: vascular pedicle nasoseptal flap. Laryngoscope 2006;116(10):1882–6.

70. Hegazy HM, Carrau RL, Snyderman CH, et al. Transnasal endoscopic repair of cerebrospinal fluid rhinorrhea: a meta-analysis. Laryngoscope 2000; 110(7):1166–72.

71. Soudry E, Turner JH, Nayak JV, et al. Endoscopic reconstruction of surgically created skull base defects: a systematic review. Otolaryngol Head Neck Surg 2014;150(5):730–8.

72. DeConde AS, Suh JD, Ramakrishnan VR. Treatment of cerebrospinal fluid rhinorrhea. Curr Opin Otolaryngol Head Neck Surg 2015;23(1):59–64.

73. Alsaffar H, Sowerby L, Rotenberg BW. Postoperative nasal debridement after endoscopic sinus surgery: a randomized controlled trial. Ann Otol Rhinol Laryngol 2013;122(10):642–7.

74. Green R, Banigo A, Hathorn I. Postoperative nasal debridement following functional endoscopic sinus surgery, a systematic review of the literature. Clin Otolaryngol 2014;40(1):2–8.

75. Komotar RJ, Starke RM, Raper DM, et al. Endoscopic endonasal versus open repair of anterior skull base CSF leak, meningocele, and encephalocele: a systematic review of outcomes. J Neurol Surg A Cent Eur Neurosurg 2013;74(4):239–50.

Endoscopic Endonasal Approach for Removal of Tuberculum Sellae Meningiomas

Leo F.S. Ditzel Filho, MD[a], Daniel M. Prevedello, MD[a,b],*,
Ali O. Jamshidi, MD[a], Ricardo L. Dolci, MD[b],
Edward E. Kerr, MD[a], Raewyn Campbell, MD[b],
Bradley A. Otto, MD[a,b], Ricardo L. Carrau, MD[a,b]

KEYWORDS

- Endonasal • Endoscopic • Meningioma • Skull base • Tuberculum sellae

KEY POINTS

- Nearly all tuberculum sellae meningiomas are amenable to endonasal resection; lateral extension beyond the internal carotid arteries is the major limitation to resection.
- Vascular encasement or optic canal invasion increases the complexity of the surgery but is not a limitation of the approach.
- Potential advantages of the approach include the absence of neurovascular retraction or displacement, increased visibility underneath the optic apparatus, and removal of infiltrated hyperostotic bone.
- The main disadvantages include the risk for cerebrospinal fluid leakage, need for dedicated training and equipment, and steep learning curve.
- The endonasal approach for removal of tuberculum sellae meningiomas requires a wide transnasal corridor, with removal of the right middle turbinate, posterior ethmoidectomies, resection of the posterior third of the septum for creation of a single working cavity, and elevation of a pedicled nasoseptal flap.

INTRODUCTION

Tuberculum sellae meningiomas are challenging lesions; located in the suprasellar space, they can displace and distort the superjacent optic apparatus causing visual impairment, encase critical neurovascular structures, and promote hyperostosis and optic canal invasion.[1] These features render their safe resection a daunting task. Historically, this has been accomplished through open transcranial approaches, especially the classic pterional-transsylvian route[2] or through more complex skull base approaches, such as the cranio-orbito-zygomatic[3] and its variants and even the fronto-basal interhemispheric technique.[4] More recently, less invasive methods also have been proposed, including the lateral supraorbital[5] and the "eyebrow" subfrontal[6–8] craniotomies. Regardless of which technique is chosen, all transcranial routes require a certain degree of cerebral retraction; in some instances, even some manipulation of the optic apparatus is necessary for tumor removal, especially the component located underneath the chiasm and ipsilateral optic nerve, often demanding "blind"

[a] Department of Neurological Surgery, Wexner Medical Center, The Ohio State University, 410 West 10th Avenue, Columbus, OH 43210, USA; [b] Department of Otolaryngology – Head & Neck Surgery, Wexner Medical Center, The Ohio State University, 410 West 10th Avenue, Columbus, OH 43210, USA
* Corresponding author. Department of Neurological Surgery, Wexner Medical Center, The Ohio State University, 410 West 10th Avenue, N-1049 Doan Hall, Columbus, OH 43210.
E-mail address: Daniel.Prevedello@osumc.edu

Neurosurg Clin N Am 26 (2015) 349–361
http://dx.doi.org/10.1016/j.nec.2015.03.005
1042-3680/15/$ – see front matter © 2015 Elsevier Inc. All rights reserved.

curettage of that space. Furthermore, given the pattern of growth typical of these lesions, rising from the tuberculum arachnoid and projecting upward and posteriorly, the superior hypophyseal arteries are often displaced along with the tumor capsule and are thus directly in the surgeon's angle of attack, demanding the dissection to take place within an even tighter window.

The past decade witnessed several technological advances in skull base surgery, the most important of which arguably is the rise of endoscopic endonasal surgery.[9–23] When applied to tuberculum sellae meningiomas,[24] expanded endoscopic endonasal approaches (EEAs) seem to present several advantages: the need for cerebral retraction is obviated, given the ventral angle through which the surgeon tackles these lesions; because the optic apparatus is displaced superiorly and posteriorly, it is involved only in dissection at the end stages of surgery, during release of the tumor capsule from the optic nerves themselves, thus lowering the amount of optic manipulation. Moreover, because the superior hypophyseal arteries are also typically dislodged toward the optic chiasm, freeing them from the tumor capsule is also facilitated and takes place only at the end of tumor removal, with minimal handling. Based on these potential features, EEAs have become the workhorse for the authors in nearly all suprasellar tumors, meningiomatous or otherwise.

Hence, herein we describe our current indications and contraindications, surgical technique and anatomy, as well as complication management and avoidance strategies for the endoscopic endonasal resection of tuberculum sellae meningiomas.

INDICATIONS/CONTRAINDICATIONS

For indications and contraindications, see **Table 1**.

SURGICAL ANATOMY

The surgical anatomy and spatial relations of the ventral skull base and the suprasellar space have been described in detail[25–27]; the main pertinent structures and landmarks are depicted in **Fig. 1**.

SURGICAL TECHNIQUE
Preoperative Planning

All patients submitted to endonasal resection of tuberculum sellae meningiomas undergo the following:

- Anesthesia evaluation with nasal swab and culture; if positive for methicillin-resistant *Staphylococcus aureus* (MRSA), the patient

is treated in the morning of surgery with a single nasal application of a povidone-iodine solution at 5% (3M, St. Paul, MN).
- Magnetic resonance imaging (MRI) of the brain and computed axial tomography (CT) scan, both thinly sliced (<3 mm) and fused for intraoperative navigation. Special attention is given to the position of the pituitary stalk, the anterior cerebral arteries, and the presence of hyperostosis and/or optic canal invasion.
- Full pituitary hormone serum sampling, including growth hormone, prolactin, thyroid-stimulating hormone, cortisol, adrenocorticotrophic hormone, testosterone, follicle-stimulating hormone, and luteinizing hormone. This aims to establish preoperative endocrine dysfunction, if any.
- Ophthalmologic evaluation with visual field testing.
- Otolaryngology evaluation, to detect sinonasal abnormalities, especially signs of infection.

Preparation and Patient Positioning

Preparation

- General anesthesia with orotracheal intubation: *no cerebrospinal fluid (CSF) diversion is used.*
- Prophylactic antibiotics: cefepime if MRSA negative, cefepime and vancomycin if MRSA positive.
- Urinary catheter placement.
- Copious nasal irrigation with oxymetazoline hydrochloride solution and facial/nasal decontamination with iodine solution; the abdomen is also prepped in case a fat graft is necessary.
- The navigation tower and at least 2 monitors are positioned according to the otolaryngologist's hand dominance (**Fig. 2**).

Positioning

- Supine position, with the head fixed on the Mayfield 3-pin headholder. The neck is slightly extended and the head turned to the right, with the whole body tilted to the left (see **Fig. 2**). The body is secured and protected with foam and tape; the navigation transmitter is attached to the headholder.

Surgical Approach

The surgical approach is composed of the following sequential steps (**Fig. 3**):

1. Right middle turbinectomy, performed with curved strong sinus scissors.

Table 1
Indications and contraindications

| Indications | Contraindications | |
	Relative	Absolute
• Tuberculum sellae meningiomas with optic apparatus compression and/or documented growth and/or endocrine dysfunction, *despite size*	• Presence of sinonasal infection[a] • Significant tumor component lateral to the ICA(s) and lateral to the anterior clinoids[b]	• Clinical instability that prevents general anesthesia • Lack of appropriate personnel and/or equipment

Note that vascular (superior hypophyseal arteries, anterior cerebral arteries)/pituitary stalk encasement or optic canal involvement increase the complexity of the approach tremendously; however they *are not contraindications to endonasal surgery.*

Abbreviation: ICA, internal carotid artery.

[a] Treat for 3 weeks (if bacterial) or 6 weeks (if fungal) before proceeding with endonasal surgery.

[b] Endonasal surgery may be an option if optic decompression is the goal in cases in which total resection is not feasible (ie, bilateral cavernous sinus invasion); if extension beyond the ICA is unilateral and there is no cavernous sinus invasion, consider transcranial surgery.

2. Bilateral posterior ethmoidectomies, performed with microdebrider.

3. Elevation of the nasoseptal flap[28] and storing in the nasopharynx (side is decided based on local anatomy but preferably on the right side to avoid conflict with power instruments on the left nostril from a right-handed surgeon).

4. Posterior septectomy.

5. Incision and rotation of the now-exposed contralateral septal mucosa to cover the denuded septum.[29,30]

6. Wide bilateral opening of the sphenoid sinus with Kerrison rongeurs and high-speed drill; extreme care is taken not to damage the pedicle of the nasoseptal flap.

Surgical Procedure

The surgical procedure is composed of the following sequential steps (**Fig. 4**):

1. Drilling of the sphenoidal septae and skull base; the bone is drilled down to eggshell thickness and elevated from the dura. This starts at the

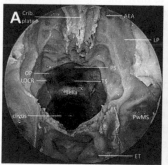 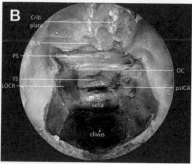 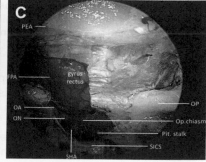

Fig. 1. Anatomic overview of the transsphenoidal transsellar/transtubercular/transplanum approach. (*A*) Panoramic view of a wide sphenoidotomy and bilateral posterior ethmoidectomies revealing the main landmarks of the posterior sphenoidal wall. AEA, anterior ethmoidal artery; Crib. plate, cribriform plate; ET, Eustachian tube; LOCR, lateral optic-carotid recess; LP, lamina papyracea; OP, optic protuberance; PS, planum sphenoidale; PwMS, posterior wall of the maxillary sinus; TS, tuberculum sellae. (*B*) Bone removal; note that the exposure extends from the cribriform plate and the posterior ethmoidal artery superiorly to the sellar floor inferiorly and from lamina papyracea to lamina papyracea laterally. Also note that the left optic canal has been partially removed to allow exploration within the optic sheath. Crib. plate, cribriform plate; LOCR, lateral optic-carotid recess; OC, optic canal; PEA, posterior ethmoidal artery; PS, planum sphenoidale; psICA, parasellar internal carotid artery; TS, tuberculum sellae. (*C*) Exposure of the suprasellar space and right optic canal; the dura has been partially removed on the right side along with the right optic canal to reveal the contents of the suprasellar space. FPA, frontopolar artery; OA, ophthalmic artery; ON, optic nerve; OP, optic protuberance; Op. chiasm, optic chiasm; PEA, posterior ethmoidal artery; Pit. stalk, pituitary stalk; SHA, superior hypophyseal artery; SICS, superior intercavernous sinus.

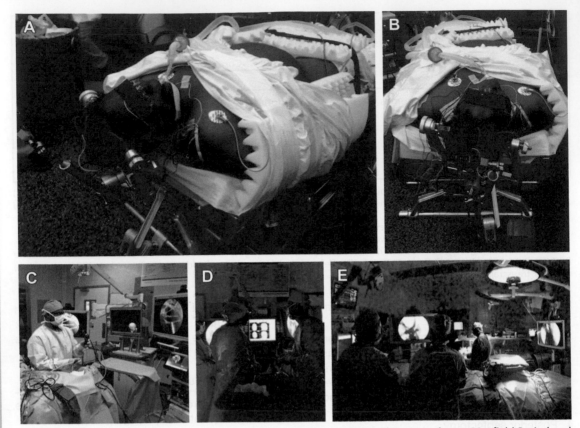

Fig. 2. Patient and room positioning. (*A, B*) Patient positioning. The head is secured on a Mayfield 3-pin head-holder and slightly turned to the right; the neck is gently extended to improve the operating angle. Note that the abdomen is prepped in case a fat graft is necessary and the extensive foaming and taping to secure the patient. (*C, D*) Monitor positioning when the otolaryngologist is left-handed; 2 monitors flank the navigation tower at the head of the bed. The otolaryngologist stands to the left of the patient to drive the endoscope while the neurosurgeon, on the patient's right, performs the tumor dissection. (*E*) Monitor positioning when the otolaryngologist is right handed; a monitor is placed to the left of the patient and another at the patient's feet and both the otolaryngologist and neurosurgeon stand to the patient's right.

sella, followed by the planum sphenoidale (a trapezoid-shaped osteotomy is performed and the planum is elevated in a single piece) and finally the tuberculum.

2. Coagulation of enlarged dural vessels to promote tumor devascularization (there are often large McConnell capsular arteries associated with tuberculum sellae meningiomas).

3. Dural opening starts at the midline of the suprasellar space and is carried superiorly to the SICS, which is visualized but not ligated. The dural opening is extended laterally above the SICS to expose the base of the tumor and to determine the position of the pituitary gland. This plane is followed posteriorly to encounter the pituitary stalk.

4. Tumor biopsy and debulking can be achieved with microscissors and aspiration or with the use of side-cutting aspiration devices.[31] We

have decreased the use of ultrasonic aspirators in endonasal surgery because of the risk of heat damage to the nostrils.

5. Extracapsular dissection: microsurgical principles are always respected and the arachnoid envelope of the tumor is used to protect critical surrounding neurovascular structures, namely the superior hypophyseal arteries, the pituitary stalk, the optic nerves, and chiasm. Once the tumor remnant has been freed from these structures, it is "delivered" into the sphenoid cavity and removed. If too adherent or too voluminous, the tumor remnant may be resected in piecemeal fashion. It is imperative to ensure that the anterior cerebral arteries are not attached to the tumor capsule before mobilizing it.

6. If optic canal involvement is present, the optic sheath (now exposed after drilling during the approach) is opened with angled scissors

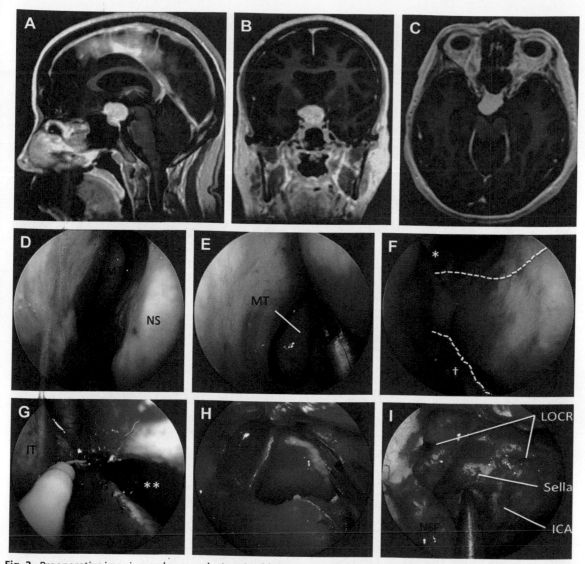

Fig. 3. Preoperative imaging and approach. A sagittal (*A*), coronal (*B*), and axial (*C*) contrast T1-weighted brain MRI reveals a large suprasellar tumor promoting optic chiasm compression, suggestive of a tuberculum sellae meningioma. (*D*) Nasal landmarks on the right nostril. IT, inferior turbinate; MT, middle turbinate; NS, nasal septum. (*E*) The middle turbinate (MT) is resected with strong, sinus scissors and detached downward; care is taken not to avulse it from its implantation because of the risk of a premature CSF leak from the anterior cranial fossa. (*F*) The nasoseptal flap (*dashed line*) is elevated on the right, with the pedicle located between the sphenoid sinus (*asterisk*) and the choana (*dagger*). Once harvested, the flap may be stored within the ipsilateral maxillary sinus or at the choana. (*G*) The contralateral septal mucosa is incised and mobilized anteriorly to cover the denuded cartilaginous septum, revealing the left nasal corridor (*double asterisk*). IT, inferior turbinate. (*H*) The sphenoid sinus is widely opened bilaterally, thus creating a single operating chamber at the posterior end of the nasal pathway. (*I*) The sphenoid sinus and its landmarks are exposed, including the sella, the left carotid protuberance (ICA) and the lateral optic-carotid recesses (LOCR); note the nasoseptal flap (NSF) mobilized inferiorly toward the choana.

under angled endoscopic visualization; care is taken not to damage the ophthalmic arteries during dissection of this tumor component.
7. Copious irrigation with warm saline clears the surgical field of blood and debris while promoting hemostasis.

8. Multilayered reconstruction concludes the procedure; although several methods have been described, the authors currently use the following sequence: inlay collagen matrix, onlay nasoseptal flap, sphenoid filling with synthetic foam.

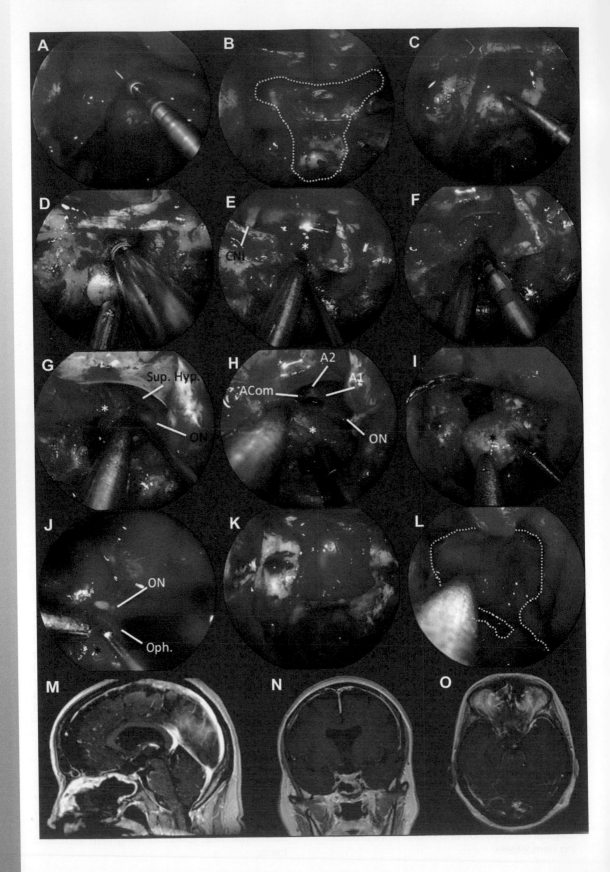

COMPLICATIONS AND MANAGEMENT

- The main complication is by far postoperative CSF leakage,[32] usually brought on by flap displacement or technical error. It is considered a medical urgency and the patient is always brought back to the operation room for flap repositioning and/or bolstering with abdominal fat. Lumbar drains are reserved for the rare occasion of a recurrent leak after a new surgical correction. Acetazolamide is used if transient increased intracranial pressure (ICP) is present; if perennial, the increased ICP is permanently managed with ventriculo-peritoneal shunting.
- Meningitis is extremely rare,[33] even in the setting of a CSF leak. If present, it is managed with wide-spectrum antibiotics aimed to cover the sinonasal flora.
- Sinonasal infection and scarring are uncommon and addressed as a typical sinus surgery postoperative recovery.
- Unless intraoperative vascular damage occurs, neurologic deterioration is not expected. If visual worsening is present, a surgical site hematoma should be suspected and the patient submitted to a stat noncontrast head CT. If the patient is nonarousable or presents with seizures, hypertensive pneumocephalus must be ruled out, also with a head CT. In both instances, emergent drainage is necessary.
- Manipulation of the pituitary stalk may incur diabetes insipidus; if the patient is awake and accepting fluids, oral intake is encouraged to replace the fluid loss. If ineffective, desmopressin is started. Cortisol insufficiency or syndrome of inappropriate antidiuretic hormone secretion is extremely rare.
- Clinical complications (respiratory and urinary infections, deep vein thrombosis) occur in the same rates as transcranial surgeries and must be addressed accordingly.

POSTOPERATIVE CARE

All patients submitted to endonasal resection of tuberculum sellae meningiomas undergo the following:

- Immediate postoperative care in an intensive care unit environment.
- Prophylactic intravenous antibiotics for the initial 24 hours after surgery (the same regimen started before the operation is maintained; oral antibiotics are then started until the packing is removed, typically at postoperative day 5).
- Electrolyte monitoring, especially to rule out diabetes insipidus.
- Serum prolactin and cortisol levels are measured in the morning of the first postoperative day to ensure pituitary function is preserved.
- Noncontrast head CT is performed as soon as possible to rule out immediate complications; a brain MRI is typically performed in the first postoperative day to confirm the degree of resection and establish a baseline for future comparisons.
- Regular postoperative measures are taken as with any transcranial surgery, including deep

Fig. 4. Tumor resection, closure, and postoperative imaging. (*A*) Septations within the sphenoid are drilled down. (*B*) The sella, planum sphenoidale, and tuberculum sellae are drilled down, in this sequence, to complete the exposure (*dashed line*). If necessary, the bone covering the optic canal also may be removed with a more delicate drill and copious irrigation. (*C*) Once eggshell thick, the bone is elevated from dura with a Cottle dissector. (*D*) Before dural opening, large vessels on the tuberculum dura are coagulated with a single shaft bipolar device (*dagger*). (*E*) The dura is opened to reveal a fibrous tumor (*asterisk*) obliterating the suprasellar space. CNI, olfactory tract. (*F*) The tumor is debulked with the combination of microscissors, dissectors, and a side-cutting aspiration device. (*G*) Once enough volume reduction is achieved, the tumor (*asterisk*) collapses onto itself and extracapsular dissection takes place. Initially, the lateral edges are detached from the surrounding structures, including the superior hypophyseal arteries (Sup. Hyp.) and the optic nerves (ON). (*H*) The superior limit of the tumor (*asterisk*) is carefully dissected from the optic chiasm and the vessels of the anterior communicating complex. A1, first segment of the anterior cerebral artery; A2, second segment of the anterior cerebral artery; ACom, anterior communicating artery; ON, optic nerve. (*I*) Once released from the surrounding arachnoid and neurovascular elements, the tumor (*asterisk*) is "delivered" into the sphenoid cavity. (*J*) The right optic canal and sheath are opened to remove tumor invasion (*asterisk*); note that an angled endoscope pointing to the left is necessary to obtain this view. ON, optic nerve; Oph., ophthalmic artery. (*K*) The dural defect is plugged with a partial inlay sheet of collagen matrix, which is secured at the center by a second sheet of the same material. (*L*) The nasoseptal flap (*dashed line*) is positioned over the entire defect. Postoperative sagittal (*M*), coronal (*N*), and axial (*O*) T1-weighted brain MRI confirms a total resection. Note the enhancement of the nasoseptal flap on the sagittal and coronal views.

vein thrombosis prophylaxis and adequate pain management.

- No nasal catheters are permitted and straining is strictly avoided to prevent flap displacement; this includes proscribing incentive spirometry or the use of straws, sneezing and coughing with the mouth open, use of stool softeners, and avoiding bending or lifting completely.
- While in the hospital, the patient is challenged daily for a CSF leak by tilting the head forward; if clear fluid is present and a CSF leak is not obvious, a head CT is performed (to detect pneumocephalus). Collecting fluid to test for beta-2-transferrin is not helpful in this phase because the nasal cavity has been recently exposed to CSF during surgery and false positives are common. If present, the CSF leak is managed with surgery in an urgent fashion.
- Provided no complications arise, patients are typically discharged on postoperative day 2. On postoperative day 5, they return to the otolaryngology clinic for removal of nasal packing/splints and evaluation. During the initial 3 months after surgery these consults may vary in frequency, according to the degree of nasal scarring and crusting present. The patient is followed at the neurosurgical clinic at 30 days after surgery and onward accordingly, depending mainly on the meningioma grade confirmed by pathology. A postoperative ophthalmologic evaluation with visual field testing is also performed within the first 30 days to establish the visual patterns for future comparison.

OUTCOMES

Given the recent development of the technique, studies on purely endoscopic endonasal resection of tuberculum sellae meningiomas are still somewhat scarce; typically studies tend to cluster these lesions along with other meningiomas of the anterior cranial base, especially those of the olfactory groove and planum sphenoidale, often making it impossible to differentiate them solely based on the data provided in these articles, and therefore negatively impacting proper analysis. Moreover, variations on the definitions of resection rate among investigators further hinder this examination. Finally, some investigators published several studies within a short period with a similar number of patients but focused on different aspects of the technique and outcomes; this could mean that the same population was represented more than once and therefore it could influence the analysis. It is the authors' opinion that, despite the anatomic

proximity, these are completely different entities and should be discussed as such. Hence, **Table 2** summarizes the findings of the most recent studies related *specifically* to tuberculum sellae meningiomas; those articles focused on describing technical modifications, such as reconstruction strategies rather than clinical outcomes, were thus excluded from this review.

As expected, these studies depict initial experiences and relatively small series, ranging from single cases to a more robust 37-patient cohort. In brief, 203 patients were reported in 29 studies; tumor dimensions varied greatly among articles, both in their description as in their availability. Resection rates were also not displayed in a uniform fashion; gross total resection rates ranged from 54% to 100% among those studies in which it was described (81% overall). Of the available data, the most common complication was CSF leakage (19% overall); other advert events included transient (2.6%) or permanent diabetes insipidus (1.9%) and postoperative panhypopituitarism (3.3%). There were 2 major vascular injuries (1.3%) and 2 deaths (1.3%), from intraventricular hemorrhage and deep vein thrombosis/pulmonary embolism. Anosmia occurred in 2 patients (1.3%). Regarding visual complications, 3 patients (1.9%) presented transient visual deterioration and 2 (1.3%) were left with a permanent postoperative deficit.

There were 3 meta-analysis studies that contemplated the endonasal endoscopic technique applied to tuberculum sellae meningiomas. Komotar and colleagues[22] compared EEAs with open approaches series, but did also include planum meningiomas in their analysis. The open group presented a larger mean maximal diameter (2.83 vs 2.7 cm) as well as higher gross total resection rates (84.1% vs 74.7%, $P = .041$) but also a slightly higher visual deterioration rate (14.2% vs 12.7%); conversely, CSF leak rates were higher in the endoscopic group (21.3% vs 4.3%). Nonetheless, visual improvement was significantly higher in the endoscopic cohort (73.5% vs 58.7%, $P = .039$). Clark and colleagues[34] also compared series of open and endonasal approaches. In groups of patients with similar tumor dimensions, they found that although related to a higher rate of CSF leak (21% vs 5%, $P<.05$) the endoscopic cohort was also associated with a significantly higher rate of visual improvement (50%–100% vs 25%–78%, $P<.05$); in this study, both groups presented similar gross total resection rates. Finally, Graffeo and colleagues[35] performed a systematic review of open and endoscopic approaches. Once again, the endoscopic cohort was associated with a higher CSF leak rate (21.5% vs 4.4%, $P<.001$) but also with higher visual improvement (87% vs 61%,

Table 2
Studies on endoscopic endonasal resection of tuberculum sellae meningiomas

Authors/Year	No. of Cases	Average Tumor Dimensions	Rate of Resection	Complications
Jho,[36] 2001	1	10 × 15 mm	1/1 (100%) GTR	None
de Divitiis et al,[37] 2007	2	Not available	2/2 (100%) GTR	None
Laufer et al,[23] 2007	3	3.5 cm (largest diameter on MRI)	2/3 (67%) GTR 1/3 (33%) STR	1/3 (33%) with CSF leak and permanent DI
Prevedello et al,[38] 2007	1	6.8 cm^3	1/1 (100%) GTR	None
de Divitiis et al,[39] 2007	6	13.7 cm^3	5/6 GTR (83.3%) 1/6 STR (16.7%)	2/6 (33.4%) with CSF leak 1/6 (16.7%) with Intraventricular hemorrhage and death 1/6 (16.7%) with permanent DI 2/6 (33.4%) with temporary vision deterioration
Cappabianca et al,[40] 2008	4	Not available	4/4 GTR (100%)	None
de Divitiis et al,[20] 2008	7	2 cases <2 cm greatest diameter 5 cases 2–4 cm greatest diameter	6/7 (85.7%) GTR 1/7 (14.2%) STR	1/7 (14.2%) with permanent DI 1/7 (14.2%) with intraventricular hemorrhage and death 1/7 (14.2%) with CSF leak
Gardner et al,[24] 2008	13	12.03 cm^3	11/13 (84.6%) GTR 1/13 (7.7%) NTR (>95%) 1/13 (7.7%) STR (<95%)	8/13 (62%) with CSF leak
Fatemi et al,[6] 2009	12	25 ± 8 mm greatest diameter	7/12 (58%) GTR 3/12 (25%) NTR 2/12 (16%) STR	1 (7%) with visual deterioration 4/12 (33%) with CSF leakage 1 (7%) postoperative panhypopituitarism
Wang et al,[41] 2009	7	15.36 cm^3	6/7 (85.7%) GTR 1/7 (14.3%) STR	None
Dehdashti et al,[42] 2009	1	Not available	1/1 (100%) GTR	1/1 (100%) CSF leak
Ceylan et al,[43] 2009	2	2 cm and 4 cm greatest diameter	1/2 (50%) GTR 1/2 (50%) STR	Not available
Wang et al,[44] 2010	12	15.4 cm^3	11/12 (91.7%) GTR 1/12 (8.3%) subtotal	1/12 (8.3%) with CSF leak 1/12 (8.3%) with transient DI
Kurschel et al,[45] 2011	8	Not available	Not available	Not available
Van Gompel et al,[19] 2011	13	N/A 24.3 ± 6.6 mm greatest diameter	7/13 (54%) GTR 6/13 (46%) STR (3/6 planned decompression)	1 (7.7%) visual deterioration 1 (7.7%) ACA infarction

(continued on next page)

Table 2
(continued)

Authors/Year	No. of Cases	Average Tumor Dimensions	Rate of Resection	Complications
Liu et al,[46] 2011	2	2.7 cm and 3 cm greatest diameter	2/2 (100%) GTR	1/2 (50%) with CSF hypotension due to use of lumbar drain
Fernandez-Miranda et al,[47] 2012	1	Not available	1/1 (100%) GTR	None
Chowdhury et al,[48] 2012	6	3 cases 3 × 3 cm 3 cases 4 × 4 cm	5/6 GTR (83.3%) 1/6 (16.7%) subtotal	1 (16.7%) with CSF leakage 1 (16.7%) with transient visual deterioration
Attia et al,[21] 2012	4	2.0 cm greatest diameter	3/4 (75%) GTR 1/4 (25%) STR (1 planned decompression)	1/4 (12.5%) with anosmia
Padhye et al,[49] 2012	2	Not available	Not available	Not available
Lee et al,[50] 2013	2	2.3 cm greatest diameter	2/2 (100%) GTR	1/2 (50%) with CSF leak
Monaco et al,[51] 2013	1	Not available	1/1 (100%) GTR	1/1 (100%) with CSF leakage, DVT, PE and death
Gadgil et al,[52] 2013	5	6.3 cm^3	4/5 (80%) GTR 1/5 (20%) STR	3/5 (60%) with transient DI 1/5 (20%) with CSF leakage
Khan et al,[53] 2014	17	10.14 cm^3	11/17 (64.7%) GTR 6/17 (35.3%) subtotal	2/17 (11.8%) with CSF leakage 4/17 with postoperative endocrine dysfunction
Ottenhausen et al,[54] 2014	9	11.98 cm^3	16/20 GTR (80%) 4/20 (20%) subtotal	2/20 (10%) with CSF leakage
Koutourousiou et al,[55] 2014	37	Not available	32/37 GTR (86.5%)	Not available specifically for tuberculum sellae meningiomas
Yano et al,[56] 2014	12	Not available	Not available specifically for tuberculum sellae meningiomas	1/12 (8.4%) with vascular injury 1/12 (8.4%) with delayed deficit 1/12 (8.4%) with infection 2/12 (16.8%) with CSF leakage
Ishii et al,[57] 2014	6	Not available	5/6 (83.3%) GTR 1/6 (16.7%) subtotal	1/6 (16.7%) with anosmia 1/6 (16.7%) with CSF leakage
Brunworth et al,[58] 2014	7	Not available	Not available	Not available

Abbreviations: ACA, anterior cerebral artery; DI, diabetes insipidus; DVT, deep vein thrombosis; GTR, gross total resection; NTR, near total resection; PE, pulmonary embolism; STR, subtotal resection.
  Data from Refs.[6,19–21,23,24,36–58]

$P<.001$) and lower visual deterioration (2.1% vs 11.4%, $P = .009$) rates.

These studies, along with the results presented in the current review, confirm the intuitive notion that EEAs offer superior results in terms of visual recovery and preservation at the cost of higher CSF leak rates. However, one must be mindful that a significant component of this complication is associated with results from studies that were published before the nasoseptal flap reconstruction era; hence, future comparisons with the outcomes from more recent EEA series should reflect considerable improvement in this regard.

SUMMARY

Endoscopic endonasal resection of tuberculum sellae meningiomas is a feasible technique that enables tumor removal without the need for retraction or displacement of neurovascular structures; nonetheless, it requires dedicated training and equipment, with a steep learning curve. Postoperative CSF leakage remains the main complication. Optic canal invasion also may be addressed from a ventral perspective; these potential advantages seem to positively influence the visual outcomes of these patients.

REFERENCES

1. Al-Mefty O, Smith R. Tuberculum sellae meningiomas. In: Al-Mefty O, editor. Meningiomas. New York: Raven Press; 1991. p. 395–411.
2. Fahlbusch R, Schott W. Pterional surgery of meningiomas of the tuberculum sellae and planum sphenoidale: surgical results with special consideration of ophthalmological and endocrinological outcomes. J Neurosurg 2002;96(2):235–43.
3. Mortini P, Barzaghi LR, Serra C, et al. Visual outcome after fronto-temporo-orbito-zygomatic approach combined with early extradural and intradural optic nerve decompression in tuberculum and diaphragma sellae meningiomas. Clin Neurol Neurosurg 2012;114(6):597–606.
4. Ganna A, Dehdashti AR, Karabatsou K, et al. Frontobasal interhemispheric approach for tuberculum sellae meningiomas; long-term visual outcome. Br J Neurosurg 2009;23(4):422–30.
5. Romani R, Laakso A, Kangasniemi M, et al. Lateral supraorbital approach applied to tuberculum sellae meningiomas: experience with 52 consecutive patients. Neurosurgery 2012;70(6):1504–18 [discussion: 1518–9].
6. Fatemi N, Dusick JR, de Paiva Neto MA, et al. Endonasal versus supraorbital keyhole removal of craniopharyngiomas and tuberculum sellae meningiomas.
Neurosurgery 2009;64(5 Suppl 2):269–84 [discussion: 284–6].
7. McLaughlin N, Ditzel Filho LF, Shahlaie K, et al. The supraorbital approach for recurrent or residual suprasellar tumors. Minim Invasive Neurosurg 2011;54(4):155–61.
8. Reisch R, Perneczky A. Ten-year experience with the supraorbital subfrontal approach through an eyebrow skin incision. Neurosurgery 2005;57(4 Suppl):242–55.
9. Kassam A, Snyderman CH, Mintz A, et al. Expanded endonasal approach: the rostrocaudal axis. Part I. Crista galli to the sella turcica. Neurosurg Focus 2005;19(1):E3.
10. Kassam A, Snyderman CH, Mintz A, et al. Expanded endonasal approach: the rostrocaudal axis. Part II. Posterior clinoids to the foramen magnum. Neurosurg Focus 2005;19(1):E4.
11. Kassam AB, Gardner P, Snyderman C, et al. Expanded endonasal approach: fully endoscopic, completely transnasal approach to the middle third of the clivus, petrous bone, middle cranial fossa, and infratemporal fossa. Neurosurg Focus 2005;19(1):E6.
12. Kassam AB, Gardner PA, Snyderman CH, et al. Expanded endonasal approach, a fully endoscopic transnasal approach for the resection of midline suprasellar craniopharyngiomas: a new classification based on the infundibulum. J Neurosurg 2008;108(4):715–28.
13. Kassam AB, Prevedello DM, Thomas A, et al. Endoscopic endonasal pituitary transposition for a transdorsum sellae approach to the interpeduncular cistern. Neurosurgery 2008;62(3 Suppl 1):57–72 [discussion: 72–4].
14. Kassam AB, Vescan AD, Carrau RL, et al. Expanded endonasal approach: vidian canal as a landmark to the petrous internal carotid artery. J Neurosurg 2008;108(1):177–83.
15. Kassam AB, Prevedello DM, Carrau RL, et al. The front door to Meckel's cave: an anteromedial corridor via expanded endoscopic endonasal approach—technical considerations and clinical series. Neurosurgery 2009;64(3 Suppl):71–82 [discussion: 82–3].
16. Kassam A, Carrau RL, Snyderman CH, et al. Evolution of reconstructive techniques following endoscopic expanded endonasal approaches. Neurosurg Focus 2005;19(1):E8.
17. Frank G, Pasquini E, Doglietto F, et al. The endoscopic extended transsphenoidal approach for craniopharyngiomas. Neurosurgery 2006;59(Suppl 1):ONS75–83.
18. Frank G, Sciarretta V, Calbucci F, et al. The endoscopic transnasal transsphenoidal approach for the treatment of cranial base chordomas and chondrosarcomas. Neurosurgery 2006;59(1 Suppl 1):ONS50–7 [discussion: ONS50–7].
19. Van Gompel JJ, Frank G, Pasquini E, et al. Expanded endonasal endoscopic resection of anterior fossa meningiomas: report of 13 cases and meta-analysis of the literature. Neurosurg Focus 2011;30(5):E15.

20. de Divitiis E, Esposito F, Cappabianca P, et al. Tuberculum sellae meningiomas: high route or low route? A series of 51 consecutive cases. Neurosurgery 2008; 62(3):556–63 [discussion: 556–63].

21. Attia M, Kandasamy J, Jakimovski D, et al. The importance and timing of optic canal exploration and decompression during endoscopic endonasal resection of tuberculum sella and planum sphenoidale meningiomas. Neurosurgery 2012;71(1 Suppl Operative):58–67.

22. Komotar RJ, Starke RM, Raper DM, et al. Endoscopic endonasal versus open transcranial resection of anterior midline skull base meningiomas. World Neurosurg 2012;77(5–6):713–24.

23. Laufer I, Anand VK, Schwartz TH. Endoscopic, endonasal extended transsphenoidal, transplanum transtuberculum approach for resection of suprasellar lesions. J Neurosurg 2007;106(3):400–6.

24. Gardner PA, Kassam AB, Thomas A, et al. Endoscopic endonasal resection of anterior cranial base meningiomas. Neurosurgery 2008;63(1):36–52 [discussion: 52–4].

25. Rhoton AL Jr. The sellar region. Neurosurgery 2002; 51(4 Suppl):S335–74.

26. Wang J, Bidari S, Inoue K, et al. Extensions of the sphenoid sinus: a new classification. Neurosurgery 2010;66(4):797–816.

27. Peris-Celda M, Kucukyuruk B, Monroy-Sosa A, et al. The recesses of the sellar wall of the sphenoid sinus and their intracranial relationships. Neurosurgery 2013;73(2 Suppl Operative):ONS117–31 [discussion: ONS131].

28. Kassam AB, Thomas A, Carrau RL, et al. Endoscopic reconstruction of the cranial base using a pedicled nasoseptal flap. Neurosurgery 2008;63(1 Suppl 1):ONS44–52 [discussion: ONS52–3].

29. Caicedo-Granados E, Carrau R, Snyderman CH, et al. Reverse rotation flap for reconstruction of donor site after vascular pedicled nasoseptal flap in skull base surgery. Laryngoscope 2010;120(8): 1550–2.

30. Kasemsiri P, Carrau RL, Otto BA, et al. Reconstruction of the pedicled nasoseptal flap donor site with a contralateral reverse rotation flap: technical modifications and outcomes. Laryngoscope 2013; 123(11):2601–4.

31. McLaughlin N, Ditzel Filho LF, Prevedello DM, et al. Side-cutting aspiration device for endoscopic and microscopic tumor removal. J Neurol Surg B Skull Base 2012;73(1):11–20.

32. Kassam AB, Prevedello DM, Carrau RL, et al. Endoscopic endonasal skull base surgery: analysis of complications in the authors' initial 800 patients. J Neurosurg 2011;114(6):1544–68.

33. Kono Y, Prevedello DM, Snyderman CH, et al. One thousand endoscopic skull base surgical procedures demystifying the infection potential: incidence and description of postoperative meningitis and brain abscesses. Infect Control Hosp Epidemiol 2011;32(1):77–83.

34. Clark AJ, Jahangiri A, Garcia RM, et al. Endoscopic surgery for tuberculum sellae meningiomas: a systematic review and meta-analysis. Neurosurg Rev 2013;36(3):349–59.

35. Graffeo CS, Dietrich AR, Grobelny B, et al. A panoramic view of the skull base: systematic review of open and endoscopic endonasal approaches to four tumors. Pituitary 2014;17(4):349–56.

36. Jho HD. Endoscopic endonasal approach to the optic nerve: a technical note. Minim Invasive Neurosurg 2001;44(4):190–3.

37. de Divitiis E, Cavallo LM, Cappabianca P, et al. Extended endoscopic endonasal transsphenoidal approach for the removal of suprasellar tumors: Part 2. Neurosurgery 2007;60(1):46–58 [discussion: 58–9].

38. Prevedello DM, Thomas A, Gardner P, et al. Endoscopic endonasal resection of a synchronous pituitary adenoma and a tuberculum sellae meningioma: technical case report. Neurosurgery 2007;60(4 Suppl 2):E401 [discussion: E401].

39. de Divitiis E, Cavallo LM, Esposito F, et al. Extended endoscopic transsphenoidal approach for tuberculum sellae meningiomas. Neurosurgery 2007;61(5 Suppl 2):229–37 [discussion: 237–8].

40. Cappabianca P, Cavallo LM, Esposito F, et al. Extended endoscopic endonasal approach to the midline skull base: the evolving role of transsphenoidal surgery. In: Pickard JD, Akalan N, Di Rocco C, et al, editors. Advances and technical standards in neurosurgery. New York: Springer Wien; 2008. p. 152–99.

41. Wang Q, Lu XJ, Li B, et al. Extended endoscopic endonasal transsphenoidal removal of tuberculum sellae meningiomas: a preliminary report. J Clin Neurosci 2009;16(7):889–93.

42. Dehdashti AR, Ganna A, Witterick I, et al. Expanded endoscopic endonasal approach for anterior cranial base and suprasellar lesions: indications and limitations. Neurosurgery 2009;64(4):677–87 [discussion: 687–9].

43. Ceylan S, Koc K, Anik I. Extended endoscopic approaches for midline skull-base lesions. Neurosurg Rev 2009;32(3):309–19 [discussion: 318–9].

44. Wang Q, Lu XJ, Ji WY, et al. Visual outcome after extended endoscopic endonasal transsphenoidal surgery for tuberculum sellae meningiomas. World Neurosurg 2010;73(6):694–700.

45. Kurschel S, Gellner V, Clarici G, et al. Endoscopic rhino-neurosurgical approach for non-adenomatous sellar and skull base lesions. Rhinology 2011;49(1): 64–73.

46. Liu JK, Christiano LD, Patel SK, et al. Surgical nuances for removal of tuberculum sellae meningiomas with optic canal involvement using the endoscopic endonasal

extended transsphenoidal transplanum transtuberculum approach. Neurosurg Focus 2011;30(5):E2.

47. Fernandez-Miranda JC, Pinheiro-Nieto C, Gardner PA, et al. Endoscopic endonasal approach for a tuberculum sellae meningioma. J Neurosurg 2012;32(Suppl):E8.

48. Chowdhury FH, Haque MR, Goel AH, et al. Endoscopic endonasal extended transsphenoidal removal of tuberculum sellae meningioma (TSM): an experience of six cases. Br J Neurosurg 2012;26(5):692–9.

49. Padhye V, Naidoo Y, Alexander H, et al. Endoscopic endonasal resection of anterior skull base meningiomas. Otolaryngol Head Neck Surg 2012;147(3):575–82.

50. Lee JY, Barroeta JE, Newman JG, et al. Endoscopic endonasal resection of anterior skull base meningiomas and mucosa: implications for resection, reconstruction, and recurrence. J Neurol Surg A Cent Eur Neurosurg 2013;74(1):12–7.

51. Monaco BA, Ramos HF, Gomes MQ, et al. Expanded endonasal approach to skull base meningiomas. Arq Neuropsiquiatr 2013;71(5):330–1.

52. Gadgil N, Thomas JG, Takashima M, et al. Endoscopic resection of tuberculum sellae meningiomas. J Neurol Surg B Skull Base 2013;74(4):201–10.

53. Khan OH, Krischek B, Holliman D, et al. Pure endoscopic expanded endonasal approach for olfactory groove and tuberculum sellae meningiomas. J Clin Neurosci 2014;21(6):927–33.

54. Ottenhausen M, Banu M, Placantonakis DG, et al. Endoscopic endonasal resection of suprasellar meningiomas: the importance of case selection and experience in determining extent of resection, visual improvement and complications. World Neurosurg 2014;82(3–4):442–9.

55. Koutourousiou M, Fernandez-Miranda JC, Stefko ST, et al. Endoscopic endonasal surgery for suprasellar meningiomas: experience with 75 patients. J Neurosurg 2014;120(6):1326–39.

56. Yano S, Hide T, Shinojima N, et al. Endoscopic endonasal skull base approach for parasellar lesions: initial experiences, results, efficacy, and complications. Surg Neurol Int 2014;5:51.

57. Ishii Y, Tahara S, Teramoto A, et al. Endoscopic endonasal skull base surgery: advantages, limitations, and our techniques to overcome cerebrospinal fluid leakage: technical note. Neurol Med Chir (Tokyo) 2014;54(12):983–90.

58. Brunworth J, Padhye V, Bassiouni A, et al. Update on endoscopic endonasal resection of skull base meningiomas. Int Forum Allergy Rhinol 2015;5(4):344–52.

Endoscopic Endonasal Approach for Craniopharyngiomas

Jörg Baldauf, MD[a], Werner Hosemann, MD[b],
Henry W.S. Schroeder, MD[a],*

KEYWORDS

- Endoscopic endonasal approach • Craniopharyngiomas • Retrochiasmatic tumor

KEY POINTS

- The endoscopic endonasal approach for the management of craniopharyngiomas has increasingly been used as an alternative to microsurgical transsphenoidal or transcranial approaches.
- This approach is a major step forward in the treatment of these difficult lesions because of improved resection rates and better visual outcome.
- Especially in retrochiasmatic tumors, the endonasal approach provides better access to the lesion and reduces the degree of manipulations of the optic apparatus.
- The panoramic view offered by endoscopy and the use of angulated optics allows the removal of lesions extending far into the third ventricle avoiding microsurgical brain splitting.

 A video of the endoscopic endonasal resection of an intraventricular craniopharyngeoma accompanies this article at http://www.neurosurgery.theclinics.com/

INTRODUCTION

Craniopharyngiomas (CPs) represent one of the most challenging tumor entities in neurosurgery. Because of its critical vicinity to important neurovascular structures, the surgery is demanding and requires a thorough understanding of the anatomy of the suprasellar region.

CPs are benign epithelial tumors of the sellar region originating from remnants of Rathke's cleft. They are classified by the World Health Organization as grade I neoplasms.[1] The papillary form is almost exclusively found in the adult population and the adamantinomatous subtype mainly occurs in children.[2,3] There is a bimodal age distribution of the incidence of CPs with a higher amplitude in childhood. However, the prognosis of these tumors in particular is a matter of growth pattern. The extent of the tumor in relation to the optic chiasm, pituitary gland and stalk, hypothalamus, carotid artery, and anterior cerebral artery complex as well as the location of the tumor with respect to the sella and diaphragm, is important for surgical planning. In addition to the tumor size and the multilobulated characteristics with solid and cystic components, it is of significant interest whether the lesion does extend into the third ventricle or not and its relation to it. To solve the problem of choosing the right surgical strategy for individual cases, a variety of topographic and clinical classifications of CPs have been transferred into surgical practice parallel to

Disclosure: H.W.S. Schroeder is consultant to Karl Storz GmbH & Co KG (Tuttlingen, Germany).
[a] Department of Neurosurgery, Ernst Moritz Arndt University, Sauerbruchstrasse, Greifswald 17475, Germany;
[b] Department of Otorhinolaryngology, Ernst Moritz Arndt University, Walter-Rathenau-Strasse 43-45, Greifswald 17475, Germany
* Corresponding author.
E-mail address: henry.schroeder@uni-greifswald.de

Neurosurg Clin N Am 26 (2015) 363–375
http://dx.doi.org/10.1016/j.nec.2015.03.013
1042-3680/15/$ – see front matter © 2015 Elsevier Inc. All rights reserved.

technological progress of instrumentation and equipment.[2,4–7]

Albert E. Halsted has been credited with the first successful transsphenoidal resection of a CP performed in 1909.[8] The transsphenoidal approach for tumors of the sellar region is strongly related to Harvey Cushing and Oskar Hirsch.[9] In 1909, Cushing described his first surgery through the transsphenoidal route for partial removal of the pituitary gland in a patient with acromegaly.[10] A detailed historical review concerning the endonasal approach for CPs written by Gardner and colleagues[11] mentioned that Cushing abandoned the approach for CPs for safety reasons given by technological and visualization limitations. In contrast, Hirsch developed and kept to the endonasal transsphenoidal approach and reported his first small series of 12 patients treated for tumors of the pituitary gland in 1911 at the third international laryngo-rhinological congress in Berlin.[12] Ten of the patients improved in clinical outcome and 2 died. The latter were subjected to autopsy. In one, a large tumor of the pituitary gland was found that mainly extended into the intracranial space and third ventricle. Hirsch made 2 important statements about his experience regarding the transsphenoidal approach. First, an improvement of clinical symptoms can be expected if the tumor is located exclusively inside the sella and reveals cystic components. Second, if a tumor is mainly growing intracranially, the endonasal approach and all other extracranial methods will not succeed. Fortunately, the introduction of the operating microscope opened a new door to neurosurgery in general, as well as to the transsphenoidal endonasal route particularly. Hardy stressed the importance of the microsurgical approach for pituitary adenomas and CPs in 1971 and mentioned that "the intrasellar subdiaphragmatic type of CP can be totally removed transphenoidally."[13] Laws improved the microsurgical technique for CPs and expressly underlined that if "the sella turcica is enlarged, transsphenoidal microsurgery can be the procedure of choice, even when significant intracranial extension is present."[14,15]

The stepwise technological progress extended the transsphenoidal access, initially described by Weiss,[16] to reach the suprasellar/supradiaphragmatic space. However, transcranial approaches to CPs with intraventricular growth have also been used via pterional, transcortical, interhemispheric, transcallosal, and transforaminal routes.[2]

The microsurgical–endonasal resection of sellar tumors was successfully complemented by the use of an endoscope by Apuzzo and colleagues[17] in 1977 after Guiot had already introduced the endoscope to transsphenoidal surgery more than a decade earlier.[18] Two decades later, Carrau and Jho reported their first series of purely endoscopic endonasal removal of pituitary adenomas.[19,20] The continuous advancement of the endoscope, in addition to the development of specific instruments and sophisticated endoscopic studies of the parasellar and anterior skull base anatomy allowed the extension of the spectrum of indications for the technique. This initial work was spearheaded by "The original Pittsburgh group" with Carrau, Kassam and co-workers as well as the Naples group with Cappabianca and De Divitiis, and also the Bologna group with Frank and Pasquini, who promoted the endoscopic extended endonasal approach in the early years of the 21st century.[21–24] Nowadays, the endoscopic approach is widely accepted and is used regularly. However, there is a long learning curve and cadaver studies are recommended. Additionally, close cooperation between an ENT-head and neck surgeon and neurosurgeon is necessary. Based on their extraordinary experience, Kassam and colleagues[24] specified a V-level scale of complexity of endoscopic endonasal skull base procedures that provides a useful guide. According to their scale, the endoscopic endonasal approach to CPs is a level IV category referring to the fact that intradural surgery is usually required. Several studies have demonstrated already excellent results for CP patients.[25–30] Compared with the transcranial microscopic approach, the endoscopic approach promises a higher rate of gross total resection (GTR) and improved visual outcome because there is less manipulation of the optic apparatus, especially in retrochiasmatic lesions.[31]

INDICATIONS AND LIMITATIONS FOR ENDOSCOPIC EXTENDED ENDONASAL APPROACH

Patients with CPs can present with a great variety of symptoms including headache, visual symptoms, hormonal disorders such diabetes insipidus and hypopituitarism, mental and memory disturbances, gait difficulties, and hypothalamic disturbances such as the Fröhlich's syndrome (adiposogenital dystrophy). The typical symptoms of increased intracranial pressure are commonly related to an associated hydrocephalus owing to tumor extension into the third ventricle.

All symptomatic CPs are an indication for surgery. Asymptomatic lesions can be followed with MRI. However, growing lesions should be treated before they become symptomatic.[32] If the patient presents with acute hydrocephalus owing to obstruction of the foramina of Monro by a cystic component of the tumor, an initial transcranial transventricular endoscopic cyst fenestration can be performed before the endonasal tumor resection to release the increased intracranial pressure.

The goal of surgery for CPs is GTR or near total resection, if feasible. However, tumor removal has to be restricted to subtotal resection or even partial resection when the risk of neurovascular damage is expected to be high to avoid unacceptable postoperative morbidity. The surgical approach depends on the individual growth pattern of the tumor. Important essentials for the endoscopic extended endonasal approach are listed in **Table 1** and limitations are presented in **Box 1** with respect to the recent literature.[6,25,27,30] Categories A through G try to display an increase of the necessary surgical expertise according to certain pathologic conditions. Each surgical case must be assessed individually for the endoscopic extended endonasal approach or should be alternatively considered for a primary or second stage transcranial approach. Type IV CP isolated to the third ventricle and/or optic recess according Kassam and colleagues[6] is stressed to be not feasible by extended endonasal approach. In our opinion, the endonasal approach is especially useful and superior to any transcranial approach when the lesion is retrochiasmatic with a prefixed chiasm. Compared with the transcranial approach, manipulation of the optic apparatus is reduced, as is the risk of visual deterioration. The success of tumor removal depends on the consistency and characteristics of the lesion (solid, cystic, or multilobular) as well as the invasion of the hypothalamic area.

Box 1
Limitations and unfavorable factors of the endoscopic extended endonasal approach
1. Hypoplastic sphenoid sinus
2. Narrow sellar floor/reduced intercarotid artery distance
3. Combined prechiasmatic and retrochiasmatic tumor extension
4. Significant lateral tumor extension
5. Predominantly solid component in large tumors
6. Type IV lesions according to Kassam[6]

The latter has to be thoroughly assessed in all kind of CPs involving the third ventricle and represents the main reason for preventing a GTR.

SURGICAL MANAGEMENT
Preoperative Planning

Taking a case history and performing a neurologic examination are the first steps in the patient evaluation. Additionally, endocrinologic and visual assessment (visual acuity and visual field) is mandatory before and after surgery. An early consultation with an ENT is advisable to define details of the individual surgical strategy. We strongly recommend neuropsychological testing for adults and children before surgery, if the condition of the patient allows, because behavioral or cognitive problems can already be present before intervention or might occur after tumor resection.[33,34] Furthermore, the body mass index and eating behavior are of interest because of the possibility of postoperative obesity and hyperphagia owing to hypothalamic damage.[35]

Sophisticated preoperative imaging is of utmost importance and includes CT and MRI. CT reveals calcifications within solid nodules and rim or capsule of cystic parts. Thin layer bone window CT demonstrates the bony anatomy of the paranasal sinuses, nasal cavity, clivus, and anterior skull base. It discloses nasal septum deviations, conchal abnormalities, and provides an exact map of the intrasphenoid septations, which are important for anatomic orientation. MRI demonstrates tumor extension in every plane including differentiation in solid and cystic components of the tumor. It provides the basis to evaluate the surgical corridor as mentioned in **Table 1** and **Box 1**. Neurovascular conflicts such as distortions of the optic chiasm or branches of the Circle of Willis

Table 1	
Categories of surgical expertise of endoscopic extended endonasal approach for craniopharyngiomas regarding tumor location/extension according to recent literature	
Category	Tumor Location/Extension
A	Intrasellar + infradiaphragmatic
B	Intrasuprasellar + infradiaphragmatic
C	Suprasellar + infradiaphragmatic; preinfundibular
D	Supradiaphragmatic; preinfundibular, transinfundibuar
E	+ Ventricle floor compression
F	+ Ventricular invasion
G	Pure intraventricular

Data from Refs.[6,25,27,30]

are well visualized on T2 sequences. These authors agree with others that a special meaning is related to the axial and coronal fluid-attenuated inversion recovery or T2 sequences regarding hypothalamic invasion by the tumor.[32] Our illustrative case presents typical MRI features (**Fig. 1**).

Depending on the imaging findings, an approach is selected. The decision to approach the lesion transcranially or endonasally depends on several factors. One of the most important considerations is the position of the chiasm in relation to the tumor. If the tumor is located retrochiasmatic, pushing the chiasm anteriorly (prefixed chiasm), the endonasal approach provides better access to the lesion avoiding unnecessary manipulations of the chiasm. This is especially true in smaller tumors, which only elevate the floor of the third ventricle but are not located intraventricularly. In these lesions, the lamina terminalis approach should not be chosen. If the tumor is located anteriorly to the chiasm causing a postfixed chiasm like in tuberculum sellae meningiomas, the lesion can be approached transcranially or endonasally. However, in most CPs, there is a prefixed chiasm. If the tumor has significant lateral extension (>1 cm lateral to the carotids), it might be impossible to remove these parts totally through the nose when they are stuck to the

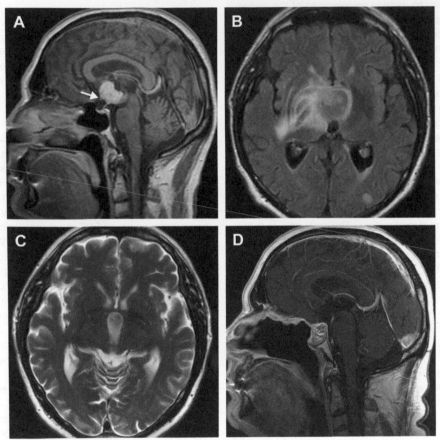

Fig. 1. This 61-year-old man presented with a 6-month history of progressive mental deterioration including decrease of short-term memory. Ten days before admission, he developed a disturbance of consciousness, disorientation, and bladder dysfunction. Endocrinologic evaluation demonstrated panhypopituitarism and diabetes insipidus. A typical Addisonian crisis was observed. MRI revealed a suprasellar contrast enhancing tumor extending into the third ventricle with solid components (*A*). The optic chiasm was displaced anteriorly (*arrow*). Pituitary gland and sella seemed to be normal. Hypothalamic invasion of the lesion was suspected because of the perifocal edema on T2 and fluid-attenuated inversion recovery images with lateral extension into the basal ganglia on the right side (*B*). Gross total resection was performed, including section of the pituitary stalk, which was already infiltrated and destroyed by the tumor. The sphenoid and intradural phases of the extended endonasal approach is shown in **Figs. 2** and **3**. Postoperatively, the patient was very confused, but recovered soon regarding conscious level and cognitive function. Surprisingly, body weight remained stable. Hormonal substitution is required. There is no recurrence of the tumor on MRI 2 years after surgery (*C, D*). The edema has resolved completely (*C*). Image (*D*) also demonstrates covering of the skull base defect by the nasoseptal flap.

surrounding structures. Tumors with large lateral extension should undergo removal via craniotomy. However, tumor extension into the third ventricle, even when they fill the entire ventricle, can be removed endonasally, provided there is communication with the suprasellar space and no ventricular wall invasion. The axis of the approach is ideal to get even the tumor parts in the posterior third ventricle.

Usually, a transsellar–transtuberculum–transplanum approach is sufficient to remove a CP. In tumors with retroclival tumor extension, an addition transclival approach has to be added. In giant tumors with extension in all directions, a combined endonasal–transcranial approach may be necessary. In the rare instance of a purely intrasellar craniopharyngeoma, a simple transsellar approach is sufficient. The approach, steps, and goal of the surgery should be discussed between rhinosurgeon and neurosurgeon at least the day before the surgery.

Perioperative Care and Patient Positioning

After induction of general anesthesia, the endotracheal tube is positioned and fixed in the left corner of the mouth. The nasal surgical part may be characterized by mucosal bleeding. Therefore, a throat pack is inserted to the oral cavity to protect the oropharynx from accumulation of blood and irrigation solution during the surgical procedure. Xylometazoline 0.1% or epinephrine (1:1000) is applied to the nasal mucosa before surgery with the aid of cotton pads. Preoperative antibiotics (cefuroxime 1.5 g) are administered intravenously. The application is repeated when the surgery lasts longer than 6 hours. If a major cerebrospinal fluid (CSF) leak is expected, a lumbar drain is inserted, but is kept closed until the end of the surgery. Postoperative CSF diversion diminishes tension on the skull base reconstruction avoiding CSF leakage.

Perioperatively, 100 mg hydrocortisone is given intravenously within the first hour of surgery followed by 100 mg hydrocortisone administered over the first 24 hours. Oral medication is then continued. The dose depends on the clinical situation of the patient.

The position of the patient is supine and the back elevated to 30° to reduce the venous pressure within the cavernous sinus. The neck is tilted gently to the left and the head slightly extended and turned toward the surgeon fixed to a Mayfield clamp. If required, the navigational image guidance is set up and patient registration is performed using CT and MRI data.

Beside the preparation of nose and nasal cavity with iodine solution, the periumbilical region is disinfected in case a fat graft is needed. Then the patient is draped and the ceiling-mounted boom arm that houses all videoendoscopic equipment needed during surgery is positioned. The 2 right-handed surgeons stand on the right side of the patient. The operating nurse stands on the opposite side to allow easy change of the surgical instruments. The ventilator and the anesthesiologist are positioned on the left side of the patient at the foot level.

SURGICAL APPROACH
General Aspects

Our endoscopic endonasal surgery is a 2-surgeon, 3- or 4-handed technique as proposed by Kassam and colleagues.[6] This technique enables 1 surgeon to work bimanually in the depth while the other surgeon is moving the endoscope like a "mobile" endoscope holder (Video 1). The advantage is the flexible mobility of the endoscope with respect to the operating field, which is somehow missing with a fixed holding device. Sometimes, a third instrument is used by the second surgeon helping in the dissection, but usually he irrigates frequently to clean the lens and the surgical field. We use 18-cm-long rigid rod–lens Hopkins endoscopes with a diameter of 4 mm (Karl Storz GmbH & Co KG, Tuttlingen, Germany). For very narrow nostrils or nasal cavities, 2.7-mm scopes are available; however, they are rarely required. Most of the surgery is performed under view of a 0° endoscope. However, the 30° and 45° endoscopes are also frequently used to work around a corner and to visualize intraventricular tumor extensions. In our opinion, a prerequisite for extended endonasal surgery for CPs is a high-definition video camera. High definition provides a brilliant image that allows easily the differentiation of the various tissues like, for example, the tumor, hypothalamus, and gliotic plane, which can be difficult with a standard progressive addition lens or NTSC (National Television System Committee) camera.[36] Usually, the ENT–head and neck surgeon starts the procedure. However, the neurosurgeon should be able to perform this part of the surgery as well. This is important in a case of emergency when the ENT is not available.

In our opinion, the endoscopic extended endonasal approach can be divided in different steps, which have been described and mentioned by others.[6,32,37]

The Nasal Phase

The initial nasal phase of the approach is characterized by binostril endoscopic inspection of the nasal cavity to visualize the nasal anatomy. The choana as the main landmark, the turbinates, and, if possible, the sphenoid ostium are identified on both sides. Then, the lower and middle turbinates are lateralized to create some working space. To protect the mucosa, we place cotton pads soaked in with xylometazoline on the turbinates. The main working nostril is on the right side because the endoscope is placed here together with another instrument or suction device. We try to avoid resection of the right middle turbinate, but excision may be necessary if lateral dislocation does not provide enough space. Then, a nasoseptal flap is created and stored in the nasopharynx. The size of the flap depends on the size of the skull base defect expected for the approach. Usually, we harvest the flap on the right side, but if there are major bony spurs or other unsuitable anatomic conditions, we elevate the flap on the left side. It is important to preserve at least 1 cm of the septal mucosa near the skull base so as to not endanger the sense of olfaction. It is also important to preserve the vascular pedicle (nasoseptal artery) of the flap at the site of the posterior septal artery. After having stored the flap in the nasopharynx, the posterior bony parts of the septum are removed and a reverse flap of the contralateral mucosa is created to cover the anterior parts of the ipsilateral denuded septum. This flap is fixed with 2 sutures to the anterior cartilaginous septum.[38]

The Sphenoid Phase

The sphenoid phase starts using both nostrils for bimanual manipulation. The rostrum of the sphenoid sinus is removed with the aid of a high-speed drill. The sphenoid sinus is opened wide in all directions. Great care has to be taken to preserve the vascular pedicle of the flap when opening the sphenoid sinus on the side of the flap. On the contralateral side, the mucosal branches of the sphenopalatine artery (posterior septal artery) should be coagulated to avoid postoperative hemorrhage. A posterior ethmoidectomy is performed until the tuberculum sellae and the planum sphenoidale are exposed sufficiently. The mucosa of the sphenoid sinus is removed and the intrasphenoidal bony septa are drilled flat to provide a good bed for the nasoseptal flap.[6,39] The created space must guarantee an optimal dissection within the sphenoid cavity avoiding collisions of the instruments during surgical maneuvers. When the sphenoid sinus is well pneumatized, important anatomic landmarks can easily be identified, such as the optic canals, carotid protuberances of the clival and cavernous carotid artery, clivus, and lateral and medial opticocarotid recesses. When the sphenoid sinus is not well-pneumatized, neuronavigation is helpful to stay oriented during the necessary bone removal.

The next step is the drilling of the skull base. We routinely create a wide opening in the skull base to provide ample room for dissection. The bony sellar floor, the tuberculum sellae, and the posterior planum are removed from carotid to carotid and optic nerve to optic nerve, respectively. The drilling technique is characterized by eggshell thinning of the bone with diamond drills and gentle elevation of the remaining layer with a plate dissector (**Fig. 2**A–C). Continuous irrigation is required while drilling because it keeps the vision clear and avoids heat injury to the underlying neurovascular structures. The medial aspects of the optic canals and the cavernous carotids are unroofed partially. If the tumor has significant retroclival extension, the upper clivus is drilled as well. Significant venous bleeding is rarely encountered during the transsellar–transplanum–transtuberculum approach. If it occurs, it can easily be managed by application of FloSeal hemostatic sealant (Baxter Healthcare Corporation, Hayward, CA) especially if the cavernous or intercavernous sinus are involved.

The Intradural Phase

The intradural step starts with horizontal dural incisions below and above the superior intercavernous sinus to facilitate coagulation of the sinus (see **Fig. 2**D–F). Alternatively, the sinus can be occluded with titanium clips.[37] After transection of the superior intercavernous sinus, the upper dural incision is extended in a V-shaped fashion anteriorly in the direction of the optic nerves. The anteriorly based dural flap can be excised or simply coagulated if it is falling back and obscuring the access to the suprasellar region. Thereafter, the diaphragma sellae is cut until the pituitary stalk is reached. Early identification of the pituitary stalk is a major advantage of the endonasal approach. Before the arachnoid is opened, the superior hypophyseal arteries have to be identified. It is of utmost importance to preserve the vessels because they represent the major blood supply to the chiasm and stalk (**Fig. 3**A, B). Then, the arachnoid is cut to expose the tumor.

The relation of the tumor to the stalk is explored. When a patient presents with panhypopituitarism and the stalk is infiltrated (especially transinfundibular type II lesions according to Kassam and colleagues),[6] we do not hesitate to sacrifice it. If it is still functioning, all efforts are taken to preserve the stalk. We agree that, in type II transinfundibular CPs, a high stalk section is recommended to achieve a GTR.[32,40]

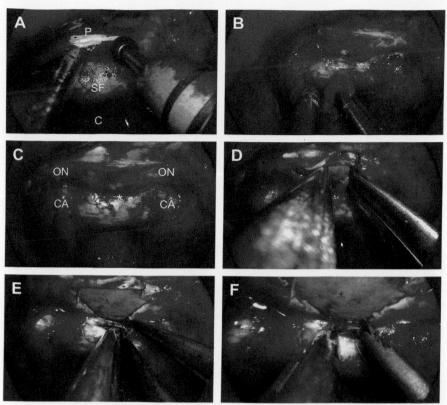

Fig. 2. Sphenoid phase. (*A*) Eggshell drilling of the sella floor (SF) and planum sphenoidale (P) within in the sphenoid cavity. (*B*) Thin bone layers are removed. (*C*) Panoramic view on the exposed dura after complete bone removal. Location of the optic nerve (ON), carotid artery (CA), and superior intercavernous sinus (SIS [*asterisk*]) are labeled. (*D*) Dura opening of the suprasellar space. (*E*) Coagulation of the SIS. (*F*) Section of the SIS.

The concept of CP surgery is characterized by initial debulking of the tumor and identification of the interface between the tumor and adjacent anatomic structures and especially the hypothalamus, which is frequently only a paper thin membrane. After a sharp incision of the tumor capsule, cystic parts of the lesion are evacuated by suction, and solid tumor tissue is removed with the aid of grasping forceps, curettes, or ultrasonic aspirator (see **Fig. 3**C–F). If the tumor is very calcified, all techniques are insufficient and the tumor has to be removed in a time-consuming piecemeal fashion with cutting instruments. After debulking, the dissection plane between hypothalamus and tumor is identified. The dissection is performed around the tumor, before it is removed. It is ill-advised to simply pull on the tumor, because it can be adherent to the basilar artery, perforators, and hypothalamus. Cystic components of the tumor located within the third ventricle are frequently not adherent to the ventricular wall, and can be removed easily. Sometimes, the CSF pressure pushes the cystic part spontaneously out of the ventricle. When the tumor is collapsed,

an extracapsular dissection along the gliotic cleavage plane is done bimanually by gentle traction–countertraction using 2 grasping forceps. The most difficult decision to be made during the resection is how radical of a dissection to undertake. No general recommendation can be given. It is a very individual decision that is made while resecting the lesion. We usually attempt a GTR of the lesion. However, when we cannot identify a dissection plane between the craniopharyngeoma and the hypothalamus, we perform a near total resection, leaving a thin layer of tumor on the hypothalamus. Usually, there is a good arachnoid dissection plane between the tumor and the neurovascular structures of the interpeduncular fossa. Sharp dissection is preferred in this area. If the tumor is not coming down spontaneously, 30° or even 45° endoscopes have to be used to dissect the tumor from the upper third ventricle. The tumor is expected to be adherent to the hypothalamus and columns of the fornix. Consequently, visual control while working around the corner is mandatory at this point of surgery to avoid forniceal damage or venous bleeding caused by traction injury.

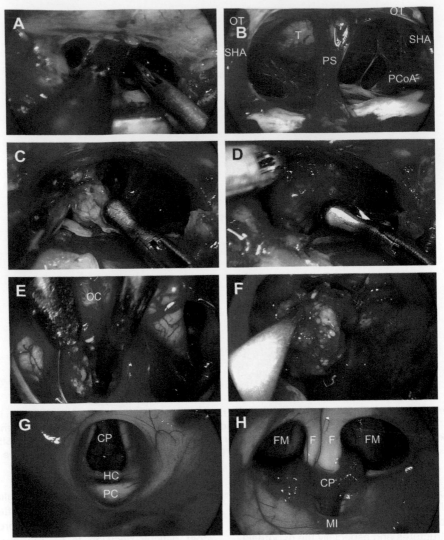

Fig. 3. Intradural phase. (*A*) Supradiaphragmatic sharp dissection of arachnoid membranes. (*B*) The supradiaphragmatic area is exposed. Pituitary stalk (PS), posterior communicating artery (PCoA), superior hypophyseal artery (SHA), optic tract (OT), and tumor (T) are visualized. (*C*) Debulking of the tumor. (*D*) Bimanual extracapsular dissection with grasping and dissection forceps. The PS is lateralized to the left. (*E*) Switching to a 30° endoscope enables safe retrochiasmatic tumor debulking (optic chiasm [OC]). (*F*) A large piece of tumor is mobilized from the third ventricle to the sphenoid cavity. (*G*) Final inspection of the dorsal part of the third ventricle after complete tumor removal (choroid plexus [CP], habenular commissure [HC], posterior commissure [PC]). (*H*) Inspection of the anterior part of the third ventricle with the 45° endoscope (choroid plexus [CP], fornix [F], foramen of Monro [FM], and massa intermedia [MI]).

After tumor resection, the surgical field is irrigated thoroughly to remove blood and tumor debris. The third ventricle is inspected using a 45° endoscope (see **Fig. 3**G, H).

Closure

Endonasal approaches for craniopharyngiomas usually result in a major CSF leak, particularly if the tumor extends into the third ventricle. Therefore, a sophisticated skull base closure technique is mandatory to avoid a postoperative CSF leak.[31] We usually avoid any foreign material and prefer fat, fibrin glue, and the nasoseptal flap (**Fig. 4**). We put a piece of fat in the skull base defect so that it cannot fall intradurally into the resection cavity of the tumor. A larger part of the fat graft remains extradural between the planum

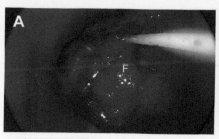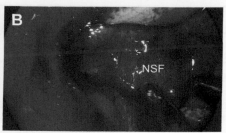

Fig. 4. Closure of the skull base defect. (*A*) Insertion of a fat graft (F) on dural level with intradural extension. Fibrin glue application on boarder area. (*B*) Covering the bony margins with a pedicled, vascularized nasoseptal flap (NSF).

and the sella. If the clivus is indented deeply, a fat graft is placed for a better fit of the nasoseptal flap. The fat is fixed with a little bit fibrin glue. Thereafter, the nasoseptal flap is mobilized from the nasopharynx and carefully positioned over the defect avoiding any foldings in the flap. The flap should be at least 5 to 8 mm larger than the defect in all directions because it will shrink a bit. Utmost care has to be taken to place the correct (periosteal) surface of the flap on the exposed skull base. Additionally, fibrin glue is applied around the edge of the flap. The flap is then covered with Surgicel (oxidized cellulose; Ethicon, Inc, Somerville, NJ) and gel foam to protect the flap. Finally, nasal tamponades are placed to support the flap. They remain in place for 3 to 5 days. The lumbar drainage is opened immediately after surgery to secure CSF diversion and prevent increases in intracranial pressure. It remains open for 5 days continuously at the level of the external auditory canal. In rare cases presenting preoperatively with hydrocephalus, a CSF leak may persist and ultimately require a ventriculoperitoneal shunt to stop the leakage.

COMPLICATIONS AND MANAGEMENT

Complications may occur intraoperatively or postoperatively. Intraoperative complications include injury to neurovascular structures, which may lead to major hemorrhage, brain infarction, and cranial nerve palsies. Nerve palsies occur fortunately only rarely, and are mostly transient affecting the III and IV nerves.[26,41] Utmost care has to be taken when the tumor is adherent to the basilar artery and perforators arising from the basilar tip. Rupture of the perforators may lead to coma and death. Dissection of an adherent lesion to the chiasm may result in decline of visual acuity and visual field cut. Preservation of the superior hypophyseal arteries is essential in preserving vision.

The most frequent postoperative complication seen after endoscopic extended endonasal

approach for CPs is a CSF leak. It has been reported to occur in 3.8% to 69%.[25,26] Cavallo and colleagues[30] observed that the risk of CSF leakage increases in patients with third ventricle involvement. We agree that placing a lumbar drain to reduce CSF pressure over the skull base reconstruction is advisable in cases with wide opening of the third ventricle. Because of routine application of the vascularized pedicled nasoseptal flap, the CSF leak rate after extended endonasal approach with intraarachnoidal dissection has decreased dramatically.[39,42] The prolonged postoperative discomfort with crusting and discharge resulting from harvesting of the nasoseptal flap can be reduced with the reverse mucosal flap covering the donor site. Headache and reduced olfaction leading to a reduced quality of life have been reported as well.[43]

Other complications of the endoscopic extended endonasal approach in CPs are meningitis and hydrocephalus.[25,26,28–30,41] Complications, causes, and their management are presented in **Table 2**. In terms of worsening of pituitary function diabetes insipidus is mostly seen. Up to 46% permanent diabetes insipidus was observed by Koutourousiou and colleagues.[28] The study also demonstrated that 78% of the children were affected and only 32% of the adults.

Similar to diabetes insipidus, hypopituitarism often exists preoperatively or may deteriorate after surgery. Newly diagnosed panhypopituitarism after endoscopic intervention has been reported in up to 67% of patients postoperatively.[44]

Consequences of hypothalamic injury represent an important factor to patients' quality of life. An increase in body mass index of more than 9% underlines the problem of hyperphagia.[26] Mental disorders after extended endonasal approach for CP may be discovered as well.[26,41]

OUTCOME

The rate of GTR of endoscopic extended endonasal approach reaches around 70% in several

Table 2
Complications after endoscopic extended endonasal approach for craniopharyngiomas

Complication	Cause	Management
CSF leakage	Insufficient closure Hydrocephalus	Lumbar drainage; reexploration and repair Shunting[a]
Hydrocephalus	Preexisting hydrocephalus; hemorrhage	Shunting
Hemorrhage	Tumor adherent to neurovascular structures	Hematoma evacuation External drainage in case of hydrocephalus
Subdural hematoma[30]	Loss of CSF, pneumocephalus	Hematoma evacuation Subdural drainage
Cranial nerve palsy	Manipulation, dissection	Wait and see
Intraoperative vascular damage[24,25]	Injury owing to dissection/vascular attachment	Irrigation, diathermy, application of hemostatic agents, compression
Infection of fat graft[26]	Suspected pick up of bacteria during fat passage through a contaminated nasal corridor	Reoperation, endonasal washout, antibiotics
Meningitis	Bacterial infection	Antibiotics
Diabetes insipidus/ hypopituitarism/ SIADH/ hypernatremia	Manipulations of the stalk/ hypothalamus; stalk sacrifice; damage to pituitary or hypothalamic blood supply, vasospasm	Medical treatment
Visual decline	Manipulation; vascular Hydrocephalus	Wait and see Shunting
Hyperphagia, weight gain, obesity	Hypothalamic injury	Dietary restriction
Memory disturbance	Hypothalamic injury	Wait and see
Psychoorganic syndrome	Hypothalamic injury	Medical treatment
Rhinologic sequelae (crusting/synechiae/ sinusitis/hyposmia– anosmia)	Inappropriate resection of nasal mucosa; laceration of functional narrow passes and ostia	Rhinologic aftercare (douching, ointments, surgery for reventilation)

Abbreviations: CSF, cerebrospinal fluid; SIADH, syndrome of inappropriate antidiuretic hormone.
[a] Shunt treatment is also indicated for recurrent CSF leakage.
Data from Refs.[24–26,30]

studies.[25,29,30,45] The extent of tumor resection is related to tumor location, consistency, and mainly adherence to neurovascular structures in particular to the hypothalamus. In the cohort reported by Koutourousiou and colleagues,[28] the overall GTR rate was only 37.5%. However, they stated that "GTR was not considered safe and was therefore not attempted in every patient." It is, therefore, necessary to recognize that subtotal resection in combination with adjuvant radiotherapy may lower the risk of perioperative morbidity in a certain number of patients.[46] A systematic review by Komotar and colleagues[31] revealed an advantage of the endoscopic extended endonasal approach and transsphenoidal microscopic approach compared with open transcranial approaches to achieve GTR in CPs. Additionally, improvement of vision after extended endonasal approach (56%) is significantly better in contrast with transcranial approaches (33%) and tends to be superior to microscopic transsphenoidal approach (44%). The same study demonstrated that deterioration of vision is less pronounced in extended endonasal approach than in the other approaches.

Outcome regarding degree of tumor resection and visual improvement in studies with at least 20 patients is documented in **Table 3**.

Table 3
Outcome in studies on extended endonasal approach greater than 20 patients regarding GTR/NTR/vision improvement

Author, Year	No Patients/Surgeries	GTR/NTR	Vision Improvement
Koutourousiou et al,[28] 2013	64	24 (37.5)/22 (34.4)	38 (86.4)
Leng et al,[26] 2012	26	18 (69)/2 (7.9)	20 (77)
Kalinin et al,[41] 2013	56	39 (69.4)/—	32 (57.4)
Cavallo et al,[30] 2014	103	71 (68.9)/—	59 (74.7)

GTR/NTR/vision improvement presented as number of patients (%).
Abbreviations: GTR, gross tumor resection; NTR, near total resection.
Data from Refs.[26,28,30,41]

SUMMARY

The introduction of the endoscopic endonasal extended approach is a major step forward in the management of craniopharyngeomas. It has improved the resection rate and the visual outcome. Especially in retrochiasmatic lesions pushing the chiasm anteriorly (prefixed chiasm), the endonasal approach provides a better access to the lesion and reduces the degree of manipulations of the optic apparatus. The panoramic view offered by endoscopy and the use of angulated optics allows the removal of lesions extending far into the third ventricle avoiding microsurgical brain splitting such as translamina terminalis or transcallosal approaches. Of course, there is a significant learning curve in this demanding surgery, requiring intensive training before performing this intervention.

ACKNOWLEDGMENTS

The authors thank M. Matthes, MSc, for his help in preparing the illustrations.

SUPPLEMENTARY DATA

Supplementary data related to this article can be found online at http://dx.doi.org/10.1016/j.nec.2015.03.013.

REFERENCES

1. Louis DN, Ohgaki H, Wiestler OD, et al. The 2007 WHO classification of tumours of the central nervous system. Acta Neuropathol 2007;114(2):97–109.

2. Adamson TE, Wiestler OD, Kleihues P, et al. Correlation of clinical and pathological features in surgically treated craniopharyngiomas. J Neurosurg 1990; 73(1):12–7.

3. Larkin SJ, Ansorge O. Pathology and pathogenesis of craniopharyngiomas. Pituitary 2013;16(1):9–17.

4. Fukushima T, Hirakawa K, Kimura M, et al. Intraventricular craniopharyngioma: its characteristics in magnetic resonance imaging and successful total removal. Surg Neurol 1990;33(1):22–7.

5. Pascual JM, Gonzalez-Llanos F, Barrios L, et al. Intraventricular craniopharyngiomas: topographical classification and surgical approach selection based on an extensive overview. Acta Neurochir (Wien) 2004;146(8):785–802.

6. Kassam AB, Gardner PA, Snyderman CH, et al. Expanded endonasal approach, a fully endoscopic transnasal approach for the resection of midline suprasellar craniopharyngiomas: a new classification based on the infundibulum. J Neurosurg 2008;108(4):715–28.

7. Hoffman HJ, De SM, Humphreys RP, et al. Aggressive surgical management of craniopharyngiomas in children. J Neurosurg 1992;76(1):47–52.

8. Halstead AE. Remarks on operative treatment of tumors of the hypophysis. Trans Am Surg Assoc 1910; 28:73–93.

9. Hirsch O. Ueber endonasale Operationsmethoden bei Hypophysis-Tumoren mit Bericht über 12 operierte Fälle. Berl Klin Wschr 1911;48:1933–5.

10. Cushing H III. Partial hypophysectomy for acromegaly: with remarks on the function of the hypophysis. Ann Surg 1909;50(6):1002–17.

11. Gardner PA, Prevedello DM, Kassam AB, et al. The evolution of the endonasal approach for craniopharyngiomas. J Neurosurg 2008;108(5):1043–7.

12. Liu JK, Cohen-Gadol AA, Laws ER Jr, et al. Harvey Cushing and Oskar Hirsch: early forefathers of modern transsphenoidal surgery. J Neurosurg 2005; 103(6):1096–104.

13. Hardy J. Transsphenoidal hypophysectomy. 1971. J Neurosurg 2007;107(2):458–71.

14. Laws ER Jr. Transsphenoidal removal of craniopharyngioma. Pediatr Neurosurg 1994;21(Suppl):157–63.

15. Laws ER Jr. Transsphenoidal microsurgery in the management of craniopharyngioma. J Neurosurg 1980;52(5):661–6.

16. Weiss MH. The transnasal transsphenoidal approach. In: Apuzzo MJ, editor. Surgery of the third

ventricle. Baltimore (MD): Williams & Wilkins; 1987. p. 476–94.

17. Apuzzo ML, Heifetz MD, Weiss MH, et al. Neurosurgical endoscopy using the side-viewing telescope. J Neurosurg 1977;46(3):398–400.

18. Guiot G, Thibaut B, Bourreau M. Extirpation of hypophyseal adenomas by trans-septal and trans-sphenoidal approaches. Ann Otolaryngol 1959;76:1017–31 [in French].

19. Carrau RL, Jho HD, Ko Y. Transnasal-transsphenoidal endoscopic surgery of the pituitary gland. Laryngoscope 1996;106(7):914–8.

20. Jho HD, Carrau RL. Endoscopic endonasal transsphenoidal surgery: experience with 50 patients. J Neurosurg 1997;87(1):44–51.

21. Cappabianca P, Cavallo LM, Esposito F, et al. Extended endoscopic endonasal approach to the midline skull base: the evolving role of transsphenoidal surgery. Adv Tech Stand Neurosurg 2008;33: 151–99.

22. De Divitiis E, Cavallo LM, Cappabianca P, et al. Extended endoscopic endonasal transsphenoidal approach for the removal of suprasellar tumors: Part 2. Neurosurgery 2007;60(1):46–58.

23. Frank G, Pasquini E, Mazzatenta D. Extended transsphenoidal approach. J Neurosurg 2001;95(5):917–8.

24. Kassam AB, Prevedello DM, Carrau RL, et al. Endoscopic endonasal skull base surgery: analysis of complications in the authors' initial 800 patients. J Neurosurg 2011;114(6):1544–68.

25. Gardner PA, Kassam AB, Snyderman CH, et al. Outcomes following endoscopic, expanded endonasal resection of suprasellar craniopharyngiomas: a case series. J Neurosurg 2008;109(1):6–16.

26. Leng LZ, Greenfield JP, Souweidane MM, et al. Endoscopic, endonasal resection of craniopharyngiomas: analysis of outcome including extent of resection, cerebrospinal fluid leak, return to preoperative productivity, and body mass index. Neurosurgery 2012;70(1):110–23.

27. Cavallo LM, Solari D, Esposito F, et al. The endoscopic endonasal approach for the management of craniopharyngiomas involving the third ventricle. Neurosurg Rev 2013;36(1):27–37.

28. Koutourousiou M, Gardner PA, Fernandez-Miranda JC, et al. Endoscopic endonasal surgery for craniopharyngiomas: surgical outcome in 64 patients. J Neurosurg 2013;119(5):1194–207.

29. Bosnjak R, Benedicic M, Vittori A. Early outcome in endoscopic extended endonasal approach for removal of supradiaphragmatic craniopharyngiomas: a case series and a comprehensive review. Radiol Oncol 2013;47(3):266–79.

30. Cavallo LM, Frank G, Cappabianca P, et al. The endoscopic endonasal approach for the management of craniopharyngiomas: a series of 100 patients. J Neurosurg 2014;121(1):100–13.

31. Komotar RJ, Starke RM, Raper DM, et al. Endoscopic endonasal compared with microscopic transsphenoidal and open transcranial resection of craniopharyngiomas. World Neurosurg 2012;77(2): 329–41.

32. Conger AR, Lucas J, Zada G, et al. Endoscopic extended transsphenoidal resection of craniopharyngiomas: nuances of neurosurgical technique. Neurosurg Focus 2014;37(4):E10.

33. Ondruch A, Maryniak A, Kropiwnicki T, et al. Cognitive and social functioning in children and adolescents after the removal of craniopharyngioma. Childs Nerv Syst 2011;27(3):391–7.

34. Bellhouse J, Holland A, Pickard J. Psychiatric, cognitive and behavioural outcomes following craniopharyngioma and pituitary adenoma surgery. Br J Neurosurg 2003;17(4):319–26.

35. Roth CL. Hypothalamic obesity in patients with craniopharyngioma: profound changes of several weight regulatory circuits. Front Endocrinol (Lausanne) 2011;2:49.

36. Schroeder HW, Nehlsen M. Value of high-definition imaging in neuroendoscopy. Neurosurg Rev 2009; 32(3):303–8.

37. Cappabianca P, Frank G, Pasquini E, et al. Extended endoscopic endonasal transsphenoidal approaches to the suprasellar region, planum sphenoidale & clivus. In: De Divitiis E, Cappabianca P, editors. Endoscopic endonasal transsphenoidal surgery. Wien (Austria); New York: Springer; 2003. p. 176–82.

38. Kasemsiri P, Carrau RL, Otto BA, et al. Reconstruction of the pedicled nasoseptal flap donor site with a contralateral reverse rotation flap: technical modifications and outcomes. Laryngoscope 2013; 123(11):2601–4.

39. Hadad G, Bassagasteguy L, Carrau RL, et al. A novel reconstructive technique after endoscopic expanded endonasal approaches: vascular pedicle nasoseptal flap. Laryngoscope 2006; 116(10):1882–6.

40. Liu JK, Christiano LD, Patel SK, et al. Surgical nuances for removal of retrochiasmatic craniopharyngioma via the endoscopic endonasal extended transsphenoidal transplanum transtuberculum approach. Neurosurg Focus 2011;30(4):E14.

41. Kalinin PL, Fomichev DV, Kutin MA, et al. Endoscopic endonasal anterior extended transsphenoidal approach in craniopharyngioma surgery. Zh Vopr Neirokhir Im N N Burdenko 2013;77(3):13–20 [in Russian].

42. Kassam AB, Thomas A, Carrau RL, et al. Endoscopic reconstruction of the cranial base using a pedicled nasoseptal flap. Neurosurgery 2008;63(1 Suppl 1):ONS44–52.

43. Georgalas C, Badloe R, van Furth W, et al. Quality of life in extended endonasal approaches for skull base tumours. Rhinology 2012;50(3):255–61.

44. Jane JA Jr, Kiehna E, Payne SC, et al. Early outcomes of endoscopic transsphenoidal surgery for adult craniopharyngiomas. Neurosurg Focus 2010; 28(4):E9.

45. Frank G, Pasquini E, Doglietto F, et al. The endoscopic extended transsphenoidal approach for craniopharyngiomas. Neurosurgery 2006;59(1 Suppl 1):ONS75–83.

46. Schoenfeld A, Pekmezci M, Barnes MJ, et al. The superiority of conservative resection and adjuvant radiation for craniopharyngiomas. J Neurooncol 2012;108(1):133–9.

Endoscopic Endonasal Approach for Olfactory Groove Meningiomas
Operative Technique and Nuances

James K. Liu, MD[a,b,*], Ellina Hattar, BA[a],
Jean Anderson Eloy, MD[a,b]

KEYWORDS

- Olfactory groove meningioma • Endoscopic skull base surgery • Endoscopic endonasal approach
- Transcribriform • Anterior skull base

KEY POINTS

- Olfactory groove meningiomas are midline skull base lesions that represent approximately 10% of all intracranial meningiomas.
- Radical resection including the dural attachment and involved hyperostotic bone (Simpson grade I) offers the best chance of minimizing recurrence.
- Although surgical resection via a transcranial approach remains the mainstay of treatment, in carefully selected cases, the endoscopic endonasal approach via the transcribriform corridor provides direct access to the tumor blood supply (ethmoidal arteries) for early devascularization and removal of the underlying hyperostotic bone at the cranial base, so that radical Simpson grade I resection can be achieved without additional brain retraction or manipulation.

INTRODUCTION

Olfactory groove meningiomas represent approximately 10% of all intracranial meningiomas.[1–6] These midline skull base lesions arise from the dura of the cribriform plate and planum sphenoidale. Hyperostosis of the adjacent underlying bone is not uncommon, and occasionally, tumor extension can be found in the ethmoid sinuses and nasal cavity in approximately 15% to 25% of cases.[5,7–15] Radical resection, including the dural attachment and involved hyperostotic bone (Simpson grade I), offers the best chance of minimizing recurrence. Incomplete removal can result in tumor recurrence, usually at the cribriform plate, ethmoid sinuses with extension into the paranasal sinuses.[3–5,9,16–18]

The most common surgical approaches for resecting olfactory groove meningiomas are the bifrontal transbasal approaches and pterional approaches.[3–5,19–22] Additional cranial base extensions may be used, if desired, such as orbital rim (orbitopterional or modified orbitozygomatic) or supraorbital bar removal (extended transbasal) to minimize brain retraction and gain additional exposure. These transcranial approaches generally require some degree of brain retraction or manipulation, but can adequately access and resect the tumor. Complications can include cerebral edema, venous infarction, hematoma, cerebrospinal fluid (CSF) leakage, bone flap infection, with a mortality of up to 5%.[3]

[a] Department of Neurological Surgery, Center for Skull Base and Pituitary Surgery, Neurological Institute of New Jersey, Rutgers New Jersey Medical School, 90 Bergen Street, Suite 8100, Newark, NJ 07103, USA;
[b] Department of Otolaryngology-Head and Neck Surgery, Center for Skull Base and Pituitary Surgery, Neurological Institute of New Jersey, Rutgers New Jersey Medical School, 90 Bergen Street, Suite 8100, Newark, NJ 07103, USA
* Corresponding author. Department of Neurological Surgery, Neurological Institute of New Jersey, Rutgers New Jersey Medical School, 90 Bergen Street, Suite 8100, Newark, NJ 07103, USA.
E-mail address: james.liu.md@rutgers.edu

Recently, there has been increased interest in the use of the endoscopic endonasal approach (EEA) via the transcribriform corridor for resection of olfactory groove meningiomas.[1,23–31] Nevertheless, this continues to be a topic of debate.[32] Because these tumors originate at the ventral skull base, the endonasal route provides direct access to the tumor blood supply (ethmoidal arteries) for early devascularization, and removal of the underlying hyperostotic bone at the cranial base so that radical Simpson grade I resection can be achieved.[29] In carefully selected patients, these tumors can be totally removed without additional brain retraction or manipulation.

In this report, we review the surgical technique and operative nuances for removal of olfactory groove meningiomas using the EEA. We also discuss the indications, limitations, complication avoidance and management, and postoperative care.

PREOPERATIVE CONSIDERATIONS, INDICATIONS, AND LIMITATIONS

The anatomic limits of the endonasal transcribriform corridor are the posterior table of the frontal sinuses anteriorly, the medial orbits (lamina papyracea) laterally, and the planum sphenoidale and tuberculum sellae posteriorly. A panoramic view of the ventral skull base can be obtained of this transcribriform corridor with a 30-degree angled endoscope aimed superiorly. Early devascularization of the tumor can be performed because the site of dural attachment and the primary tumor blood supply (anterior and posterior ethmoidal arteries) are adjacent to the paranasal sinuses. In carefully selected patients, a Simpson grade I resection of the tumor, including its dural attachment and involved hyperostotic bone, can be achieved (**Figs. 1** and **2**).

Choosing the appropriate surgical approach is largely determined by careful study of the preoperative imaging, particularly the size of the tumor, location, site and extent of the dural attachment, degree of involvement of neighboring vascular structures (tumor encasement of vascular structures), degree of T2 changes (pial invasion), and surgeon's preference. If the basal dural attachment is confined between the medial walls of the orbit, then the EEA may be considered a suitable approach. If, however, the dural attachment and

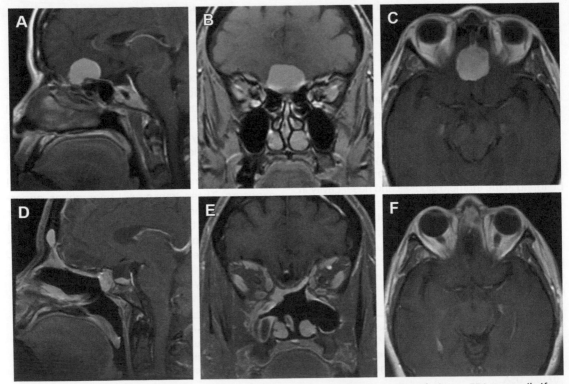

Fig. 1. (A–C) MRI showing an olfactory groove meningioma suitable for removal via an EEA transcribriform approach. The dural attachment is confined to the operative corridor and there is a "cortical cuff" protecting the anterior cerebral arteries. There is also some hyperostotic bone at the base of the tumor that is removed during the surgical approach. (D–F) Postoperative MRI shows complete Simpson grade I removal of the tumor including the hyperostotic bone. Enhancement from the nasoseptal flap can be seen at the anterior skull base.

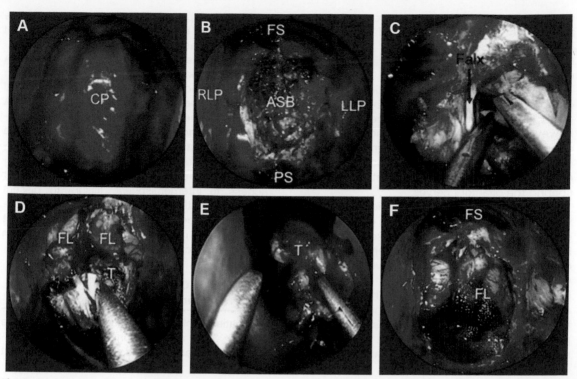

Fig. 2. Intraoperative photographs of the tumor removal from **Fig. 1**. (*A*) Endoscopic view of the cribriform plate (CP) using 30-degree endoscope pointing superiorly at the ventral skull base. (*B*) After opening the frontal sinuses (FS) via an endoscopic modified Lothrop procedure, a ventral keyhole transcribriform craniectomy has been performed from the right lamina papyracea (RLP) to the left lamina papyracea (LLP) in the coronal plane, and from the posterior table of the frontal sinus (FS) to the planum sphenoidale (PS) in the sagittal plane. The dura of the anterior skull base (ASB) has been coagulated to devascularize the tumor. (*C*) After opening the dura, the falx (*black arrow*) is divided sharply from an anterior-to-posterior direction to release the tumor from the falx cerebri. (*D–F*) The tumor (T) is carefully dissected away from the frontal lobes (FL) in an extracapsular fashion using bimanual microdissection techniques.

associated tumor extends laterally over the orbital roofs, a complete Simpson grade I resection is not feasible. Some laterally extending tumors may be difficult to access through the transcribriform corridor, which can result in residual tumor and a site for future recurrence. Although extending the bone removal laterally over the orbits can be performed, skull base reconstruction becomes more challenging and the risk of postoperative CSF leakage increases. Significant anterosuperior tumor extension behind the posterior wall of the frontal sinus may also prohibit safe complete removal, as this is often a "difficult-to-reach" area. If a radical resection is the desired goal, a transcranial approach should be considered in these cases.

The presence of tumor encasement of major vessels is very important to identify on preoperative imaging, as this may preclude complete removal regardless of surgical approach. Whether the tumor is approached transcranially or endonasally, it is often safer to leave a small tumor

remnant adherent to critical neurovascular structures to avoid a major catastrophic vascular injury. However, in the event of a vascular injury, such as a vessel tear or avulsion, it is more feasible to gain vascular control with temporary clips and perform direct vessel repair or bypass in an open approach than with an endonasal approach. Thus, in cases with vascular encasement, we strongly prefer an open transcranial approach, particularly if a near-to-gross total removal is desired. In our opinion, it is technically safer to dissect tumor off of the A2 vessels in the interhemispheric fissure from a transbasal interhemispheric approach than an endonasal approach with current instrumentation. Therefore, it is important to identify a "cortical cuff" (rim of neural tissue that separates the tumor capsule from the A2 vessels and anterior communicating artery complex) or an arachnoid CSF cleft between the tumor and the vessels, when considering an EEA for olfactory groove meningiomas.

The patient's preoperative olfactory function is also an important factor to consider when choosing the optimal surgical approach. It is paramount to counsel patients that olfactory function is invariably lost after an EEA by nature of the transcribriform approach (removal of olfactory mucosa, transection of olfactory nerves/tracts). Therefore, if preoperative olfaction is already compromised, an EEA should be considered, given all other surgical factors are favorable. If, however, olfaction is intact and the patient strongly wishes to preserve this function, a transcranial approach (pterional, transbasal) should be considered because it has a better chance at sparing the olfactory nerves.

The EEA also is suitable for patients presenting with recurrent meningiomas at the cribriform plate extending into the paranasal sinuses (**Fig. 3**). This is not uncommon in patients who have had previous craniotomy for olfactory groove meningiomas where the cribriform plate was not previously drilled out at the initial surgery. The EEA has the advantage of removing the sinonasal portion of the tumor, drilling out the hyperostotic cribriform plate, and providing a solution for skull base reconstruction with the vascularized pedicled nasoseptal flap, especially in patients who have had previous craniotomy where the pericranial flap is unavailable for reconstruction.

In some cases, a combined transcranial/EEA strategy can be considered for some tumors with significant tumor extension laterally and paranasal sinus involvement (**Fig. 4**).[29,33,34] Although an EEA alone offers the advantage of removing the sinonasal tumor and hyperostotic cribriform plate, the addition of a transcranial approach (bifrontal transbasal approach) offers wider exposure of the anterior skull base over both orbital roofs and shorter access to interhemispheric fissure to dissect tumor off of critical vessels. Conversely, the visualization afforded by the endoscope can detect tumor in the nasal cavity that is often hidden from the transcranial view from above.

SURGICAL TECHNIQUE
Preparation and Patient Positioning

The patient is placed in the supine position with the head in 3-pin skull fixation under general anesthesia. The head is rotated slightly toward the right

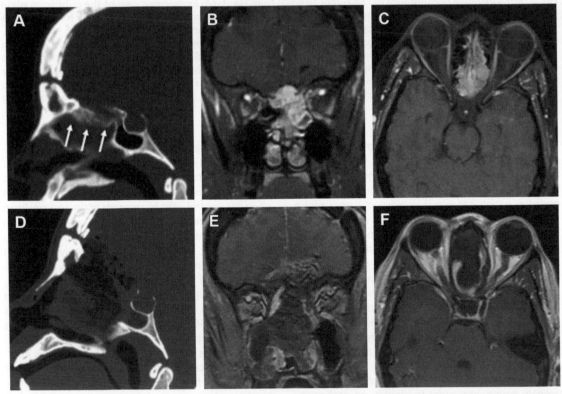

Fig. 3. (*A–C*) CT and MRI showing a recurrent olfactory meningioma arising at the cribriform plate with extension inferiorly into the paranasal sinuses. The patient had a previous bifrontal craniotomy with a gross total removal; however, the cribriform plate was not completely drilled out. Note the hyperostotic bone at the cribriform plate (*A, white arrows*). An EEA transcribriform approach was performed to completely remove the tumor recurrence. (*D–F*) Postoperative CT and MRI show complete removal.

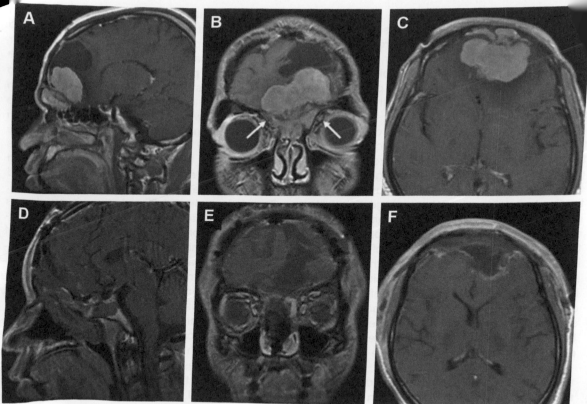

Fig. 4. (*A–C*) Preoperative MRI showing a recurrent olfactory meningioma with invasion into the frontal sinuses and anterior ethmoid sinuses. Because of the broad dural attachment over the orbital roofs (*white arrows*) and significant hyperostosis of the frontal bone and posterior table of the frontal sinuses, a combined transcranial (bifrontal craniotomy) and EEA was performed with complete resection of the tumor. Because the pericranial flap was no longer available (because of previous usage in the initial craniotomy), a pedicled nasoseptal flap was used endonasally for the reconstruction. (*D–F*) Postoperative MRI showing complete resection.

side to facilitate comfortable access to the nose when the surgeon stands on the patient's right side. In addition, the neck is extended slightly to facilitate access to the cribriform region. We generally do not use lumbar drains in EEA transcribriform procedures. Intravenous antibiotics, antiepileptics for seizure prophylaxis, and 10 mg dexamethasone are administered at the start of the operation. Intraoperative navigation is used with either an MRI, computed tomography angiography (CTA), or both modalities merged. This is helpful in determining the extent of bony opening along the sagittal and coronal planes, as well as predicting the proximity of critical neighboring vasculature.

The nose and nares are prepped with betadine solution, and Oxymetazoline (Afrin)-soaked pledgets are placed into the nasal cavity to decongest the nasal mucosa. The thigh is also prepped for harvesting of an autologous fascia lata graft. We use a standard 2-surgeon, 3-handed to 4-handed binaural technique with a neurosurgeon and otolaryngologist. Intraoperative neurophysiologic

monitoring of somatosensory and motor evoked potentials is performed throughout the case.

Endoscopic Endonasal Transcribriform Approach

In our practice, we prefer to use a 30-degree endoscope as our workhorse for extended EEA approaches because it provides additional viewing angles in multiple directions by simply rotating the scope. Our clinical experience is consistent with the findings in an anatomic study by Batra and colleagues,[35] in which the 30-degree endoscope provided the best view of the ventral skull base from the frontal sinus to the planum sphenoidale with the least distortion in comparison with the 0-degree and 70-degree endoscopes.

The nasal septum and tail and anterosuperior attachment of the middle turbinates are injected with 1% lidocaine with epinephrine (1:100,000 dilution). The inferior turbinates are lateralized with a Goldman elevator and both middle turbinates are resected to create access to the cribriform plate. Bilateral maxillary antrostomies are performed to expose the orbital floor, an important anatomic landmark. Bilateral sphenoidotomies are performed with care taken to preserve the vascular pedicle (along the arch of the choana) to the nasal septum.

A large vascularized pedicled nasoseptal flap is then harvested from either side and rotated into the posterior nasopharynx until the reconstruction phase.[36–40] It is important to design the flap in such a manner to maximize the surface area of the flap to provide adequate coverage of the anticipated skull base dural defect. The anterior margin of the incision is made at the septocolumellar junction to maximize the sagittal reach of the flap. The incision is extended laterally along the floor of the nose to increase the coronal dimension of the flap. It is better to overestimate the defect size and oversize the flap than to have a smaller flap with suboptimal coverage. Care is taken to protect the vascular pedicle from inadvertent trauma to prevent vascular compromise of the flap.

The sphenoidotomy is widened and bilateral total ethmoidectomies are performed with a tissue microdebrider to expose the junction of the lamina papyracea with the fovea ethmoidalis. An extended frontal sinusotomy (modified Lothrop procedure) is performed to expose the anterior extent of the transcribriform corridor.[41] A superior septectomy is performed to provide a panoramic view with binostril access to the ventral cribriform plate. An additional posterior septectomy can be made to allow triangulation of instrumentation through both nostrils to the surgical target. The Lothrop cavity (common frontal sinus cavity) is widened and the nasofrontal beak is thinned down with up-angled curettes and a high-speed drill to expose the posterior frontal sinus wall. The endoscopic modified Lothrop procedure is an important step in the exposure of the transcribriform corridor because it provides exposure of the posterior table of the frontal sinus, a key landmark to delineate the anterior border of the transcribriform corridor.[29] This also serves as a ledge to tuck inlay graft material and a platform to lay down the nasoseptal flap.

Next, a transcribriform craniectomy of the ventral skull base is performed using a high-speed drill with copious irrigation (**Figs. 5** and **6**). The boundaries of the craniectomy are largely determined by the size of the tumor and the extent of the dural attachment. In general, the

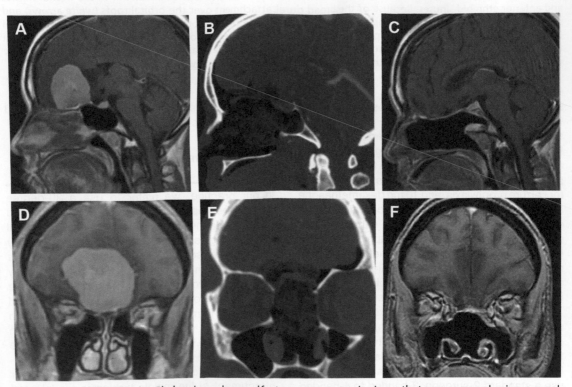

Fig. 5. Preoperative MRI (*A, D*) showing a large olfactory groove meningioma that was removed using a purely EEA transcribriform approach. Postoperative CT (*B, E*) and 1-year postoperative MRI (*C, F*) show complete resection with excellent reconstruction of the anterior cranial base.

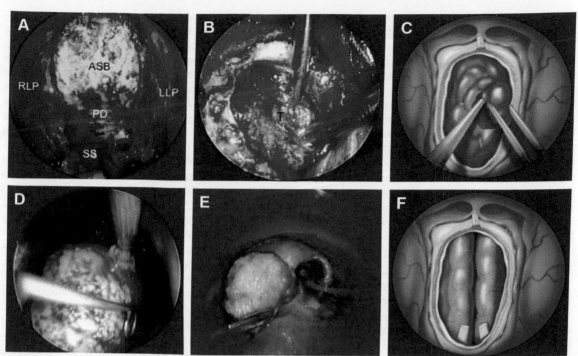

Fig. 6. Intraoperative photographs of intradural tumor removal from case in **Fig. 5**. (*A*) An endoscopic transcribriform craniectomy has been performed from the right lamina papyracea (RLP) to the left lamina papyracea (LLP) coronally to expose the dura of the anterior skull base (ASB). The dura of the planum sphenoidale (PD) is exposed due to the posterior extent of the tumor in the sagittal plane. The sphenoid sinus (SS) is also exposed. (*B, C*) After opening the dura, the tumor (T) is debulked internally using a tumor aspirator and microdebrider. (*D, E*) Careful extracapsular dissection is performed to dissect the tumor away from the frontal lobes and to deliver the tumor from the nostrils. (*F*) Illustration showing the frontal lobes after tumor removal. (Illustration by Christine Gralapp © 2012.)

craniectomy extends from the posterior wall of the frontal sinus at the level of the crista galli to the planum sphenoidale in the sagittal plane, and from lamina papyracea to lamina papyracea in the coronal plane. After thinning down the fovea ethmoidalis and cribriform plate, the crista is drilled down and dissected away from the dural reflections. The anterior and posterior ethmoidal arteries are coagulated and divided bilaterally to devascularize the tumor. Care is taken to avoid retraction of the proximal end of these arteries back into the orbit before they are adequately coagulated so as to avoid orbital hematoma and proptosis. The exposed dura is further coagulated to devascularize the basal attachment of the tumor.

Intradural Tumor Removal

The dura is opened laterally on each side just medial to the lamina papyracea in the sagittal plane. The anterior dural incision is made transversely and the falx is divided sharply in an anterior-to-posterior direction with angled scissors. The posterior incision is made transversely across the region of the planum sphenoidale. For larger tumors, intracapsular debulking of the tumor is performed with suction, ultrasonic aspiration, or with a side-cutting tumor aspirator (NICO Myriad, Indianapolis, IN). For fibrous solid tumors that are unresponsive to the aforementioned instruments, an angled rotating-suction microdebrider (Diego; Gyrus ACMI-ENT Division, Bartlett, TN) can be used.[42] It is paramount that the debulking instrument stays intracapsular without breaching the tumor capsule so as to avoid injury to neighboring neurovascular structures.

After adequate debulking of the tumor, extracapsular dissection is performed using bimanual microsurgical techniques. The tumor capsule is carefully separated from the surrounding brain by maintaining the arachnoid planes. However, in larger tumors with edema on T2-weighted imaging, there may be pial invasion and subpial dissection may be necessary to remove the tumor. Micropaddies are used to separate the tumor capsule from the surrounding brain. Although the width of the tumor may be larger than the width of the operative corridor, the tumor can be collapsed and gathered into the operative window from a lateral to medial fashion. The natural pulsations of the brain also facilitate medialization and delivery of the tumor through the transcribriform defect.

It is important to avoid premature "pulling" of the tumor before the capsule is completely dissected free from all surrounding neurovascular structures so as to avoid a catastrophic vascular avulsion or injury. Sharp dissection is performed to separate critical vasculature from the tumor, particularly the anterior cerebral arteries. If there is any tumor that is strictly adherent to neighboring vessels, it is safer to leave a small remnant of tumor so as to avoid vascular injury that could result in hemorrhage or stroke, or permanent neurologic deficit. Once the tumor is delivered out of the defect, meticulous hemostasis is achieved and a monolayer of Surgicel is placed on the resection bed.

Skull Base Reconstruction

Successful multilayered reconstruction of these transcribriform cranial base defects is paramount to prevent postoperative CSF leakage. Although initial rates of reported postoperative CSF leaks after EEA were more than 20%, the advent of the vascularized pedicled nasoseptal flap has largely decreased the incidence of this complication to less than 5%.[37,39,43]

For transcribriform defects, we have previously described a triple-layer reconstruction technique (**Figs. 7–9**).[44] This repair method consists of 3 layers. The first layer is an autologous fascia lata graft that is placed intradurally as an inlay graft. It is important to adequately tuck the edges of the graft underneath the dural margins. A layer of Surgicel is placed over the defect to hold the graft in place. Next, a layer of implantable ready-to-use acellular dermal allograft (AlloDerm; LifeCell Corp., Bridgewater, NJ) is tucked between the bony edge and the dural cuff, and wedged in by using gentamicin-soaked Gelfoam pledgets. The redundant edges of the acellular dermal allograft

are placed over the bony defect as an overlay, and the tucked portions act as an inlay (see **Figs. 7** and **8**). This creates a "gasket" effect for a watertight seal. Alternatively, for smaller defects, the first layer is either an acellular dermal allograft or autologous fascia lata layer as the initial inlay graft followed by another acellular dermal allograft as a second inlay graft (see **Fig. 9**). The final third layer of the repair is a vascularized pedicled nasoseptal flap, which is rotated into position over the transcribriform defect. Care is taken to ensure that the vascular pedicle is adequately released so that the anterior "reach" of the flap covers the posterior table of the frontal sinus without tension. The triple-layer reconstruction is bolstered with a layer of Surgicel, followed by gentamicin-soaked Gelfoam pledgets, and further buttressed by a Merocel nasal tampon (Medtronic Xomed, Minneapolis, MN) lathered in bacitracin ointment. The Merocel packing is removed at 10 to 12 days after surgery in the office setting while the patient is maintained on antibiotics. We have had only one case of postoperative CSF leakage (4%) in 24 EEA transcribriform patients when using the described triple-layered reconstruction technique (Liu JK and colleagues, unpublished results, 2015). We typically do not use tissue sealants or postoperative lumbar drainage for these defects, as this has not made any difference in postoperative CSF leaks.[45–47] With the triple-layer repair, we have found that rigid structural reconstruction of the anterior cranial base (with mesh, Medpor, or bone) is not necessary to prevent frontal lobe sagging or encephalocele formation.[48]

Postoperative Care

The patient is maintained on broad-spectrum intravenous antibiotics for approximately 48 to 72 hours, and then transitioned to oral antibiotics until the nasal packing is removed (10–12 days after surgery)

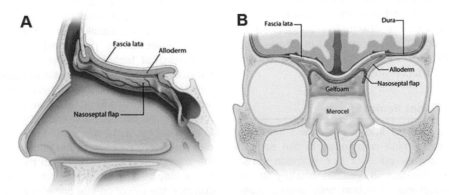

Fig. 7. Illustration (A: sagittal, B: coronal) showing the triple-layer reconstruction technique for large cribriform defects after EEA resection of anterior skull base tumors. (Illustration by Christine Gralapp © 2012.)

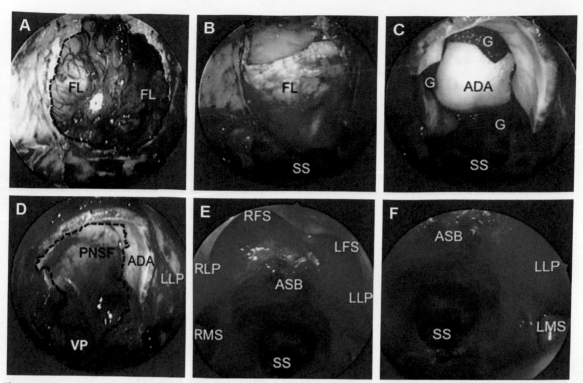

Fig. 8. Endoscopic photographs of triple-layer reconstruction of patient in **Fig. 5**. (*A*) The frontal lobes are exposed within the skull base dural defect (*dotted line*) after removal of the olfactory groove meningioma. (*B*) An initial layer of autologous fascia lata (FL) is placed as an inlay graft. (*C*) The second layer consists of an acellular dermal allograft (ADA) that is wedged between the bone of the skull base defect and the dural edge using pieces of Gelfoam (G). This creates a "gasket" effect so that a watertight seal is achieved using a combined inlay and overlay from the ADA. (*D*) The pedicle nasoseptal flap (PNSF) (*dotted line*) comprises the third layer of the repair and placed over the ADA. (*E,* *F*) Delayed 3-month nasal endoscopy shows excellent mucosalization of the anterior skull base (ASB) after triple-layered reconstruction. LFS, left frontal sinus; LLP, left lamina papyracea; LMS, left maxillary sinus; RFS, right frontal sinus; RLP, right lamina papyracea; RMS, right maxillary sinus; SS, sphenoid sinus; VP, vascular pedicle.

in the office. Deep venous thrombosis prophylaxis is composed of thromboembolism-deterrent stockings and Venodyne boots, which are used intraoperatively and immediately postoperatively. Subcutaneous heparin injection, 5000 units twice a day, is initiated at 24 hours after surgery, and then transitioned to low molecular weight heparin (Lovenox) 40 mg once a day at 48 hours after surgery, if there are no hemorrhagic complications detected on the immediate postoperative CT scan. Early ambulation with physical therapy is encouraged as early as postoperative day 1. We routinely obtain postoperative imaging with a noncontrasted CT scan in the immediate postoperative period and an MRI with and without gadolinium on postoperative day 1. If there is considerable preoperative or postoperative edema noted on T2-weighted MRI, dexamethasone is maintained and weaned off over 5 to 7 days. Prophylactic antiepileptics are maintained and weaned off at the 6-week follow-up visit if the patient remains seizure free.

Complications and Management

Postoperative CSF leakage remains a challenge with extended EEA approaches and is the most common surgical complication associated with endonasal removal of olfactory groove meningiomas. We recommend endoscopic reexploration and revision of the repair for most CSF leaks after EEA. Koutourousiou and colleagues[28] recently published the largest series to date of EEA removal of olfactory groove meningiomas. In their series of 50 patients, postoperative CSF leaks occurred in 15 patients (30%) and meningitis in 1 patient (2%). All of them were managed with return to the operating room for reexploration and revision of the repair. Two cases (2%) required an extracranial pericranial flap for reconstruction. This can be a useful strategy for recalcitrant CSF leaks despite nasoseptal flap repair, if the pericranium is available.

Avulsion or traumatic injury of any surrounding arteries (frontoorbital, frontopolar, anterior

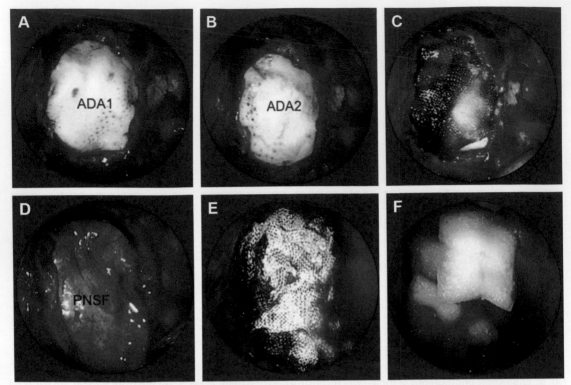

Fig. 9. Endoscopic photographs of triple-layer reconstruction of patient in **Fig. 1**. (*A*) An initial layer of acellular dermal allograft (ADA1) is placed as an inlay graft tucked underneath the anterior skull base dural defect. (*B*) A second layer of acellular dermal allograft (ADA2) is placed as another inlay graft. (*C*) A layer of Surgicel is placed over the ADA2. (*D*) The pedicled nasoseptal flap (PNSF) is rotated over the skull base defect repair as the third layer. The triple-layer repair is bolstered with a layer of Surgicel (*E*) followed by gentamicin-soaked Gelfoam pledgets (*F*).

cerebral, anterior communicating, recurrent artery of Heubner) can result in intraoperative hemorrhage, stroke, and neurologic deficit. In the event of acute intraoperative hemorrhage, vascular control and hemostasis must be obtained to prevent catastrophic hemorrhaging. For small arterial leaks (pinhole), a wisp of cotton or muscle graft can be applied to the site of bleeding. However, for arterial injuries that cannot be directly repaired, occlusion with clips may be necessary to stop further bleeding. One should be prepared for emergent craniotomy for open vascular repair and/or bypass, if necessary. Immediate and delayed catheter angiography is warranted to rule out early and delayed pseudoaneurysm formation, respectively. Vascular complications are best avoided by careful and meticulous extracapsular dissection, avoiding premature pulling of the tumor, and leaving remnants of tumor that are adherent to important vasculature.

Other potential complications include sinus infection, respiratory failure, brain abscess, postoperative seizures, hydrocephalus, deep venous thrombosis, and pulmonary embolus.[28] It is also important to inform the patient preoperatively that the EEA approach for olfactory groove meningiomas will invariably result in loss of olfaction because of the nature of the surgical approach.

SUMMARY

The endoscopic endonasal transcribriform approach offers a direct midline approach to the ventral skull base to access and remove olfactory meningiomas without brain retraction or significant manipulation of neurovascular structures. Early tumor devascularization and removal of adjacent hyperostotic bone can be achieved. Significant lateral extension of the tumor and vascular encasement may be limitations for a complete Simpson grade I resection when using an endonasal approach. Therefore, careful patient selection is critical for successful outcomes. One should be prepared to perform transcranial approaches or combined open/EEA approaches, if indicated. The triple-layer reconstruction with a nasoseptal flap is an effective repair method to prevent CSF leakage for EFA transcribriform defects.

REFERENCES

1. Adappa ND, Lee JY, Chiu AG, et al. Olfactory groove meningioma. Otolaryngol Clin North Am 2011;44(4):965–80, ix.

2. Bakay L. Olfactory meningiomas. The missed diagnosis. JAMA 1984;251(1):53–5.

3. Nakamura M, Struck M, Roser F, et al. Olfactory groove meningiomas: clinical outcome and recurrence rates after tumor removal through the frontolateral and bifrontal approach. Neurosurgery 2007; 60(5):844–52 [discussion: 844–52].

4. Obeid F, Al-Mefty O. Recurrence of olfactory groove meningiomas. Neurosurgery 2003;53(3):534–42 [discussion: 542–3].

5. Spektor S, Valarezo J, Fliss DM, et al. Olfactory groove meningiomas from neurosurgical and ear, nose, and throat perspectives: approaches, techniques, and outcomes. Neurosurgery 2005; 57(Suppl 4):268–80 [discussion: 268–80].

6. McDermott MW, Wilson CB. Meningiomas. In: Youmans J, editor. Neurological surgery. 4th edition. Philadelphia: WB Saunders; 1996. p. 2782–825.

7. Bakay L, Cares HL. Olfactory meningiomas. Report on a series of twenty-five cases. Acta Neurochir (Wien) 1972;26(1):1–12.

8. Derome PJ, Guiot G. Bone problems in meningiomas invading the base of the skull. Clin Neurosurg 1978;25:435–51.

9. Hentschel SJ, DeMonte F. Olfactory groove meningiomas. Neurosurg Focus 2003;14(6):e4.

10. Rubinstein AB, Arbit E. Intracranial meningiomas presenting with epistaxis–case report and literature review. J Otolaryngol 1985;14(4):248–50.

11. Solero CL, Giombini S, Morello G. Suprasellar and olfactory meningiomas. Report on a series of 153 personal cases. Acta Neurochir (Wien) 1983;67(3–4): 181–94.

12. Lee KF, Suh JH, Lee YE, et al. Meningioma of the paranasal sinuses. Neuroradiology 1979;17(3): 165–71.

13. Maiuri F, Salzano FA, Motta S, et al. Olfactory groove meningioma with paranasal sinus and nasal cavity extension: removal by combined subfrontal and nasal approach. J Craniomaxillofac Surg 1998; 26(5):314–7.

14. Persky MS, Som ML. Olfactory groove meningioma with paranasal sinus and nasal cavity extension: a combined approach. Otolaryngology 1978;86(5): ORL714–20.

15. Zygourakis CC, Sughrue ME, Cabero AB, et al. Management of planum/olfactory meningiomas: predicting symptoms and postoperative complications. World Neurosurg 2014;82(6):1216–23.

16. Mathiesen T, Lindquist C, Kihlstrom L, et al. Recurrence of cranial base meningiomas. Neurosurgery 1996;39(1):2–7 [discussion: 8–9].

17. Simpson D. The recurrence of intracranial meningiomas after surgical treatment. J Neurol Neurosurg Psychiatry 1957;20(1):22–39.

18. Snyder WE, Shah MV, Weisberger EC, et al. Presentation and patterns of late recurrence of olfactory groove meningiomas. Skull Base Surg 2000;10(3): 131–9.

19. Bitter AD, Stavrinou LC, Ntoulias G, et al. The role of the pterional approach in the surgical treatment of olfactory groove meningiomas: a 20-year experience. J Neurol Surg B Skull Base 2013;74(2):97–102.

20. Mielke D, Mayfrank L, Psychogios MN, et al. The anterior interhemispheric approach—a safe and effective approach to anterior skull base lesions. Acta Neurochir (Wien) 2014;156(4):689–96.

21. Pallini R, Fernandez E, Lauretti L, et al. Olfactory groove meningioma. Report of 99 cases surgically treated at the Catholic University School of Medicine, Rome. World Neurosurg 2014;83(2):219–31.e3.

22. Schaller C, Rohde V, Hassler W. Microsurgical removal of olfactory groove meningiomas via the pterional approach. Skull Base Surg 1994;4(4): 189–92.

23. de Divitiis E, Esposito F, Cappabianca P, et al. Endoscopic transnasal resection of anterior cranial fossa meningiomas. Neurosurg Focus 2008;25(6):E8.

24. Gardner PA, Kassam AB, Thomas A, et al. Endoscopic endonasal resection of anterior cranial base meningiomas. Neurosurgery 2008;63(1):36–52 [discussion: 52–4].

25. Greenfield JP, Anand VK, Kacker A, et al. Endoscopic endonasal transethmoidal transcribriform transfovea ethmoidalis approach to the anterior cranial fossa and skull base. Neurosurgery 2010;66(5): 883–92 [discussion: 892].

26. Khan OH, Sc M, Anand VK, et al. Endoscopic endonasal resection of skull base meningiomas: the significance of a "cortical cuff" and brain edema compared with careful case selection and surgical experience in predicting morbidity and extent of resection. Neurosurg Focus 2014;37(4):E7.

27. Komotar RJ, Starke RM, Raper DM, et al. Endoscopic endonasal versus open transcranial resection of anterior midline skull base meningiomas. World Neurosurg 2012;77(5–6):713–24.

28. Koutourousiou M, Fernandez-Miranda JC, Wang EW, et al. Endoscopic endonasal surgery for olfactory groove meningiomas: outcomes and limitations in 50 patients. Neurosurg Focus 2014;37(4):E8.

29. Liu JK, Christiano LD, Patel SK, et al. Surgical nuances for removal of olfactory groove meningiomas using the endoscopic endonasal transcribriform approach. Neurosurg Focus 2011;30(5):E3.

30. Padhye V, Naidoo Y, Alexander H, et al. Endoscopic endonasal resection of anterior skull base meningiomas. Otolaryngol Head Neck Surg 2012;147(3): 575–82.

31. Webb-Myers R, Wormald PJ, Brophy B. An endoscopic endonasal technique for resection of olfactory groove meningioma. J Clin Neurosci 2007; 15(4):451–5.

32. Schwartz TH. Should endoscopic endonasal surgery be used in the treatment of olfactory groove meningiomas? Neurosurg Focus 2014;37(4):E9.

33. Liu JK, Decker D, Schaefer SD, et al. Zones of approach for craniofacial resection: minimizing facial incisions for resection of anterior cranial base and paranasal sinus tumors. Neurosurgery 2003;53(5):1126–35 [discussion: 1135–7].

34. Liu JK, O'Neill B, Orlandi RR, et al. Endoscopic-assisted craniofacial resection of esthesioneuroblastoma: minimizing facial incisions–technical note and report of 3 cases. Minim Invasive Neurosurg 2003;46(5):310–5.

35. Batra PS, Kanowitz SJ, Luong A. Anatomical and technical correlates in endoscopic anterior skull base surgery: a cadaveric analysis. Otolaryngol Head Neck Surg 2010;142(6):827–31.

36. Hadad G, Bassagasteguy L, Carrau RL, et al. A novel reconstructive technique after endoscopic expanded endonasal approaches: vascular pedicle nasoseptal flap. Laryngoscope 2006;116(10):1882–6.

37. Kassam AB, Thomas A, Carrau RL, et al. Endoscopic reconstruction of the cranial base using a pedicled nasoseptal flap. Neurosurgery 2008;63(1 Suppl 1):ONS44–52 [discussion: ONS52–3].

38. Eloy JA, Patel AA, Shukla PA, et al. Early harvesting of the vascularized pedicled nasoseptal flap during endoscopic skull base surgery. Am J Otolaryngol 2013;34(3):188–94.

39. Liu JK, Schmidt RF, Choudhry OJ, et al. Surgical nuances for nasoseptal flap reconstruction of cranial base defects with high-flow cerebrospinal fluid leaks after endoscopic skull base surgery. Neurosurg Focus 2012;32(6):E7.

40. Pinheiro-Neto CD, Prevedello DM, Carrau RL, et al. Improving the design of the pedicled nasoseptal flap for skull base reconstruction: a radioanatomic study. Laryngoscope 2007;117(9):1560–9.

41. Scott NA, Wormald P, Close D, et al. Endoscopic modified Lothrop procedure for the treatment of chronic frontal sinusitis: a systematic review. Otolaryngol Head Neck Surg 2003;129(4):427–38.

42. Patel SK, Husain Q, Kuperan AB, et al. Utility of a rotation-suction microdebrider for tumor removal in endoscopic endonasal skull base surgery. J Clin Neurosci 2014;21(1):142–7.

43. Zanation AM, Carrau RL, Snyderman CH, et al. Nasoseptal flap reconstruction of high flow intraoperative cerebral spinal fluid leaks during endoscopic skull base surgery. Am J Rhinol Allergy 2009;23(5): 518–21.

44. Eloy JA, Patel SK, Shukla PA, et al. Triple-layer reconstruction technique for large cribriform defects after endoscopic endonasal resection of anterior skull base tumors. Int Forum Allergy Rhinol 2013; 3(3):204–11.

45. Eloy JA, Choudhry OJ, Friedel ME, et al. Endoscopic nasoseptal flap repair of skull base defects: is addition of a dural sealant necessary? Otolaryngol Head Neck Surg 2012;147(1):161–6.

46. Eloy JA, Choudhry OJ, Shukla PA, et al. Nasoseptal flap repair after endoscopic transsellar versus expanded endonasal approaches: is there an increased risk of postoperative cerebrospinal fluid leak? Laryngoscope 2012;122(6):1219–25.

47. Eloy JA, Kuperan AB, Choudhry OJ, et al. Efficacy of the pedicled nasoseptal flap without cerebrospinal fluid (CSF) diversion for repair of skull base defects: incidence of postoperative CSF leaks. Int Forum Allergy Rhinol 2012;2(5):397–401.

48. Eloy JA, Shukla PA, Choudhry OJ, et al. Assessment of frontal lobe sagging after endoscopic endonasal transcribriform resection of anterior skull base tumors: is rigid structural reconstruction of the cranial base defect necessary? Laryngoscope 2012; 122(12):2652–7.

Endonasal Endoscopic Management of Parasellar and Cavernous Sinus Meningiomas

Bjorn Lobo, MD[a], Xin Zhang, MD[a],
Garni Barkhoudarian, MD[a], Chester F. Griffiths, MD[a,b],
Daniel F. Kelly, MD[a],*

KEYWORDS

- Cavernous sinus meningioma • Parasellar meningioma • Endonasal endoscopic approach
- Minimally invasive neurosurgery

KEY POINTS

- Aggressive surgical resection of cavernous sinus meningiomas (CSMs) and parasellar meningiomas may result in significant morbidity.
- Multimodality treatment is required for effective treatment of CSMs and parasellar meningiomas.
- Bony sellar, cavernous sinus, and skull base decompression with conservative tumor debulking through an endonasal endoscopic approach seems a safe and effective option for initial management of invasive skull base meningiomas.

INTRODUCTION

The management of CSMs and parasellar meningiomas offers a significant challenge to skull base surgeons because of their close proximity and potential involvement of cranial nerves (CNs) II–VI, the carotid arteries, and the pituitary-hypothalamic axis. Over the past 30 years, an evolution in the treatment of these tumors has occurred. In the 1980s and 1990s, relatively aggressive lateral, anterolateral, and posterolateral skull base approaches were developed. This movement was fostered by a better understanding of skull base surgical anatomy and the rationale that extent of resection was inversely related to recurrence rates. Reports of significant rates of new CN deficits with low rates of improvement of preoperative CN deficits,[1,2] however, resulted in this aggressive approach for CSM gradually reconsidered and falling out favor at many centers. Concurrently, reports of good tumor control with stereotactic radiosurgery (SRS)[3–7] and stereotactic radiotherapy (SRT)[6] led to a paradigm shift to a more conservative surgical management of CSMs and parasellar meningiomas followed by observation and possible adjuvant radiation[8–10] or radiation alone as a first-line treatment.[4,7]

A more conservative transcranial surgical approach was described by Couldwell and colleagues[11] in 2006 who documented their management of CSMs in 11 patients using a frontotemporal craniotomy followed with planned SRS or SRT. The goal of surgery was to use selective intercavernous and extracavernous tumor removal to decompress the CNs and reduce the overall tumor volume that would be treated with postoperative radiation. Although the study had

Disclosures: D.F. Kelly receives royalties from Mizuho, Inc. The remaining authors disclose no competing financial interest.
[a] The Brain Tumor Center & Pituitary Disorders Program, Providence's Saint John's Health Center, John Wayne Cancer Institute, 2200 Santa Monica Boulevard, Santa Monica, CA 90404, USA; [b] Department of Otolaryngology, Pacific Eye & Ear Specialists, 11645 Wilshire Boulevard, Los Angeles, CA 90025, USA
* Corresponding author.
E-mail address: kellyd@jwci.org

Neurosurg Clin N Am 26 (2015) 389–401
http://dx.doi.org/10.1016/j.nec.2015.03.004
1042-3680/15/$ – see front matter © 2015 Elsevier Inc. All rights reserved.

a small sample size, 3 of 5 patients with eye motility difficulty and 2 of 4 patients with visual loss improved and no patient suffered a new CN deficit after surgery. Tumor control was achieved in all patients with a median follow-up of 22 months (range 9–39 months). Akutsu and colleagues[12] in 2009 reported their results using a similar conservative surgical from the microscopic transsphenoidal route in 21 patients with CSMs. The sellar and cavernous sinus dura was opened and modest tumor debulking was performed. Overall, 32 of 34 CN deficits improved and there was no worsening. Of endocrine abnormalities, improvement was noted 16 of 28 (57.1%). Tumor control was 100% at median follow-up of 65 months.

Kano and colleagues[13] evaluated the role of previous surgery in patients treated with SRS for CSM. Of 272 patients with CSM treated over a 23-year period with SRS, 99 patients had a previous craniotomy with microsurgery for tumor removal. Microsurgery was not found to effect overall progression-free survival, which was 83.4% at 10 years. Patients who had undergone microsurgery were less likely to have an improvement of a preoperative CN deficit after SRS than patients with SRS alone (12%–15% vs 39%, respectively). One explanation for this discrepancy is that patients who had previous microsurgery may have had CN deficits secondary to surgical injury during an aggressive surgical resection given that a large proportion of the surgical patients were treated in the early and middle 1990s. Another possible explanation is that a lateral approach to the cavernous sinus may disrupt the delicate blood flow to the CNs that reside in the lateral cavernous sinus wall. Further injury with SRS may result in nerve ischemia and failure of the existing neuropathy to improve.[14]

Therefore, as previously demonstrated by Couldwell and colleagues[11] and Akutsu and colleagues,[12] an ideal surgical approach may be one that allows for selective decompression of the cavernous sinus structures, optic apparatus, and pituitary gland, with conservative tumor debulking while minimizing direct CN manipulation. Given that most CSMs and parasellar meningiomas can be directly accessed by the transsphenoidal route, the endonasal endoscopic route may offer an excellent surgical option for these challenging tumors. This approach may also enhance the efficacy and safety of SRT. This article describes endonasal endoscopic surgical management of CSMs and parasellar meningiomas, including those involving Meckel cave.

SURGICAL GOALS AND INDICATIONS

At the authors' center, an extended endonasal endoscopic approach has been adopted for performing bony decompression and selective tumor debulking of select meningiomas involving the cavernous sinus, Meckel cave, and the petroclival region. The goals of surgery are

1. Decompression of the CNs within the cavernous sinus and Meckel cave by bony removal of the parasellar skull base
2. Maximal but safe tumor removal within the sella, Meckel cave, and cavernous sinus to further optimize CN function and pituitary gland function
3. For tumors with optic canal involvement or clival extension, bony decompression of the optic canal and clivus to reduce mass effect on optic nerve and/or brainstem
4. For large tumors with significant petroclival extension and brainstem compression, endonasal parasellar debulking can be part of a 2-stage surgery that includes a retromastoid approach then endonasal approach followed by SRT (see Fig. 6).
5. Reduce overall tumor volume for future radiotherapy.
6. Obtain a histopathologic diagnosis and tissue for genomic profiling.[15–18]

The advantages of this approach over a conventional frontotemporal craniotomy are no use of brain retraction and direct access to and visualization of the pituitary gland for removal of any sellar component of the tumor. The potential disadvantages of this approach are higher rates of postoperative cerebrospinal fluid (CSF) leakage and poor access to tumor lateral to the CNs III–VI and the carotid arteries. The main indications and contraindications for the endonasal endoscopic approach are based on anatomic considerations and are listed in Table 1.

SURGICAL TECHNIQUE/PROCEDURE
Preoperative Planning

- A detailed history and physical examination are completed on all patients, with special focus on the function of CNs II–VI as well as signs and symptoms of anterior and posterior pituitary dysfunction.
- All patients undergo a volumetric MRI with gadolinium for purposes of intraoperative navigation as well as assessment of the intercavernous/carotid corridor. Additionally, a CT angiogram is often performed to provide useful information regarding sinus

Table 1
Indications and contraindications for extended endonasal endoscopic management of cavernous sinus meningiomas and parasellar meningiomas

Indications	Contraindications
Tumor within the cavernous sinus	Asymptomatic incidental CSMs or Meckel cave meningiomas
Tumor within Meckel cave	Patients with previous endonasal surgery who have already exhausted prior endonasal flap options[a]
Tumor within the sella distorting the pituitary gland	Tumors with large bulky extensions along medial sphenoid wing[a]
Tumor involving the clivus	

[a] Denotes *relative* contraindications.

anatomy, bony hypertrophy, and vascular topography.

- For tumors invading the sella tursica, or in cases of the pituitary gland possibly requiring manipulation, a full set of pituitary function testing should be completed. These tests should include serum levels of prolactin, growth hormone, insulinlike growth factor 1, gonadotrophs, respective sex hormones, thyroid-stimulating hormone, thyroxine, and morning cortisol and adrenocorticotrophic hormone.
- Formal ophthalmologic testing, including visual field testing, is completed in patients with complaints of vision loss or with significant radiographic optic apparatus compression.

Patient Positioning, Preparation, and Workflow

- All endonasal endoscopic surgery is performed in the endoscopic operating suite, which is organized to facilitate a dual-surgeon, bimanual technique (**Fig. 1**).
- After induction of general endotracheal anesthesia, the endotracheal tube is taped to the left. Muscle relaxation is withheld in cases requiring intraoperative monitoring. Neither orogastric suction tube placement nor oral packing is performed at this time because the stomach contents are suctioned at the end of the operation with a nasogastric suction tube that is temporarily placed under direct visualization with the endoscope.
- The patient is positioned in the supine position with the head slightly rotated toward the right and the chin tilted toward the surgeon, who is standing on the right side of the patient. The head is slightly flexed for parasellar lesions and may be more flexed if lesions involve the clivus.

- Mask registration (Stryker, Kalamazoo, Michigan) to the neuronavigation system is completed.
- Leads are placed for monitoring CNs III, VI, and/or V; somatosensory evoked potentials; and motor evoked potentials.
- Oxymetazoline hydrochloride nasal solution is sprayed within each nare for mucosal decongestion.
- The nares, nasal tip, and upper lip are prepped with Povidone-iodine solution.
- The right lower abdomen is also prepped for potential fat graft.

Surgical Approach

Step 1: Local anesthetic mixed with epinephrine is injected into bilateral inferior and middle turbinates.

Step 2a: Outfracturing of the middle and inferior turbinates is completed bilaterally.

Step 2b: If needed, resection of the right middle turbinate is completed to facilitate endoscopic visualization and movement of surgical instruments.

Step 3a: Bilateral olfactory fiber sparing modified rescue flaps, as described by Griffiths and colleagues,[19] are raised in cases when a CSF leak is not expected.

Step 3b: A full nasoseptal flap is raised if a high-flow CSF leak is expected.

Step 4: A posterior septectomy is performed to create a single posterior working corridor for the surgical instruments.

Step 5: The bilateral sphenoid ostia are enlarged to create a single large sphenoidotomy.

Step 6: The sphenoid septations are removed and posterior ethmoidectomies are carried out as needed to expose the sellar face.

Step 7: Identification of the internal carotid arteries including the vertical segments and cavernous sinus segments, is completed using neuronavigation and Doppler ultrasound.[20]

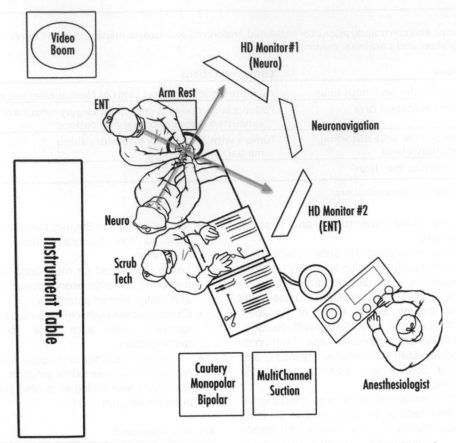

Fig. 1. The endoscopic operating suite: patient positioning is shown relative to the neurosurgeon (neuro), otolaryngologist (ENT), scrub technician (Scrub Tech), and 2 high-definition (HD) monitors. The surgical navigation screen is located between the 2 HD monitors. The scrub technician stands on the neurosurgeon's right side with the most commonly used surgical instruments over the patient. An additional back table has ancillary surgical instrumentation. The anesthesiologist and anesthesia machine are positioned immediately to patient's left-hand side with easy access to patient's airway and left-sided vascular access. (*Courtesy of* D. Kelly, MD, Santa Monica, CA.)

Step 8: Depending on tumor location, additional exposure is completed as follows:

The sella: The bone of the sellar face is thinned with a high-speed course diamond bur. The thinned bone is then removed in a piecemeal fashion with Kerrison rongeurs to expose the sellar dura.

The cavernous sinus: The ventral face of the cavernous sinus is exposed by first removing the bone over the ipsilateral sellar face using the technique discussed previously. Using Doppler ultrasound to identify the flow of the cavernous sinus and cavernous carotid artery, the bony removal is carried laterally over the anterior dural wall of cavernous sinus, including the area of the medial opticocarotid recess, as described by Labib and colleagues.[21]

Meckel cave: The approach to the Meckel cave, as described by Kassam and colleagues,[22] is used and outlined as follows:

1. The vidian nerve is identified by raising the mucosa over the rostrum laterally until the vidian nerve is seen exiting the vidian canal in the medial pterygoid plate.
2. The medial pterygoid plate is drilled to unroof the inferomedial quadrant of the vidian canal and is followed posteriorly to the genu of petrous carotid artery.
3. An ipsilateral uncinectomy is performed to gain access to the ipsilateral maxillary sinus and enlarged to facilitate surgical instrument access.
4. The sphenopalatine foramina is identified in the posterior maxillary antrum and the posterior wall of the antrum is then removed with Kerrison rongeurs to expose pterygopalatine fossa
5. The infraorbital nerve as it exits the foramen rotundum is identified and the bone superomedially is removed to expose the anterior wall of the Meckel cave.

The clivus: For tumors with clival extension and brainstem compression, a bony clivectomy can be performed (**Figs. 2**A, B and **3**). The clival recess below the sella is identified and the clival bone is removed with a combination of high-speed diamond bur and Kerrison rongeurs. In some instances the sellar floor may also be removed. For more inferior exposure, the floor of the sphenoid sinus is drilled away.

Surgical Procedure

Step 1—Bony decompression: most of the bony decompression is achieved by performing the approach to affected areas, as discussed previously. An additional site for bony decompression is the optic canal if vision loss secondary to compressive optic neuropathy is suspected.

Step 2—Dural fenestration/decompression: The dura over the compartments with tumor

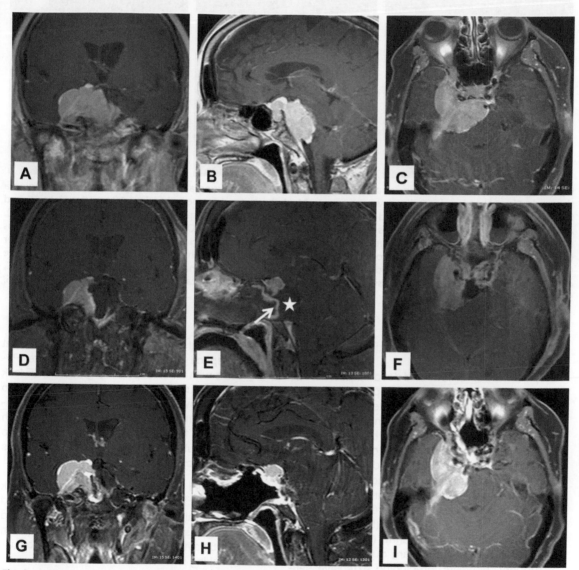

Fig. 2. A 59-year-old woman complained of dizziness and unsteady gait for 2 months. Her neurologic examination showed mild decrease of facial sensation in right V2 dermatome. Endocrinological testing revealed normal pituitary function. Preoperative coronal (*A*), sagittal (*B*), and axial (*C*) MRIs demonstrate a parasellar meningioma with extension into the right cavernous sinus, Meckel Cave, and clivus. She underwent endonasal endoscopic extended transsellar, transplanum, and transclival bony decompression and tumor debulking. Post-operative day coronal (*D*), sagittal (*E*), and axial (*F*) MRIs with fat supression MRI with gadolinium and fat-suppression showed sellar and midline clival tumor debulking and the fat graft (*star*) with nasoseptal flap (*arrow*) used for layered closure. Her 8-month post-operative coronal (*G*), saggital (*H*), and axial (*I*) MRIs showed early tumor progression predominantly in the right cavernous sinus. She remains asymptomatic and will start her 6 week course of SRT within a month.

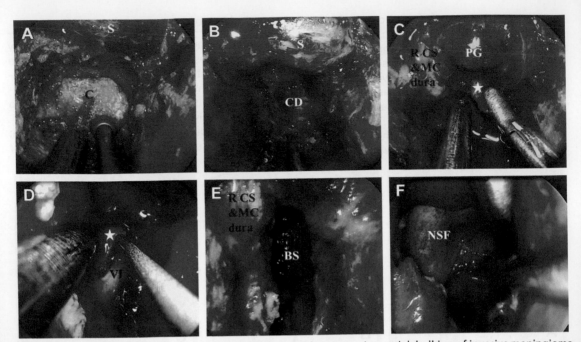

Fig. 3. Intraoperative views of endonasal endoscopic bony decompression and debulking of invasive meningioma shown in **Fig. 2** that involves sella, cavernous sinus, Meckel cave, and petroclival region. After sellar, right CS, and MC bony decompression is completed, clivectomy is performed with high-speed drill (*A*) to expose clival dural (*B*). After dural opening, sellar tumor was removed with ring curettes and NICO Myriad aspiration and tumor forceps (*C*). After removal of midline intradural prepontine meningioma, right CN VI identified running through tumor (*D*). Final view after midline meningioma removed showing brainstem with preservation of right abducens nerve (*E*). Skull base reconstruction with abdominal fat graft, collagen sponge, and nasoseptal flap (*F*). BS, brainstem; C, clivus; CD, clival dura; CS, cavernous sinus; MC, Meckel cave; NSF, nasoseptal flap; PG, pituitary gland; R, right; S, sella; VI, CN VI; star, tumor.

invasion is opened to further decompress the CNs.

Step 3—Tumor removal and decompression: Tumor within in the confined compartments of the cavernous sinus and the Meckel cave are selectively removed. Prior to any attempted tumor removal in these areas, however, especially lateral to the cavernous carotid artery, a nerve stimulator should be used to help localize the course of CN III and VI. If no nerve signal is obtained, tumor debulking can be performed with a combination of ring curettes, ultrasonic aspirator, and NICO Myriad (NICO Corporation, Indianapolis, Indiana) (see **Fig. 2**C). Many of these tumors are quite fibrous and rubbery, however, precluding extensive safe removal. Visualization of the CNs within the cavernous sinus and Meckel cave is often difficult and not indicated because this may result in further injury to the nerves during the required manipulation to expose the nerves.

Step 4—Reconstruction/closure: Large intradural potential spaces created from tumor removal are sufficiently filled with a small amount of

abdominal fat graft and with assurance that the space is not packed under pressure. Patients with an intraoperative grade 3 CSF leak have closure performed with a nasoseptal flap directly covering the dural defect and surrounding bony margin. This is then reinforced with additional fat and a collagen sponge. The flap is then buttressed with Merocel sinus packs (Medtronic, Minneapolis, Minnesota).

If a patient has no CSF leak or a low-flow CSF leak (grade 1 or 2)[23] observed intraoperatively, layered closure is usually performed with fat graft, followed by a collagen sponge and Merocel packing left in place for 5 days with continued oral antibiotics until the packing is removed.

POTENTIAL PITFALLS AND COMPLICATION AVOIDANCE
Failure of Neuronavigation

Neuronavigation registration is checked prior to the operation using several surface landmarks (nasal bridge, lateral canthi, and external auditory canals).

Additionally, it is rechecked intranasally during surgery at the keel of the sphenoid bone, a consistently midline structure. Despite these measures, neuronavigation tracking may still become inaccurate during surgery; therefore, an in-depth review of patient preoperative radiographs and a clear understanding of the anatomy are prerequisites to avoid inadvertent damage to normal structures.

Carotid Artery or Other Vascular Injury

The most common reason for vascular injury is failure to determine the course of the carotid arteries or related circle of Willis branches, which are typically encased or immediately adjacent to invasive parasellar meningiomas. The Doppler ultrasound probe is invaluable in mapping out these vessels as they course through or along the tumor. Although neuronavigation is also helpful, the use of real-time Doppler is likely more accurate, particularly as tumor is debulked and bone is removed, which may result in some shift and movement of the vessels.[20] Carotid artery injury can also occur when bone removal over the cavernous sinus and along Meckel cave is being performed. Careful use of Kerrison rongeurs and drills is mandatory. Torquing or twisting motion with rongeurs should be avoided because such maneuvers can lead to shards of bone being driven into the vessel wall resulting in laceration or avulsion injuries. Additional precautions to avoid a major vascular injury include gentle manipulation of tumor alongside the meningioma particularly because most meningiomas are relatively firm, fibrous, and rubbery. Although use of ultrasonic aspirators and the NICO instrument are sometimes helpful in removing these firm tumors, great care should be taken as the vessels are approached with these instruments and vessel location should be frequently checked with the Doppler.

Cranial Nerve Injury

CNs within the cavernous sinus and Meckel cave may be inadvertently injured secondary to surgical manipulation without knowledge of nerves close trajectory. For this reason, evoked potential monitoring of CNs 3 and 6 is used for all parasellar meningiomas with cavernous sinus invasion and prepontine extension. Intraoperative stimulation is performed during tumor dissection to further map the location of these nerves. Electrocautery in the vicinity of these nerves should be avoided to prevent thermal injury.

Postoperative Cerebrospinal Fluid Leak

The highest risk of postoperative CSF leak in patients with parasellar meningiomas is in those with a petroclival component. In such patients, a clival bony decompression and long dural opening with tumor debulking anterior to the brainstem has a high potential for postoperative CSF leak. As discussed previously, a vascularized nasoseptal flap is used for reconstruction in all such cases when a high-flow CSF leak is created. To minimize the chances of repair failure, time is taken to assure that the flap is directly opposed to the full margin of the bony opening and that no mucosa or other material, such as a collagen sponge or fibrin glue is between the flap and the bone. The flap is then reinforced with fat to provide an additional layer of organic closure. Proper buttressing is needed to prevent movement of flap during the initial perioperative period if a patient were to inadvertently perform a Valsalva maneuver. The authors commonly use Merocel packing that has a central bore through which the endoscope may be placed. By sliding the Merocel pack over the shaft of endoscope while directly visualizing the site requiring reinforcement, optimal buttressing of the flap may be accomplished. An immediate postoperative CT is completed to assure good positioning of the buttresses.

POSTOPERATIVE CARE

- An early postoperative CT scan within 2 hours of surgery is completed to assess for postoperative hematoma, alignment of Merocel packs, and extent of pneumocephalus.
- In cases of intraoperative CSF leak, patients are placed on acetazolamide for 48 hours postoperatively. Lumbar CSF drainage is rarely used.
- All patients are treated with 24 hours of perioperative intravenous antibiotic coverage followed by 5 days of oral antibiotics to prevent infection.
- Endocrinological testing is repeated postoperatively in patients with preoperative pituitary dysfunction and in patients with manipulation of their pituitary gland during surgery. Furthermore, strict records are kept of fluid intake and output to assess for postoperative diabetes insipidus.
- To achieve lasting tumor control, postoperative SRT (typically in 30 fractions over 6 weeks) is considered for patients without prior radiation who have histologically confirmed typical meningiomas. Given the slow growth rate of these tumors, SRT is typically delayed for a minimum of 3 to 6 months after surgery, and in cases of minimal residual tumor, SRT is withheld until tumor growth is seen on serial postoperative MRIs. This delay in treatment is

Table 2
Patient characteristics and clinical outcome

Case	Age, Gender	Prior Treatment	Tumor Location	World Health Organization Grade	Cranial Nerve Palsy (Before Surgery)	Pituitary Dysfunction	Postoperative Stereotactic Radiotherapy	Cranial Nerve Palsy (at Last Follow-up)	Recurrence/ Regrowth	Immediate Cranial Nerve Outcome	Long-term Cranial Nerve Outcome
1	56, F	—	CS, MC, PC, sella	I	VI	—	+	VI	S	I	I
2	71, F	—	CS, MC, PC, sella	I	II, VIII	—	—	II, VIII	S	I	I
3	53, F	—	CS, MC, PC, sella	I	III, VI	—	—	III	S	I	I
4	53, M	—	CS, MC, PC, sella	I	V1–V3, VII, VIII	+	+	V1, V2, VII, VIII	S	S	S
5	44, F	—	CS, MC, PC, sella	I	III, IV, VI	+	+	III, IV, VI	S	S	S
6	59, F	—	CS, MC, PC, sella	I	V2	—	—	V2	Pr[a]	I	I

Patient	Age, Sex	Treatment		Location							
7	49, F	—	I	CS, MC, sella	/	+	+	/	S	—	I
8	70, F	—	I	CS	/	—	—	III	S	—	S
9	69, M	—	I	CS	III	—	+	V1, V2	S	Dᵇ	S
10	56, F	—	I	MC	V1, V2	—	+	III	D	S	D
11	58, M	SRT, surgery	I	CS, MC, PC, sella	III	+	—	II, III, IV, V1–V3, VI	S	S	S
12	52, M	SRS, SRT, surgery	II	CS, MC, PC, sella	II, III, IV, V2, V3, VI	+	—	II, III, IV, V1–V3, VI	Pr	S	D
13	71, F	SRS, surgery	I	CS, MC, PC	II, V1–V3, VI, VII, VIII	—	—	II, III, VI, VII, VIII	Pr	—	S
14	58, M	SRS, SRT, surgery	I	CS, PC, sella	II	+	—	II	Pr	S	S
15	55, M	SRS, surgery	I	CS, MC, sella	/	—	—	III, IV, V2, V3	Pr	S	D

Abbreviations: CS, cavernous sinus; D, declined; I, improved; MC, Meckel cave; PC, petroclival; Pr, progression; S, stable.

ᵃ The patient has evidence of early tumor progression 8 months after surgery and will be starting SRT within a month. She is asymptomatic.

ᵇ New abducens nerve palsy after surgery, CN V2 palsy 5 months after the surgery then resolved after SRT.

done to maximize chances of CN and pituitary gland recovery. For atypical meningiomas, or tumors that show early regrowth on the 3-month postoperative MRI, SRT should be expedited. In this series, the authors encountered 1 atypical meningioma. This tumor occurred in a patient who had been previously treated with SRT and SRS and was not a candidate for more repeat radiotherapy. In patients such as this one, chemotherapy may be considered but overall has not been found effective. The hope for new targeted therapies, however, remains given the advances made in tumor genomic and proteomic profiling.[15–18]

OUTCOMES

The authors identified 15 patients in whom the endonasal approach was used to treat meningiomas involving the cavernous sinus and parasellar region. Patient characteristics and outcomes are listed in **Table 2**; 4 of the 15 patients are presented in **Figs. 2** and **4–6**.

Immediate Postoperative Cranial Nerve Function

In the authors' series, 31 preoperative CN palsies related to the tumor were documented in 12 patients (80%). After the surgery, 13 CN palsies (42%) improved or resolved, and 18 CN palsies (58%) remained stable. One patient developed a new permanent abducens nerve palsy directly related to the surgery. No other patients had worsening of an existing cranial neuropathy secondary to surgery.

Pituitary Function Outcome

Preoperative pituitary dysfunctions were found in 6 of 15 patients (40%), including 4 with central hypothyroidism, 3 with hypoadrenalism, 1 with growth

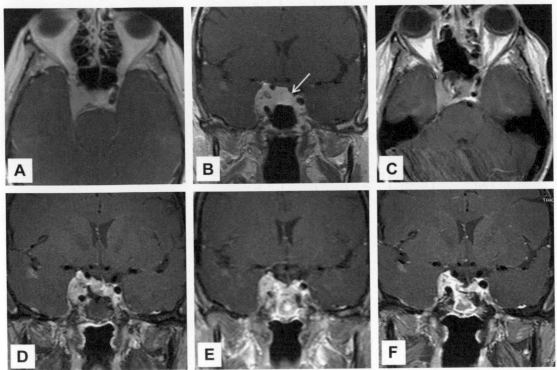

Fig. 4. A 49-year-old woman presented with increasing fatigue. Endocrinological work-up revealed low gonadotropins and hyperprolactinemia. Her neurologic examination was intact. Axial (A) and coronal (B) MRI with contrast showed a large sellar tumor with extension into the right cavernous sinus, Meckel cave and suprasellar region. The right cavernous carotid artery was completely encased with slight narrowing by the tumor. The normal pituitary gland was markedly compressed and pushed toward the left (arrow). Endonasal endoscopic skull base bony decompression and tumor debulking was performed to decompress the pituitary gland and cavernous sinus. Axial (C) and coronal (D) MRI 24 hours after the surgery showed resection of tumor along right sella and medial cavernous sinus good gland decompression. Her prolactin level normalized on postoperative day 1. Pathology confirmed a World Health Organization grade I meningioma with a Ki-67 index of 1%. The patient was subsequently treated with SRT 3 weeks after the surgery to prevent future tumor growth, with a total dose of 50.4 Gy delivered in 28 fractions. Follow-up coronal MRI 2 months after SRT (E) revealed stable tumor and at coronal MRI (F) 52 months after SRT showed tumor shrinkage. Currently, she continues to do well with no new neurologic or hormonal abnormalities.

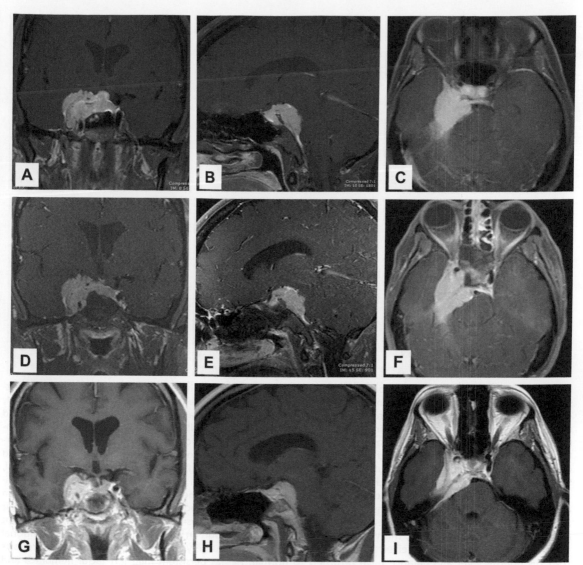

Fig. 5. A 44-year-old woman complained of progressive onset of headaches and slight diplopia for 15 months as well as irregular menstrual periods. Her neurologic examination showed mild partial palsies of right CNs III, IV, and VI. Endocrinological testing revealed an elevated prolactin level and low levels of thyroxine, corticotropin, and morning cortisol. Cornal (*A*), saggital (*B*) and axial (*C*) MRI with contrast showed a large parasellar skull base mass with extension into the right cavernous sinus, Meckel cave, and down the clivus. Endonasal endoscopic bony decompression and conservative tumor debulking was performed. The bone over the sella, right cavernous sinus, right Meckel cave, and right optic canal and upper clivus was removed. The dura was opened over the sella and medial right cavernous sinus and the fibrous tumor was debulked; additional tumor was removed from the upper clival region but no attempt was made to expose the upper brainstem. Repair of a low-pressure CSF leakage was performed using an abdominal fat graft and collagen sponge. Postoperative testing revealed transient diabetes insipidus that resolved within a week of surgery; adrenal function normalized and she has mild hyperprolactinemia. Her CN palsies remained unchanged with no new diplopia and headaches improved. Coronal (*D*), saggital (*E*), and axial (*F*) postoperative day 1 MRI with contrast showed adequate debulking of the tumor in the right cavernous sinus, sella, and clivus. Pathology confirmed a typical meningioma with Ki-67 less than 2%. The residual tumor was treated with SRT within 3 months of surgery. Coronal (*F*), saggital (*H*) and axial (*I*) MRI 4 years after surgery shows further tumor shrinkage and patient continues to do well.

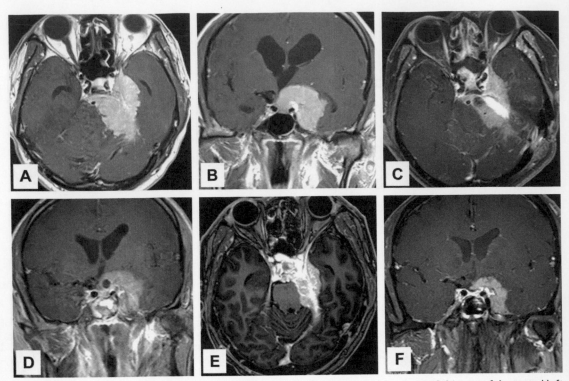

Fig. 6. Staged retrosigmoid and endonasal approach. A 52-year-old man with a 6-month history of decreased left-sided hearing, left facial numbness, imbalance, and decreased energy. Neurologic examination showed left CNs V1, V2, V3, and VIII palsies. Axial (*A*) and coronal (*B*) MRI with contrast showed a large skull base meningioma involved in the left petroclival, cerebellopontine angle, MC, and sellar and suprasellar region, which caused severe brainstem distortion and early hydrocephalus as well as encasement of the left cavernous and supraclinoid carotid artery. Staged surgery was performed to decompress the left cerebellopontine angle through a retrosigmoid craniotomy, followed by further debulking and bony decompression through an endonasal endoscopic transclival, transsellar, and transplanum approach 1 month later. Axial (*C*) and coronal (*D*) MRI after the second surgery indicated good tumor debulking with adequate brainstem decompression and resolve of hydrocephalus had been accomplished. At time of his endonasal surgery, a nasoseptal flap and abdominal fat graft were used to repair an expected grade 3 CSF leak. He developed a CSF leak, however, 12 days after surgery secondary after a bout of severe nausea and vomiting; this was repaired uneventfully through an endonasal approach with additional fat graft added. The patient received SRT 2 months after the second surgery. At last follow-up, the patient reports that his energy level and balance have returned to normal. He has persistent mild left facial numbness and decreased hearing. His axial (*E*) and coronal (*F*) MRI at 18 months after SRT shows significant tumor shrinkage.

hormone deficiency, 4 with central hypogonadism, and 4 with hyperprolactinemia. Postoperatively, pituitary dysfunctions in 4 of 6 patients (67%) improved or resolved, including 1 of the 4 (25%) with hypothyroidism, 1 of 3 (33%) with adrenal insufficiency, 2 of 4 (50%) with hypogonadism, and 1 of 4 (25%) with hyperprolactinemia. Pituitary dysfunctions in the other 2 patients persisted. One patient developed hypothyroidism 2 years after the surgery, likely related to SRT; otherwise none of the 15 patients developed new hypopituitarism after surgery.

Long-term Cranial Nerve Outcome and Tumor Control

Of the 10 patients without prior radiation (median follow-up of 24 months; range, 9–56 months), 6 received postoperative SRT and tumor control was achieved in all 6 patients (100%) with tumor shrinkage in 3 of 6 patients. Improved or stable CN outcome was observed in 9 patients (90%).

Of the 5 patients with prior surgery and SRS and/or SRT (median follow-up 18 months; range, 2–59 months), none had additional radiation. Tumor control was achieved in only 1 of 5 patients (20%), with improved or stable CN outcome in 2 patients (40%). Two of the 4 patients with tumor regrowth received another surgery for tumor debulking.

SUMMARY

CSMs and parasellar meningiomas often require multimodal treatment for effective management. Aggressive surgical resection does not necessarily translate into good tumor control and may lead to significant neurologic morbidity. Endonasal endoscopic bony skull base decompression with conservative and judicious tumor resection of these lesions seems helpful in improving or stabilizing preexisting cranial neuropathy and reversing endocrinopathy. In some instances of large petroclival tumors, the endonasal route can be combined with a retromastoid approach as a staged treatment strategy. This approach may also reduce the risk of SRT-induced tumor swelling and related complications. Additional patients treated in this manner and longer clinical follow-up are needed to better assess the efficacy of this strategy.

REFERENCES

1. O'Sullivan MG, van Loveren HR, Tew JM Jr. The surgical resectability of meningiomas of the cavernous sinus. Neurosurgery 1997;40(2):238–44 [discussion: 245–7].

2. DeMonte F, Smith HK, al-Mefty O. Outcome of aggressive removal of cavernous sinus meningiomas. J Neurosurg 1994;81(2):245–51.

3. Roche PH, Regis J, Dufour H, et al. Gamma knife radiosurgery in the management of cavernous sinus meningiomas. J Neurosurg 2000;93(Suppl 3):68–73.

4. Lee JY, Niranjan A, McInerney J, et al. Stereotactic radiosurgery providing long-term tumor control of cavernous sinus meningiomas. J Neurosurg 2002; 97(1):65–72.

5. Iwai Y, Yamanaka K, Ishiguro T. Gamma knife radiosurgery for the treatment of cavernous sinus meningiomas. Neurosurgery 2003;52(3):517–24 [discussion: 523–4].

6. Metellus P, Regis J, Muracciole X, et al. Evaluation of fractionated radiotherapy and gamma knife radiosurgery in cavernous sinus meningiomas: treatment strategy. Neurosurgery 2005;57(5):873–86 [discussion: 873–86].

7. Nicolato A, Foroni R, Alessandrini F, et al. Radiosurgical treatment of cavernous sinus meningiomas: experience with 122 treated patients. Neurosurgery 2002;51(5):1153–9 [discussion: 1159–61].

8. Pamir MN, Kilic T, Bayrakli F, et al. Changing treatment strategy of cavernous sinus meningiomas: experience of a single institution. Surg Neurol 2005;64(Suppl 2):S58–66.

9. Maruyama K, Shin M, Kurita H, et al. Proposed treatment strategy for cavernous sinus meningiomas: a prospective study. Neurosurgery 2004;55(5):1068–75.

10. Abdel-Aziz KM, Froelich SC, Dagnew E, et al. Large sphenoid wing meningiomas involving the cavernous sinus: conservative surgical strategies for better functional outcomes. Neurosurgery 2004;54(6):1375–83 [discussion: 1383–4].

11. Couldwell WT, Kan P, Liu JK, et al. Decompression of cavernous sinus meningioma for preservation and improvement of cranial nerve function. Technical note. J Neurosurg 2006;105(1):148–52.

12. Akutsu H, Kreutzer J, Fahlbusch R, et al. Transsphenoidal decompression of the sellar floor for cavernous sinus meningiomas: experience with 21 patients. Neurosurgery 2009;65(1):54–62 [discussion: 62].

13. Kano H, Park KJ, Kondziolka D, et al. Does prior microsurgery improve or worsen the outcomes of stereotactic radiosurgery for cavernous sinus meningiomas? Neurosurgery 2013;73(3):401–10.

14. Conti M, Prevedello DM, Madhok R, et al. The antero-medial triangle: the risk for cranial nerves ischemia at the cavernous sinus lateral wall. Anatomic cadaveric study. Clin Neurol Neurosurg 2008;110(7):682–6.

15. Clark VE, Serin A, Yin J, et al. Genomic analysis of non-NF2 meningiomas reveals mutations in TRAF7, KLF4, AKT1, and SMO. Science 2013;339(6123): 1077–80.

16. Brastianos PK, Horowitz PM, Santagata S, et al. Genomic sequencing of meningiomas identifies oncogenic SMO and AKT1 mutations. Nat Genet 2013;45(3):285–9.

17. Holland H, Mocker K, Ahnert P, et al. High resolution genomic profiling and classical cytogenetics in a group of benign and atypical meningiomas. Cancer Genet 2011;204(10):541–9.

18. Okamoto H, Li J, Vortmeyer AO, et al. Comparative proteomic profiles of meningioma subtypes. Cancer Res 2006;66(20):10199–204.

19. Griffiths CF, Cutler AR, Duong HT, et al. Avoidance of postoperative epistaxis and anosmia in endonasal endoscopic skull base surgery: a technical note. Acta Neurochir 2014;156(7):1393–401.

20. Dusick JR, Esposito F, Malkasian D, et al. Avoidance of carotid artery injuries in transsphenoidal surgery with the Doppler probe and micro-hook blades. Neurosurgery 2007;60(4 Suppl 2):322–8 [discussion: 328–9].

21. Labib MA, Prevedello DM, Fernandez-Miranda JC, et al. The medial opticocarotid recess: an anatomic study of an endoscopic "key landmark" for the ventral cranial base. Neurosurgery 2013;72(1 Suppl Operative):66–76 [discussion: 76].

22. Kassam AB, Prevedello DM, Carrau RL, et al. The front door to meckel's cave: an anteromedial corridor via expanded endoscopic endonasal approach- technical considerations and clinical series. Neurosurgery 2009;64(3 Suppl):71–83.

23. Esposito F, Dusick JR, Fatemi N, et al. Graded repair of cranial base defects and cerebrospinal fluid leaks in transsphenoidal surgery. Neurosurgery 2007;60(4 Suppl 2):295–303 [discussion: 303–4].

Surgical Techniques for Sinonasal Malignancies

Alexander Farag, MD[a], Marc Rosen, MD[a,b], James Evans, MD[a,b],*

KEYWORDS

- Sinonasal malignancies • Endoscopic resection • Minimally invasive • Craniofacial resection
- Endoscopic techniques

KEY POINTS

- The first chance is the best chance at an oncological cure.
- Partial resection or debulking has decreased patient overall survival.
- Piecemeal resection by tumor disassembly seems to have the same 5-year overall survival as traditional open approaches, with a marked reduction in morbidity and mortality.
- If negative margins cannot be obtained via an endoscopic approach, the surgeon must be prepared to switch to the appropriate procedures.

Sinonasal malignancies often present late because initial symptoms mimic benign disease. As a result, surgical resection can be extensive and carry a high risk due to the involvement of critical anterior cranial base structures. Traditionally, these advanced tumors were resected via potentially disfiguring open procedures with high morbidity (25%–35%) and mortality.[1] The hallmark treatment is an open craniofacial resection (oCFR), first introduced by Ketcham in 1963.[2] With the implementation of better imaging and technology, skull base surgery, is shifting toward less invasive approaches. Endoscopic resections are gaining traction, with early evidence showing equal outcomes and marked reduction in morbidity. A paradigm shift away from en bloc resection to piecemeal resection, or tumor disassembly, was seen by some as a large obstacle in this transition from open to endoscopic surgery. Opponents speculate that oncological integrity would be compromised by piecemeal resections. McCutcheon and colleagues[3] demonstrated that patients who underwent a piecemeal oCFR were equivalent to patients who were treated with an en bloc oCFR. Proponents argue that resection of

tumors involving the anterior skull base performed via an oCFR are rarely true en bloc resections.[4] Other examples of effective piecemeal resection are transoral laser surgery and Mohs micrographic surgery, which yield acceptable results.[5,6] Similarly, use of the endoscopic endonasal tumor disassembly can provide the same measure of oncological treatment as en bloc resection, if negative margins are achieved.[7]

The endoscope is a tool that has eliminated line-of-sight issues previously encountered with open techniques while providing superior definition and contrast. The implementation of angled scopes has also allowed surgeons to minimize damage or removal of uninvolved structures, greatly decreasing the morbidity and complications of these techniques in select cases.[8] Minimally invasive endoscopic resections (MIERs) have also been noted to have shorter operative time and decreased hospital stays as compared with their open counterparts.[9] However, the team must have the expertise to convert to the appropriate open approach if the tumor cannot be resected endoscopically.

[a] Department of Otolaryngology – Head and Neck Surgery, Thomas Jefferson University, 925 Chestnut Street, 6th Floor, Philadelphia, PA 19107, USA; [b] Department of Neurosurgery, Thomas Jefferson University, 909 Walnut Street, 2nd Floor, Philadelphia, PA 19107, USA
* Corresponding author.
E-mail address: James.evans@jefferson.edu

Neurosurg Clin N Am 26 (2015) 403–412
http://dx.doi.org/10.1016/j.nec.2015.03.011
1042-3680/15/$ – see front matter © 2015 Elsevier Inc. All rights reserved.

PRESENTATION

Presenting symptoms are most commonly unilateral nasal obstruction, epistaxis, or nasal mass. Patients also present with symptoms of headache, epiphora, visual disturbance, anosmia, and nasal discharge.[10–12] Unilateral symptoms are more common than bilateral symptoms.[13] Patients with advanced disease also present with paresthesias or other cranial neuropathies. These nonspecific symptoms make early diagnosis challenging as they can be attributed to other common diseases such as chronic rhinosinusitis or atypical headaches. Further complicating diagnosis, nasal endoscopy can reveal a range of findings from smooth pedunculated lesions to friable masses.

WORKUP

When a suspicious lesion is seen on endoscopy, the primary goal should be to distinguish a benign from malignant process. In most instances, an office biopsy is performed. The lesion is injected with Lidocaine hydrochloride 1 % and Epinephrine 1:100,000. If little bleeding occurs with this, a biopsy is taken. If a highly vascular lesion is suspected on endoscopy, or inadequate tissue is obtained, a biopsy is performed in the operating room after imaging is obtained with computed tomography (CT) and magnetic resonance imaging (MRI).

Debulking is avoided. Partial resections before planned oncological resections have been shown to produce poorer overall patient survival.[14] Postoperative changes from partial resection result in fibrosis and edema, which makes delineation of gross tumor boundaries and attachment sites more difficult.

Radiologic assessment of the tumor is also important for staging; it helps to characterize if the lesion is resectable. A variety of imaging modalities can help to distinguish different aspects of the tumor (**Table 1**). CT best identifies bony anatomy and bony erosion. MRI is an excellent modality to distinguish between soft tissue and inspissated secretions on T2-weighted images. Fluid-attenuated inversion recovery sequence is useful to differentiate cerebrospinal fluid from mucoceles and cystic or fluid contents. Periorbital invasion is best assessed on fat-suppressed images. Dura is best seen on T2-weighted images and postcontrast T1-weighted images. Nerve enhancement on T1-weighted images is helpful for perineural invasion.[4]

The use of fluorodeoxyglucose PET has been limited in sinonasal malignant workups, as preliminary small population studies failed to demonstrate an advantage over combined CT and MRI modalities.[15,16] In the posttreatment setting, it has been found to aid in early detection of locoregional recurrences and distant metastasis, complementary to MRI and CT.[16,17]

Table 1
Tumor features that are best assessed via their respective imaging sequence

	Imaging for Sinonasal Masses	
Tumor Features	**CT**	**MRI**
Periorbital invasion & orbital fat	Bone erosion precisely shown by CT. The perorbia is not usually distinguished from tumor signal	T1-weighted and T2-weighted sequences
Dural invasion	Contrast is useful for large areas of dural invasion. Indirect signs (skull base erosion) can correlate with small areas of dural invasion	T2-weighted and postcontrast T1-weighted sequences
Perineural invasion	Limited to indirect signs (fat effacement or enlarged foramina)	Fat-saturated T1-weighted sequences with abnormal nerve enhancement
Distinguish retained mucous secretions	Cannot be assessed with this modality	T2-weighted sequences
Communication with cisterns	—	T2-weighted sequences
Assess course of internal carotid	CT angiography with Maximum Intensity Projections (MIP) reconstructions	—
Assess neck nodal disease	CT with contrast.	—

Adapted from Harvey RJ, Winder M, Parmar P, et al. Endoscopic skull base surgery for sinonasal malignancy. Otolaryngol Clin North Am 2011;44:1080–140.

Once a malignant lesion is confirmed, a metastatic workup is performed and a definitive treatment plan is formulated. These treatment decisions occur in conjunction with an interdisciplinary tumor board, weighing tumor histology, stage, surgical resection, and adjuvant and neoadjuvant treatment.

SINONASAL MALIGNANCIES

Sinonasal malignancies account for approximately 3% of upper aerodigestive malignancies.[18,19] Squamous cell carcinoma (SCC) is the most common sinonasal malignancy, accounting for 55% to 70% (**Fig. 1**). Its most common location is the maxillary sinus (60%–70%), followed by the nasal cavity (20%–30%), ethmoid (10%–15%), and frontal and sphenoid sinus (1%). It has been associated with exposure to textile dust as well as smoking.[20,21] SCC may have an ulceration-like appearance, and nonneoplastic processes such as infections and granulomatous diseases must be excluded.

Adenoid cystic carcinoma (ACC) is the second most common sinonasal malignancy and accounts for 10% to 15% of all head and neck cancers (See **Fig. 1**).[19] This condition is most common in the maxillary sinus, followed by the nasal cavity. There are 3 histologic subtypes in which the solid pattern has a much poorer prognosis than the cribriform or tubular pattern.[22] ACC has a propensity for perineural invasion, producing significant skull base and intradural extension in late stages. Initially, these patients have a high 5-year survival but poor 10- to 15-year survivals, with locoregional recurrence reported as high as 65%.[23] Advanced disease is treated with surgery with adjuvant radiation.[23]

Adenocarcinoma is the third most common sinonasal malignancy. It comprises about 8% to 15% of sinonasal malignancies (See **Fig. 1**).[23,24] Its most common location is the ethmoid sinus (85%), and it is noted to have both a low- and high-grade subtype. It has been linked to woodworking as well as textile dust and is noted to be more common in men. It is often noted to involve the olfactory cleft, appearing as a polypoid neoplasm with well-defined boundaries. Treatment is surgical excision with adjuvant radiotherapy for advanced disease.[25]

Malignant melanoma of the sinonasal cavity comprises less than 2% of all malignant melanoma.[26] It has an extremely poor prognosis with a third of patients presenting with neck metastasis.[27] The most common location is in the nasal cavity. It can appear grayish-blue-to-white or pink-to-black.[28]

Comprising about 2% of sinonasal malignancies are esthesioneuroblastomas (ENBs), initially described by Berger and Luc in 1924 (See **Fig. 1**).[29,30] This tumor is also known as olfactory neuroblastoma, phenotypically displaying a mix of a pure neural neoplasm and a neuroendocrine epithelial tumor.[31] This rare neoplasm is estimated to have a prevalence of 0.4 cases per million individuals per year.[32]

ENBs generally originate from the olfactory neuroepithelium, which is situated mainly on the cribriform plate, superior septum, and turbinate.[33] Olfactory neuroepithelium can extend down onto the middle turbinate, with rare ectopic locations involving the inferior turbinate or maxillary sinus.[34,35] ENBs are thought to originate from the basal progenitor cells of the olfactory neuroepithelium.[34]

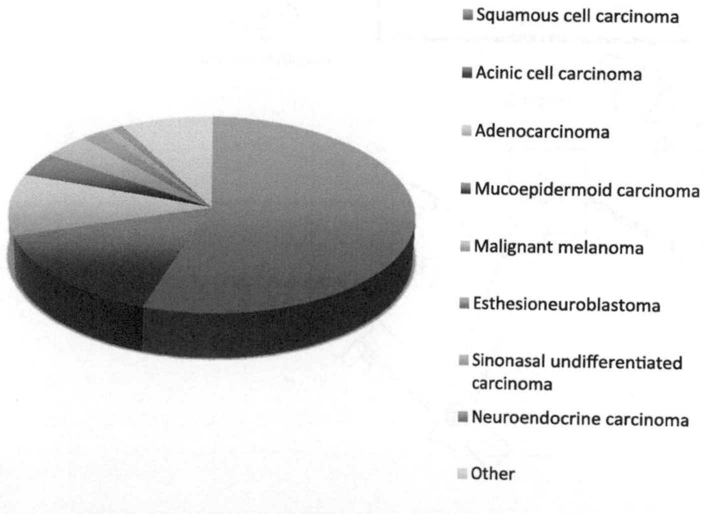

- Squamous cell carcinoma
- Acinic cell carcinoma
- Adenocarcinoma
- Mucoepidermoid carcinoma
- Malignant melanoma
- Esthesioneuroblastoma
- Sinonasal undifferentiated carcinoma
- Neuroendocrine carcinoma
- Other

Fig. 1. Proportional distribution of sinonasal malignancies.

Sinonasal undifferentiated carcinoma (SNUC) is a rare, high-grade and locally aggressive malignancy of the sinonasal tract. It was first described in 1986 by Frierson and colleagues[36] and is an aggressive ectodermally derived neoplasm originating from schneiderian epithelium in the nasal cavity and paranasal sinuses.

The cause of SNUC is unclear, and unlike undifferentiated nasopharyngeal carcinoma, recent literature does not support a definite association between SNUC and Epstein–Barr virus. There might be some correlation between smoking and SNUC, but no environmental or occupational carcinogen has been demonstrated to have strong correlation with SNUC.[36,37]

The disease is more common in men, with a male/female ratio reported to be 2:1. SNUC affects patients with an extensive age range, third to ninth decade, but it is more common in the fifth and sixth decades of life.[37]

TREATMENT

With small tumors, the goal should be identifying the attachment site and obtaining negative margins around this area. Larger tumors tend to have an element of expansive remodeling rather than frank erosion. During an oncological resection, the authors systematically disassemble the tumor as the attachment site is identified.

See **Fig. 2** for operating room topography.

PREPARING THE NOSE

- Place pledgets bilaterally in the nasal cavity soaked in Cocaine hydrochloride 4% topical solution.
- Rotate the bed 180° away from the anesthesia cart, elevating the head of the bed to 30°.
- Place the head on a donut to prevent rotation of the head.
- Calibrate the image guidance system and ensure accuracy.
- Introduce a 0° endoscope, and inject lidocaine hydrochloride 1% with epinephrine 1:100,000 into the septum, inferior and middle turbinates, and ascending process of the maxilla.
- This injection decreases bleeding, and the septal injection assists in raising a nasoseptal flap later in the procedure if needed.
- Injection of the lateral walls anterior to the uncinate aids in decreased bleeding when

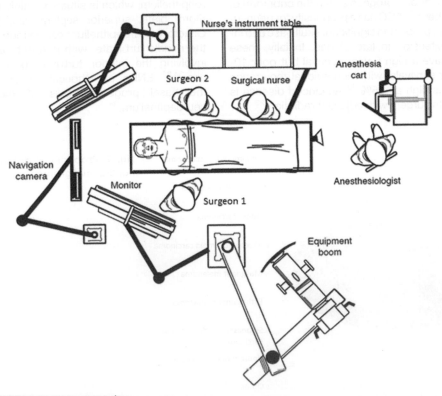

Fig. 2. Operating room topography.

instruments are repeatedly removed and inserted into the nasal cavity.

- If a nasoseptal flap is anticipated, it is often harvested at this point in time if uninvolved with tumor and stored in the nasopharynx.

MEDIAL MAXILLECTOMY

If a small tumor can be removed en bloc, this is preferred. For a larger tumor, a medial maxillectomy is performed as follows (**Fig. 3**):

- Drill along the nasal floor with a 4-mm self-irrigating diamond drill.
- Thus, the maxillary sinus should be connected via the inferior meatus to the nasal cavity.
- Extend this posteriorly to the posterior wall of the maxillary sinus and anteriorly to the nasolacrimal duct (the nasolacrimal duct is housed in the dense bone known as the ascending process of the maxilla).
- If pathology dictates, the authors resect the nasolacrimal duct anteriorly until the pyriform aperture with the 4-mm self-irrigating diamond drill.
- Endoscopically, the head of the inferior turbinate attachment marks the location of the pyriform aperture.

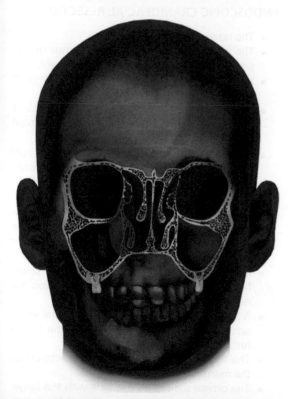

Fig. 3. Area that is commonly resected during an endoscopic medial maxillectomy.

EXTENDED ETHMOIDAL DISSECTION

- Next, an incision is made just anterior to the ascending process of the maxilla, and dissection proceeds in a subperiosteal plane along the nasal wall with the use of a freer elevator.
- Dissection is continued superiorly and laterally along the lamina papyracea to the face of the sphenoid.
- Lamina papyracea is then resected if dictated by tumor extent.
  - The blunt end of the cottle elevator is used to reflect off the thin bone. This dissection continues posteriorly until the orbital process of the palatine bone is encountered posteriorly.
- If the orbital process of the palatine bone must be cleared, then a 4-mm diamond drill is used.
- Periorbital involvement is assessed; if needed, it can be resected.
  - If an extensive dissection is required, assistance of an ophthalmologist via an orbitotomy can be extremely helpful, as the medial rectus and orbital fat can be retracted, easing the dissection and decreasing the morbidity of the procedure.
- If the tumor extends through the posterior wall of the maxillary sinus, the pterygopalatine fossa is entered.
- First, a sphenoidotomy is performed, with identification of the vidian nerve if this has not already been performed.
- In tumors in which perineural invasion is a concern, the vidian nerve may need to be extensively dissected and resected.
- Next, the mucosa of the posterior wall of the maxillary sinus is removed.
- If lateral access is required, this can be accomplished via a Caldwell-Luc incision or with removal of the nasolacrimal duct.
- A 4-mm diamond burr is then used to thin the bone of the posterior maxillary wall.
- The thin bone is removed with a 2-mm Kerrison rongeurs.
- Blunt dissection with a caudal is performed until the second and third segments of the internal maxillary artery are identified and controlled with a combination of clips and cautery.
- Control of the greater palatine artery is ensured.
- As the fat is dissected, the pterygoid muscles and venous plexus are encountered, which can be controlled with Floseal (Baxter, Deerfield, IL, USA), followed by thrombin-soaked 1 × 1 cm pledgets in addition to bipolar cautery.

- The vidian nerve is identified and dissected along the inferior portion in a 9-o'clock to 3-o'clock portion for a left-sided resection. This dissection may also be done in an anterior to posterior manner. This method prevents injury to the internal carotid artery which is located superiorly and laterally to the vidian nerve.
- Next, the pterygoid plates are drilled from the skull base attachment and removed en bloc.

If required, a medial maxillectomy can be combined with a unilateral craniofacial resection (CFR).

CRANIOFACIAL RESECTION: UNILATERAL/BILATERAL

This procedure is most commonly done for ethmoidal tumors with involvement of the skull base or masses medial to the middle turbinate. Traditionally, a unilateral CFR is described as clearing orbit to septum or orbit to orbit for a bilateral CFR (**Figs. 4** and **5**). It is classically described as extending from the frontal sinus to the planium, with resection of dura and parenchyma as needed. However, the disease always dictates the extent of resection.

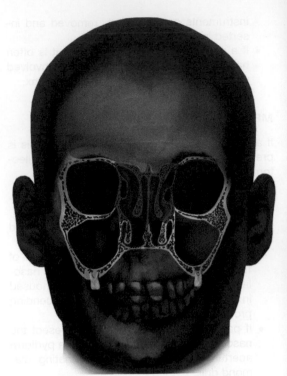

Fig. 5. Region that is typically resected via a bilateral craniofacial resection.

ENDOSCOPIC CRANIOFACIAL RESECTION

- The nose is prepared.
- The procedure is begun with a tumor disassembly to identify the site of attachment.
- Uninvolved sinuses are surgically addressed so that the margins are clearly identified.
- Common margins include the posterior wall of the frontal sinus, roof of the sphenoid, orbital lamina, and superior septum.
- Once the extent of involvement of the nasal septum has been delineated and cleared, the nasoseptal flap can be harvested from the uninvolved septum.
- If there is extensive septal involvement, the flap can be extended along the floor of the nose and laterally to under the inferior turbinate.
- In some cases, the flap will need to be sacrificed, and another type of reconstruction will need to be performed.
- A Draf III is used to address the frontal sinus and define the anterior extent of the tumor resection.
- The lateral extent of dissection is dictated by the margins.
- The orbital lamina on the side with the larger tumor burden is resected and sent for pathologic analysis.

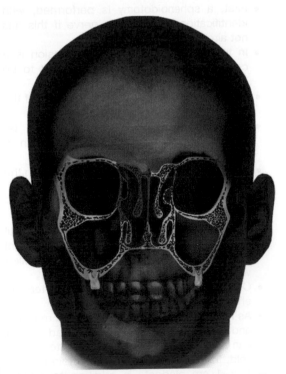

Fig. 4. Area that is typically resected during a unilateral craniofacial resection.

- The anterior and posterior septal arteries are cauterized with bipolar cautery, decreasing the vascular supply to the tumor.
- A 4-mm self-irrigating diamond bur is then used to remove the bone of the anterior cranial base, allowing for identification of dural involvement.
- Dura is then cauterized and incised lateral to the tumor.
- The falx is then dissected using blunt dissection and incised anteriorly, mobilizing the structure.
- This dissection allows access to the olfactory bulbs, which are also dissected.
- The extent of intraparenchymal disease is assessed and resected.
- Dissection continues posteriorly toward the planum. The olfactory nerves are transected

with the final posterior dural incision to remove the specimen.
- Additional dural and olfactory nerve margins are also sent for analysis at this time.

ENDOSCOPIC-ASSISTED CRANIOFACIAL RESECTION

The nasal portion is resected endoscopically, as opposed to a transfacial or midface degloving approach. A bifrontal craniotomy is performed at the same time, allowing a team to work simultaneously from above and below. The combined approach is selected when an MIER is contraindicated as described in **Table 2**.

The endoscope has revolutionized oncological techniques. Early outcomes point to overall patient survival equivalent to oCFR, with

Table 2
Indications and contraindications for common surgical procedures used to treat sinonasal malignancies

Surgical Procedure	Indications	Contraindications
Endoscopic medial maxillectomy	Sinonasal malignancy involvement of the inferior turbinate, medial maxillary wall, pterygopalatine fossa	Orbital disease Skin or palate involvement
Open total maxillectomy	Orbital fat or muscle involvement Skin or palate/teeth involvement	—
Endoscopic craniofacial resection (ECFR)	Sinonasal maligancy involving the anterior cranial base Disease limited to periosteum of lamina papyracea Disease medial or inferior to carotid and optic nerves	Skin or palatal involvement Involvement of anterior wall of frontal sinus Disease extending laterally >50% over orbital roof Disease lateral or superior to carotid or optic nerve
Endoscopic-assisted craniofacial resection	Disease extending lateral >50% over orbital roof Involvement of anterior wall of frontal sinus Disease lateral or superior to carotid or optic nerve Clear margins not able to be obtained by ECFR Skin involvement	Palatal involvement Extensive skin involvement
Open craniofacial resection (oCFR)	Disease extending lateral >50% over orbital roof Involvement of anterior wall of frontal sinus Disease lateral or superior to carotid or optic nerve Clear margins not able to be obtained by ECFR Skin involvement	—
Orbital exenteration	Traditionally combined with open maxillectomy or oCFR Extensive involvement of orbital fat Involvement of skin, nasolacrimal duct, medial rectus, optic nerve, ocular bulb	—

significantly lower morbidity.[9,38] In particular, the oCFR has limitations of visualization of the sphenoid and posterior ethmoid. It is the opinion of the authors that, given the superior definition and access attained with endoscopic techniques, open transfacial approaches are rarely needed.

POSTOPERATIVE DRESSING

For reconstruction, a fascia lata button is fashioned and placed in the typical overlay/underlay configuration (**Fig. 6**).[39]

If a flap is required, it is covered in DuraSeal (Covidien, Dublin, Ireland) and then reinforced by Nasopore (Polyganics, Groningen, Netherlands), bolstering the flap into position.

POSTOPERATIVE CARE

Postoperatively, patients are counseled to avoid Valsalva maneuvers and nose blowing practices, particularly for the first week. Patients are asked to use nasal saline spray. They use 2 sprays per

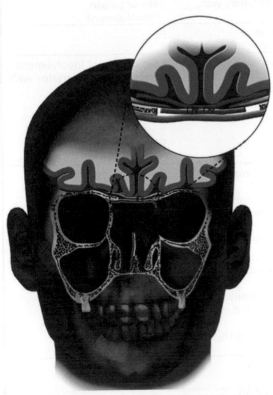

Fig. 6. Reconstruction of a bilateral craniofacial resection with a fascia lata button (*gray*) and pedicled vascularized nasoseptal flap (*pink*).

nare thrice a day. Patients are seen back on postoperative weeks 1, 3, and 8 to ensure that the wound continues to heal correctly and undergo debridement. Postoperative MRI is obtained before their first clinical visit serving as a baseline. After the first debridement, patients being irrigating the wound with normal saline thrice a day.

LIMITATIONS

Contraindications to the procedures are detailed in **Table 2**. The involvement of skin, palate, and anterior wall of the frontal sinus would preclude an MIER. Cases that also require orbital exenteration are best performed by an endoscopic assist procedure.

COMPLICATIONS AND MANAGEMENT
Cerebrospinal Fluid Leak

Cerebrospinal fluid leak is a rare occurrence in the early postoperative period. Depending on the index of suspicion, a noncontrast head CT image is obtained to assess for pneumocephalus. The threshold for surgical exploration is low.

Lumbar drains are not routinely placed. However, at the time of reexploration, a lumbar drain may be placed at the beginning of surgery. Predicated on the operative findings, it may be removed immediately after surgery or the wound drained at 5 to 10 mL/h for 2 to 3 days.

Meningitis

Meningitis is an exceedingly rare situation. Postoperatively, patients are administered antibiotics only for 24 hours. If patients have absorbable packing in place, they are administered oral antibiotics with coverage for gram-positive bacteria for 7 days. This medication provides prophylaxis against toxic shock until the absorbable packing dissolves.

Outcomes

Accurate outcomes data for sinonasal malignancies are difficult to obtain. Comparisons between studies are confounded by heterogeneous patient cohorts and treatment modality, with long-term outcomes for endoscopic approaches still under investigation. These new surgical techniques seem to have much promise in improving patient care and evolving our field (**Table 3**).

Table 3
Advantages and disadvantages for common surgical procedures commonly used to treat sinonasal malignancies

Surgical Procedure	Advantages	Disadvantages
Endoscopic medial maxillectomy	No impact on speech and swallowing	Limited access below the level of the hard palate
Open medial maxillectomy	None compared with endoscopic Not indicated in this era	Poor cosmesis
Open total maxillectomy	Wide exposure	Impact on speech and swallowing Need for free flap or obturator
Endoscopic craniofacial resection	Excellent illumination and visualization of sphenoid and frontal outflow tract Lower morbidity compared with oCFR Shorter hospitalization Equivalent short-term outcomes as oCFR in select cases	Long-term outcomes are still being investigated
Endoscopic-assisted craniofacial resection (EA-CFR)	Same as oCFR without transfacial incisions	Long-term outcomes are still being investigated
Open craniofacial resection (oCFR)	None over EA-CFR Traditional approach and current gold standard	Marked morbidity including postoperative scaring Limited visualization of sphenoid and frontal sinus outflow tract Poor cosmesis Longer hospitalization
Orbital exenteration	Improved survival in select cases	Significant psychosocial impact Poor cosmesis

SUMMARY

Given the endoscopic ability to precisely delineate tumor margins, procedures can be tailored on a case-by-case basis and are not relegated to standard ridged resections.

REFERENCES

1. Zafereo ME, Fakhri S, Prayson R, et al. Esthesioneuroblastoma: 25-year experience at a single institution. Otolaryngol Head Neck Surg 1997;123:1312–7.
2. Van Buren JM, Ommaya AK, Ketcham AS. Ten years' experience with radical combined craniofacial resection of malignant tumors of the paranasal sinuses. J Neurosurg 1986;28(4):341–50.
3. McCutcheon IE, Blacklock JB, Weber RS, et al. Anterior transcranial (craniofacial) resection of tumors of the paranasal sinuses: surgical technique and results. Neurosurgery 1996;38:471–80.
4. Harvey RJ, Winder M, Parmar P, et al. Endoscopic skull base surgery for sinonasal malignancy. Otolaryngol Clin North Am 2011;44:1080–140.
5. Jackel MC, Martin A, Steiner W. Twenty-five years experience with laser surgery for head and neck tumors: report of an International Symposium, Gottingen, Germany, 2005. Eur Arch Otorhinolaryngol 2007;264:577–85.
6. Vuyk HD, Lohuis PJ. Mohs micrographic surgery for facial skin cancer. Clin Otolaryngol Allied Sci 2001; 26:265–73.
7. Snyderman CH, Carrau RL, Kassam AB, et al. Endoscopic skull base surgery: principles of endonasal oncological surgery. J Surg Oncol 2008;97(8):658–64.
8. Devaiah AK, Andreoli MT. Treatment of esthesioneuroblastoma: a 16 year meta-analysis of 361 patients. Laryngoscope 2009;119(7):1412–6.
9. Eloy JA, Vivero RJ, Hoang K, et al. Comparison of transnasal endoscopic and open craniofacial resection for malignant tumors of the anterior skull base. Laryngoscope 2009;119:834–40.
10. Loy AH, Reibel JF, Read PW, et al. Esthesioneuroblastoma: continued follow-up of a single institution's experience. Arch Otolaryngol Head Neck Surg 2006;132:134–8.
11. Resto VA, Eisele DW, Forastiere A, et al. Esthesioneuroblastoma: the impact of treatment modality. Head Neck 2001;23:749–57.
12. Diaz EM Jr, Johnigan RH III, Pero C, et al. Olfactory neuroblastoma: the 22-year experience at one comprehensive cancer center. Head Neck 2005; 27:138–49.

13. Bachar G, Goldstein DP, Shah M, et al. Esthesio-neuroblastoma: The Princess Margaret Hospital experience. Head Neck 2008;30(12):1607–14.

14. Hanna E, Demonte F, Ibrahim S, et al. Endoscopic resection of sinonasal cancers with and without craniotomy: oncology results. Arch Otolaryngol Head Neck Surg 2009;135:1219–24.

15. Gil Z, Even-Sapir E, Margalit N, et al. Integrated PET/CT system for staging and surveillance of skull base tumors. Head Neck 2007;29:537–45.

16. Wild D, Eyrich GK, Ciernick IF, et al. In-line 18FDG-PET/CT in patients with carcinoma of the sinus/nasal area and orbit. J Craniomaxillofac Surg 2006;34:9–16.

17. Harvey RJ, Pitzer G, Nissman DB, et al. PET-CT in the assessment on previously treated skull base malignancies. Head Neck 2010;32:76–84.

18. Le QT, Fu KK, Kaplan M, et al. Treatment of maxillary sinus carcinoma: a comparison of the 1977 and 1977 American Joint Committee on cancer staging systems. Cancer 1999;86:1700–11.

19. Tiwari R, Hardillo JA, Mehta D, et al. Squamous cell carcinoma of maxillary sinus. Head Neck 2000;22:164–9.

20. Zhu K, Levine RS, Brann EA, et al. Case-control study evaluating the homogeneity and heterogeneity of risk factors between sinonasal and nasopharyngeal cancers. Int J Cancer 2002;99(1):119–23.

21. Luce D, Leclerc A, Morcet JF, et al. Occupational risk factors for sinonasal cancer: a case-control study in France. Am J Ind Med 1992;21(1):32–41.

22. Seong SY, Hyun DW, Kim YS, et al. Treatment outcomes of sinonasal adenoid cystic carcinoma: 30 cases from a single institution. J Craniomaxillofac Surg 2014;42:e171–5.

23. Lupinetti AD, Roberts DB, Williams MD, et al. Sinonasal adenoid cystic carcinoma: the M.D. Anderson Cancer Center experience. Cancer 2007;110(12):2726–31.

24. Orvidas LJ, Lewis JE, Weaver AL, et al. Adenocarcinoma of the nose and paranasal sinuses: a retrospective study of diagnosis, histological characteristics, and outcomes in 24 patients. Head Neck 2005;27(5):370–5.

25. Roush GC. Epidemiology of cancer of the nose and paranasal sinuses: current concepts. Head Neck Surg 1979;2(1):3–11.

26. Van Gerven L, Jorissen M, Nuyts S, et al. Long-term follow-up of 44 patients with adenocarcinoma of the nasal cavity and sinuses primarily treated with endoscopic resection followed by radiotherapy. Head Neck 2011;33(6):898–904.

27. Freedman HM, DeSanto LW, Devine KD, et al. Malignant melanoma of the nasal cavity and paranasal sinuses. Arch Otolaryngol 1973;97(4):322–5.

28. Lund VJ. Malignant melanoma of the nasal cavity and paranasal sinuses. Ear Nose Throat J 1980;72(4):285–90.

29. Bell D, Saade R, Roberts D, et al. Prognostic utility of Hyams histological grading and Kadish-Morita staging systems for esthesioneuroblastoma outcomes. Head Neck Pathol 2015;9:51–9.

30. Platek ME, Merzianu M, Mashtare TL, et al. Improved survival following surgery and radiation therapy for olfactory neuroblastoma: analysis of the SEER database. Radiat Oncol 2011;6:41.

31. Theilgaard SA, Buchwald C, Ingeholm P, et al. Esthesioneuroblastoma: a Danish demographic study of 40 patients registered between 1978 and 2000. Acta Otolaryngol 2003;123:433–9.

32. Moran DT, Rowley J, Jafek BW. Electron microscopy of human olfactory epithelium reveals a new cell type: the microvillar cell. Brain Res 1982;253:39–46.

33. Faragalla H, Weinreb I. Olfactory neuroblastoma: a review and update. Adv Anat Pathol 2009;16(5):322–31.

34. Ow TJ, Bell D, Kupferman ME, et al. Esthesioneuroblastoma. Neurosurg Clin N Am 2013;24(1):51–65.

35. Carney ME, O'Rilly RC, Cholevar B, et al. Expression of the human Achaete-scute 1 gene in olfactory neuroblastoma (esthesioneurblastoma). J Neurooncol 1995;26:35–43.

36. Frierson H Jr, Mills S, Fechner R, et al. Sinonasal undifferentiated carcinoma. An aggressive neoplasm derived from Schneiderian epithelium and distinct from olfactory neuroblastoma. Am J Surg Pathol 1986;10:771–9.

37. Jeng YM, Sung MT, Fang CL, et al. Sinonasal undifferentiated carcinoma and nasopharyngeal-type undifferentiated carcinoma: two clinically, biologically, and histopathologically distinct entities. Am J Surg Pathol 2002;26(3):371–6.

38. Higgins TS, Thorp B, Rawlings BA, et al. Outcome results of endoscopic vs craniofacial resection of sinonasal malignancies: a systemic review and pooled-data analysis. Int Forum Allergy Rhinol 2011;1(4):255–61.

39. Luginbuhl AJ, Campbell PG, Evans J, et al. Endoscopic repair of high-flow cranial base defects using a bilayer button. Laryngoscope 2010;120(5):876–80.

Endoscopic Endonasal Approach to Ventral Posterior Fossa Meningiomas
From Case Selection to Surgical Management

André Beer-Furlan, MD[a,b],
Eduardo A.S. Vellutini, MD, PhD[a,b],*,
Leonardo Balsalobre, MD[a,c], Aldo C. Stamm, MD, PhD[a,c]

KEYWORDS

- Endoscopic endonasal approach • Endoscopy • Meningioma • Posterior fossa meningioma
- Clival meningioma • Petroclival meningioma • Foramen magnum meningioma

KEY POINTS

- Clival, petroclival, and foramen magnum meningiomas are challenging lesions to manage independently of the selected surgical approach.
- Current literature involving the endoscopic management of ventral posterior fossa meningioma is scant mainly because of rarity of the pathologic condition, limited indications, and technical difficulties in tumor resection and skull base reconstruction.
- The main challenge in the management of ventral posterior fossa meningioma is the surgical approach selection.
- Careful anatomoradiologic evaluation, patient's clinical condition, and surgical team's expertise must guide the surgical route selection.
- Nuances of the endoscopic transclival approach and skull base reconstruction are highlighted.

INTRODUCTION

Clival, petroclival, and foramen magnum meningiomas are challenging lesions to manage independently of the selected surgical approach and represent approximately 5%[1,2] of all intracranial meningiomas. Despite reports of radiation therapy in its management, surgical resection continues to be the first and best treatment method aiming permanent tumor eradication.[3,4]

The advances in the microsurgical technique, intraoperative monitoring, and radiologic imaging drastically improved surgical outcomes of meningiomas treated through posterior skull base approaches; however, the morbidity associated with the surgical resection of these tumors is still significant. New cranial nerve (CN) palsies or persisting/worsening of preexisting palsies is the most common morbidity, and it has been reported to range from 39% to 76% of the patients.[5–8]

Disclosure of Funding: None.
Financial Support, Industry Affiliations, Grants, and/or Financial Disclosures: None. No financial disclosures for any author.
[a] Neurosurgical Department, São Paulo Skull Base Center, Rua Adma Jafet, 74 - cj. 121, São Paulo 01308, Brazil;
[b] DFV Neuro Neurosurgical Group, Rua Adma Jafet, 74 – cj.121, São Paulo 01308, Brazil; [c] ENT Department, São Paulo ENT Center, Professor Edmundo Vasconcelos Hospital, Rua Afonso Brás, 525 - cj. 13, São Paulo 04511, Brazil
* Corresponding author. Rua Dona Adma Jafet, 74 – cj.121, São Paulo 05018-000, Brazil.
E-mail address: evellu@terra.com.br

Neurosurg Clin N Am 26 (2015) 413–426
http://dx.doi.org/10.1016/j.nec.2015.03.006
1042-3680/15/$ – see front matter © 2015 Elsevier Inc. All rights reserved.

Driven by the revolution of endoscopic pituitary surgery, the development of the expanded endoscopic endonasal approach (EEA) and the associated surgical tools have pushed the limits of transnasal access to the ventral skull base. The EEA rapidly became a safe alternative on the armamentarium of skull base approaches and has been increasingly used in the management of ventral intradural posterior fossa tumors. It provides the advantage of direct access to pathologies with near-field magnification while minimizing manipulation of neurovascular structures and avoiding brain retraction, ultimately decreasing morbidity.[9–13]

Nevertheless, unlike the EEA to sellar pathology, there is a relative paucity of literature regarding endoscopic management of meningiomas, more specifically, the ventral posterior cranial fossa meningiomas. The probable reason is the combination of limiting factors, including rarity of the pathologic condition, limited indication of approaching it through an EEA, technical challenges in tumor resection and skull base reconstruction, expertise of the surgical team, and available resources.

The current literature involving the endoscopic management of these meningiomas consists in the collective experience of an approach rather than experience with the particular type of tumor.[14–21] Based on clinical experience and literature review, the authors highlight important aspects in choosing a surgical approach and managing ventral posterior fossa meningiomas through the EEA.

INDICATIONS/CONTRAINDICATIONS

Independent of the surgical route, there are prerequisites that must be met before surgery. Patient, disease, and surgeon factors must be considered, as described in **Box 1**.

The difficulty in the management of ventral posterior fossa meningiomas is not deciding when to surgically treat it, but weighting the risks and benefits when selecting the surgical approach. Thus, appropriate case selection is vital to a successful outcome.

Indications

The indications for the surgical treatment of posterior fossa meningiomas are symptomatic lesions, asymptomatic lesion with a large volume, and tumor growth on radiologic follow-up. Among these cases, in ventral posterior fossa meningiomas, the main indication for an expanded EEA is the midline location of the dural base. The more medial the dural attachment, posterior the

---

Box 1
Prerequisites for surgery

Patient factors include

- A suitable candidate for prolonged general anesthesia
- A patient with no significant comorbidities (eg, coagulopathy)
- An informed patient who is accepting of potential complications and resulting morbidity
- A patient who is motivated and compliant

Disease factors include

- Ability to surgically resect or decompress the disease
- Favorable anatomy

Surgeon factors include

- Appropriate experience and expertise
- Availability of equipment
- Intensive care or high-dependency neurosurgical postoperative care

---

brainstem dislocation, and lateral the CN displacement, the better is the indication of approaching the tumor through an anterior route. In these cases, the transclival approach is the direct route to the tumor without the need of any brainstem retraction or crossing the plane of the CNs (**Fig. 1**).

Clival meningiomas

Clival meningiomas have their primary base at the midline. They tend to displace CN V laterally and superiorly; CN VI laterally and posteriorly; CNs VII, VIII, IX, X, and XI posteriorly; CN XII posteriorly and inferiorly; and the brainstem posteriorly. The primary base and pattern of displacement makes clival meningiomas ideal for the EEA.

Petroclival meningiomas

Petroclival meningiomas have their primary base at the petroclival fissure and have a particular displacement pattern of surrounding structures. They tend to dislocate the CNs V, VII, VIII, IX, X, XI posteriorly; the CN VI medially; and the brainstem medially and posteriorly. The main advantage of approaching these tumors through an anterior route is the posterior displacement of most of the CNs. However, the medial displacement of CN VI may pose a significant surgical difficulty, and its injury risk must be weighted in the case selection. The midline component of these tumors is prone for an EEA resection. Nevertheless, petroclival meningiomas are unlikely to be completely removed through an endoscopic

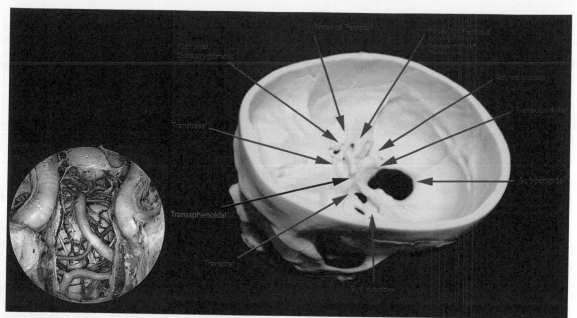

Fig. 1. Surgical approaches to the posterior cranial fossa. The transsphenoidal transclival surgical route provides significant anatomic advantage for approaching the ventral posterior fossa. (*Courtesy of* Luiz Felipe Ulrich de Alencastro, MD, Brazil.)

transclival approach because of their paramedian origin. It should be considered in combination with a posterior or lateral surgical route or when the surgical goal is brainstem decompression.

Foramen magnum meningiomas

Foramen magnum meningiomas may be cranial or spinocranial lesions. The spinocranial tumors have their origin below the foramen magnum and thereby displace the CNs and the vertebral arteries to the superior pole of the tumor. On the other hand, the cranial lesions may have its origin anywhere at the foramen magnum with different patterns of structures dislocation. The anterior cranial lesions originating at the anterior border of the foramen magnum are suited for the EEA. Their origin is medial to the hypoglossal and jugular foramen, so all the CNs are displaced posteriorly and laterally. However, the cervical extension of these tumors may pose a limitation for the EEA because of the craniocervical instability associated with the removal of the anterior arch of the C1, C2 odontoid process and its ligamentous complex. Therefore, a posterior approach is usually the choice for a single or first-stage surgery for ventral foramen magnum meningiomas that extend inferiorly to C1 and C2 levels.

Jugular tubercle meningiomas

The jugular tubercle meningiomas have their primary base at lateral location and tend to dislocate

the CNs of the jugular foramen posteriorly and CN VI superiorly. In rare cases, the medial extension to the clivus makes the endonasal resection a possibility.[18]

Contraindications

- Patient comorbidities precluding them from prolonged general anesthesia
- Lateral dural base of the meningioma
- Vascular encasement
- Unfavorable anatomy for transsphenoidal surgery
- No multidisciplinary service
- Lack of specialized equipment/instruments

SURGICAL TECHNIQUE/PROCEDURE
Preoperative Planning

Radiologic investigation

The evolution of imaging studies improved the preoperative information on the pathologic anatomy of the tumors, enabling surgeons to plan the intraoperative setting in greater detail. The radiologic preoperative investigation for a meningioma should always include computed tomography (CT) and MRI for bone and soft-tissue assessment, respectively.[22–25]

Primary base of the tumor

Identifying the primary base of the meningioma is essential to understand the growth pattern of the tumor and its relationship to surrounding neurovascular structures, which may help predict intraoperative difficulties due to pathologic anatomy.[1,26–28]

The T1-weighted with gadolinium-enhanced contrast imaging is the best MRI sequence to define the dural attachment site (dural tail) of the meningioma. Although MRI provides superior soft-tissue assessment, the CT scan with bone window remains the tool of choice for identifying calcification, hyperostosis, and osseous anatomy. Frequently, a hyperostotic bone is found at the primary base of the tumor. In addition, the CT scan bone assessment provides a better idea of the surgical corridor available and allows planning of the extent of bone removal necessary for tumor resection.

Vascular relationship

Angiographic studies (CT, MRI, or conventional) are also important to understand the vascular relationship in and around the tumor, including arterial encasement, blood supply, and venous drainage.[29]

The presence of arterial encasement must be assessed before surgery so the internal debulking of the tumor can proceed safely (**Fig. 2**). Arterial narrowing is highly suggestive of adventitia invasion, which hinders a total resection when the encased artery cannot be sacrificed.

Conventional angiography may also help to define whether sacrifice of the encased artery is possible by defining collateral flow and the patient's tolerance to balloon test occlusion.

Regarding venous assessment, the patency of a venous sinus should be known if the posterior fossa meningioma is near one of them. Preoperative diagnosis of venous sinus occlusion makes the sacrifice of the involved segment a possibility.

Cranial nerve relationship

As mentioned previously, the primary base of the meningioma determines the pattern of CN displacement, hence the surgical corridors available for tumor resection. The evolution of MRI (steady-state free precession imaging/fast imaging employing steady-state acquisition) permitted clear identification of the CNs, instead of assuming their position based on the origin of the tumor.[30,31]

Hydrocephalus

Posterior fossa meningiomas may cause obstructive hydrocephalus. In the presence of significant ventricular dilation and signs of elevated intracranial pressure, a temporary or permanent cerebrospinal fluid (CSF) diversion may be necessary before the surgical management of the tumor. In these cases, the insertion of CSF shunt immediately before addressing the meningioma may facilitate the intraoperative management of the posterior fossa tumor and may help prevent postoperative CSF leakage.

Nasosinusal assessment

Once the choice for EEA is made, the preoperative radiologic assessment of the nasosinusal region is imperative (**Box 2**). A CT scan with slice thickness of no more than 3 mm (and preferably less) and coronal, axial, and parasagittal images of the paranasal sinuses and skull base are essential before surgery.

Equipment and instrumentation

Adequate instrumentation is paramount for the endoscopic approach to the clivus and posterior fossa, and a lack of instrumentation is considered a contraindication to performing the procedure.

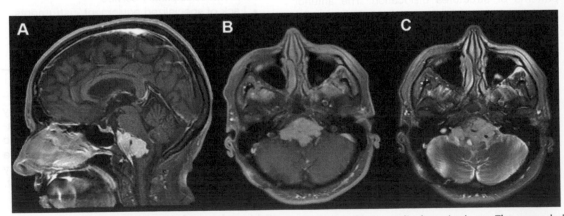

Fig. 2. MRI of a patient with brainstem compression symptoms secondary to a clival meningioma. The expanded EEA was contraindicated because of encasement of the right vertebral artery. (*A*) Sagittal preoperative T1-weighted (T1W) gadolinium-enhanced contrast imaging. (*B*) Axial T1W gadolinium-enhanced contrast imaging. (*C*) Axial T2-weighted imaging.

Box 2
Preoperative radiologic assessment of the nasosinusal region

- Nasal septum deviations
- Integrity and degree of aeration of the paranasal sinuses (particularly the sphenoid sinus)
- Location and presence of intersinus septae
- Presence of an Onodi cell
- Presence and extent of bone erosions, dehiscence, or hyperosteosis of the skull base
- Position of the internal carotid arteries (especially the paraclival segment)
- Thickness and incline of the clivus (basal angle)

The equipment includes the following:

- High-quality endoscopes (0° and 45°)
- Video equipment (camera and monitor)
- Long endoscopic bipolar forceps
- Long and delicate drills
- Long dissection instruments
- Long ultrasonic surgical aspirator
- Hemostatic materials

Preparation and Patient Positioning

The surgery is performed under hypotensive general anesthesia with total intravenous anesthetic, using propofol and remifentanil.

The patient is placed in a supine position on the operating table, head elevated 30°, neck slightly flexed, and head extended and turned toward the surgeon.

Neurophysiologic monitoring is mandatory when approaching the posterior fossa through a transnasal route. As a rule, CN VI-, motor-, and somatosensory-evoked potentials are monitored. The remaining CNs are monitored according to the tumor size and location.

Neuropatties soaked in adrenaline 1:1000 are placed in the nasal cavity for 10 minutes before the surgical procedure begins. The septum is infiltrated with lidocaine with adrenaline 1:100,000.

Surgical Approach

The endoscopic transnasal access to the posterior fossa is through a transclival approach. The clivus separates the nasopharynx from the posterior cranial fossa. It is composed of the posterior portion of the sphenoid body (basisphenoid) and the basilar part of the occipital bone (basiocciput) and is further subdivided into upper, middle, and lower thirds:

- Upper clivus is at the level of the sphenoid sinus and is formed by the basisphenoid bone including the dorsum sella.
- Middle clivus corresponds to the rostral part of the basiocciput and is located above a line connecting the caudal ends of the petroclival fissures.
- Lower clivus is formed by the caudal part of the basiocciput.

Approaching the posterior fossa through the upper two-thirds of the clivus requires the opening of the sphenoid sinus. When the posterior fossa is approached at the lower clivus, bone removal may be done solely below the sphenoid rostrum.

The intracranial surface of the upper two-thirds of the clivus faces the pons and is concave from side to side. The extracranial surface of the clivus gives rise to the pharyngeal tubercle at the junction of the middle and lower clivus. The upper clivus faces the roof of the nasopharynx that extends downward in the midline to the level of the pharyngeal tubercle.

The upper and middle clivus are separated from the petrous portion of the temporal bone on each side by the petroclival fissure. The basilar venous plexus is situated between the 2 layers of the dura of the upper clivus and is related to the dorsum sella and the posterior wall of the sphenoid sinus. It forms interconnecting venous channels between the inferior petrosal sinuses laterally, the cavernous sinuses superiorly, and the marginal sinus and epidural venous plexus inferiorly. The basilar sinus is the largest communicating channel between the paired cavernous sinuses.[32]

Surgical Procedure

Nasosinusal preparation

The access initiates with the combined transnasal/transseptal binostril approach[33]:

- Using anterior septoplasty incision, mucoperichondrial/mucoperiosteal flaps are created bilaterally.
- Most of the septal cartilage and bone are removed, preserving an L-shaped cartilage strut to support the nasal dorsum and tip.
- The mucosal flaps are lifted until both natural sphenoid ostia are on view.
- Rectangular sphenopalatine artery–based nasal septal mucosal flaps are created.
- The resulting mucosal flaps can be rotated and placed on the nasal floor back toward the choana or safely placed into the maxillary sinus cavity through a large middle meatus antrostomy.
- A wide opening of the anterior sphenoid sinus wall is created with a micro-Kerrison punch, and a drill is used to lower the sphenoid rostrum.

- The sinus mucosa that lines the clival area is reflected carefully, exposing the clival bone.

This approach allows 2 surgeons to simultaneously manipulate surgical instruments using both nostrils, has a robust tissue pedicle to help in the closure of skull base defects, and preserves the nasal septal mucosa of one side, avoiding nasal septal perforation.

Multiple modifications regarding length and width are possible, and the flap should be created according to the size and shape of the planned defect.[34]

Transclival approach

The clival bone is fully exposed, and its removal is initiated with a diamond burr drill and continued carefully with a micro-Kerrison punch if necessary. The extent of bone removal must be tailored to the size and location of the tumor, with the following limits:

- Superiorly: Floor of the sella
- Inferiorly: Foramen magnum
- Laterally: Internal carotid arteries, hypoglossal canal, and occipital condyles

The outer layer of the dura is first incised, and the basilar venous plexus is encountered. Bleeding in the plexus cannot be cauterized safely but is usually controlled with packing using hemostatic gelatin paste. Large lesions that infiltrate the dura mater often encroach on and obliterate much of the plexus, but if the lesion is not large or if the plexus is not completely compressed, profuse and intense bleeding can occur. Judicious packing,

time, patience, and experience are required to control it.[35] The interdural segment of CN VI is located laterally in this space, and lateral openings should be performed carefully with intraoperative monitoring and nerve stimulation.

The opening of the internal layer of the dura at the level of the middle and superior clivus must be accomplished with great care to avoid injury to the underlying basilar artery. Once the dura is opened, minor bleeding is stopped by bipolar coagulation, and it is finally possible to introduce the 0° endoscope carefully into the intradural space and to identify the following:

- Vertebral arteries
- Basilar artery and branches
- Anteroinferior cerebellar arteries
- Superior cerebellar arteries
- Posterior cerebral arteries
- Intradural course of CNs III, IV, V, and VI
- Brainstem
- Mamillary bodies

With angled endoscopes, it is also possible to visualize the following:

- Cerebellopontine angle
- CNs VII, VIII, IX, X, XI, and XII
- Retrosellar region

Once the anatomy is appreciated, meticulous dissection is required to remove the tumor. To optimize the surgeon's view, persistent hemostasis of the tissues of the nasal cavity and sphenoid needs to be maintained to minimize soiling of the endoscopes. Frequent irrigation and suction with

---

Box 3
Nuances and pitfalls of the technique

- The vidian nerves are important landmarks to the identification of the lacerum segment of the internal carotid artery (ICA).
- Neuronavigation tools are helpful in defining the limits of bone removal, especially in cases in which the pneumatization sphenoid sinus is not favorable or in reoperations.
- Parapharyngeal ICA must be evaluated when approaching the inferior clival region.
- It is recommended to leave a thin bone overlying the paraclival ICA as a protection during deep clival bone drilling.
- The bone drilling required to create an adequate intradural exposure must be completely finished before opening the dura.
- Early CN VI identification is important for complete and safe dural opening and tumor resection.
- The incline of the clivus (basal angle) must be considered when planning the skull base reconstruction. When the basal angle is obtuse, the nasal septal flap may be too short to cover the inferior region of the skull base defect.
- Multilayer reconstruction of the posterior fossa is imperative.
- Hydrocephalus associated with posterior fossa meningioma should be addressed before endoscopic resection of the tumor.

neurosurgical tip protected low suction is used to maintain good vision.

A 4-handed microsurgical technique is used to resect the tumor:

- Identification of the limits of the tumor and normal anatomy
- Debulking of the meningioma using microsurgical scissors and ultrasonic surgical aspirator
- Microsurgical dissection around the tumor preserving the arachnoid interface

Reconstruction

Dural repair in the region of the clivus is difficult and performed as follows:

- If the defect is large, it is first occluded with abdominal fat and then covered with grafts of fascia lata or a synthetic dural substitute.
- These grafts are covered by the sphenopalatine-based pedicled nasal septal flaps, as described previously. Fibrin glue is not typically necessary but may be used to hold the graft and flap in position.
- Spongostan powder (Ethicon, Somerville, NJ, USA) and Gelfoam (Pfizer, New York, NY, USA) are layered directly over the flap, followed by gauze packing soaked in antibiotic paste.
- A silastic splint is inserted into the nose on the side from which the graft was taken to promote reepithelialization.
- The packing is supported by a Rapid Rhino 900 (Arthrocare, Austin, TX, USA) or similar pack.
- Lumbar drain is not used routinely.
- Broad-spectrum antibiotics are used for 10 days or as long as necessary.

Nuances and Pitfalls of the Technique

Box 3 lists the nuances and pitfalls of the surgical technique.

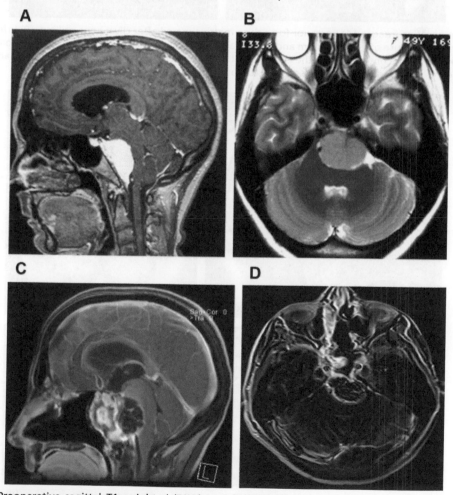

Fig. 3. (*A*) Preoperative sagittal T1-weighted (T1W) gadolinium-enhanced contrast imaging. (*B*) Preoperative axial T2-weighted (T2W) imaging. (*C*) Immediate postoperative sagittal T1W gadolinium-enhanced contrast imaging. (*D*) Immediate postoperative axial T2W imaging with fat suppression.

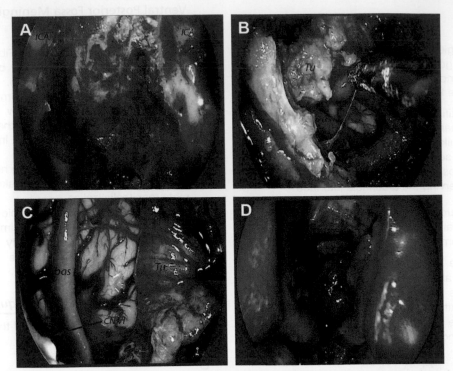

Fig. 4. Intraoperative images. (*A*) Posterior fossa dura mater exposed after clival bone drilling. (*B*) Inferior end of the tumor with exposure of the brainstem and vertebral and basilar arteries. (*C*) The tumor rotated to the left side after debulking. (*D*) Reconstruction of the clival defect using bilateral nasal septal flap. bas, basilar artery; CN VI, abducens nerve; ICA, internal carotid artery; Tu, tumor; vert, vertebral artery.

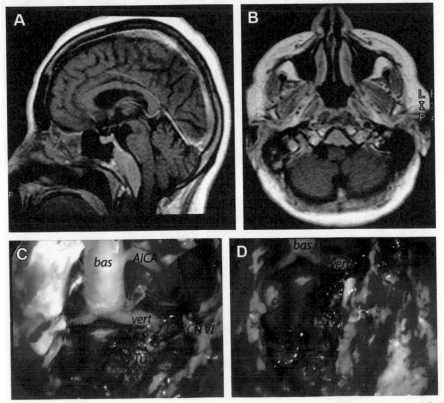

Fig. 5. (*A*) Preoperative sagittal T1-weighted (T1W) gadolinium enhanced contrast imaging (*B*) Preoperative axial T1W gadolinium-enhanced contrast imaging. (*C*) Intradural exposure of the posterior fossa and pontobulbar transition. (*D*) Residual tumor at the inferior and lateral left side. AICA, anteroinferior cerebellar artery; bas, basilar artery; CN VI, abducens nerve; Tu, tumor; vert, vertebral artery.

COMPLICATIONS

The complications are classified according to severity as minor or major and according to time of appearance as immediate or delayed.

Minor complications present little morbidity and do not compromise the patient's life, although they may be annoying and troublesome. Most of the minor complications resolve with time and conservative treatment.[32]

However, major complications present significant morbidity and the possibility of mortality.

Intracranial complications can result from direct injury to brain, CNs, meninges, blood vessels, or venous sinuses. The following are the resulting deficits:

- Loss of function of the surgical damaged structures (brain and/or CNs)
- Loss of vascular supply to critical areas
- Mass compressive effects (hematoma, others)

In addition, CSF leakage can cause symptoms directly, as well as predispose to meningitis and

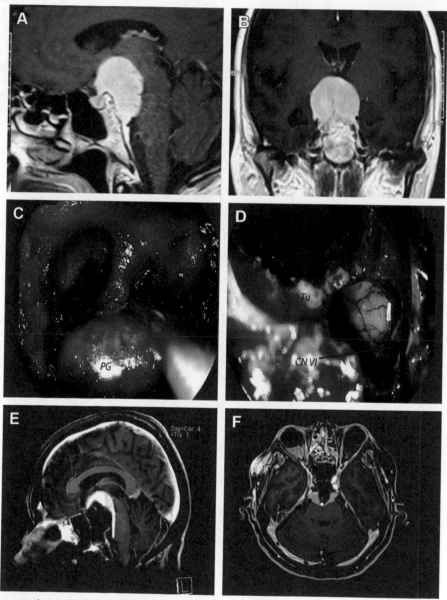

Fig. 6. (A) Preoperative sagittal T1-weighted (T1W) gadolinium-enhanced contrast imaging. (B) Preoperative coronal T1W gadolinium-enhanced contrast imaging. (C) Intradural pituitary transposition. (D) Inferior end of the tumor and exposure of the left CN VI. (E) Postoperative sagittal T1W gadolinium-enhanced contrast imaging. (F) Postoperative axial T1W gadolinium-enhanced contrast imaging. CN VI, abducens nerve; PG, pituitary gland; Tu, tumor.

Table 1
Ventral posterior fossa meningiomas resected through an EEA

Series	Number of Cases	Age/Sex	Presenting Symptoms	Location	Resection After EEA	Number of Procedures	Complications
Garcner et al,[14] 2008	2	38/F	Headache	Petroclival with parasellar involvement	Subtotal	2-stage EEA	CSF leak
		43/M	Headache, bitemporal hemianopsia, right ptosis, right facial involvement, numbness/tingling, cranial tumor embolization complicated by right carotid artery occlusion with left hemiparesis, CN VI palsy, pituitary dysfunction	Petroclival with parasellar involvement	Subtotal	3-stage EEA	CSF leak
Fraser et al,[15] 2010	1	70/F	Headache, diplopia and visual loss	Petroclival	Near total	NA	Stroke
Alexander et al,[16] 2010	1	54/M	Left CN VI palsy and ataxia	Clival	Near total	1-stage EEA	CSF leak
Prosser et al,[17] 2012	1	21/F	Headache and visual changes	Clival	Near total	2-stage EEA; 1-stage FOZ craniotomy	Bilateral CN VI palsy

Fernandez-Miranda et al,[18] 2012	1	52/F	Headache	Jugular tubercle	Total	1-stage EEA	None
Fernandez-Miranda et al,[19] 2014	5	60/F	NA	Petroclival	NA	NA	NA
		44/F	NA	Petroclival	NA	NA	NA
		58/M	NA	Petroclival	NA	NA	NA
		54/F	NA	Petroclival	NA	NA	NA
		23/F	NA	Petroclival	NA	NA	NA
Simal Julian et al,[20] 2014	1	16/F	None. CPA meningioma recurrence	Clival (without dural attachment)	Total	1-stage EEA	None
Iacoangeli et al,[21] 2014	2	NA	NA	Clival	Total	NA	None
		NA	NA	NA	NA	NA	NA
Present series	3	50/F	Headache	Clival	Near total	1-stage EEA	CSF leak; bilateral CN VI palsy
		60/F	Ataxia	Clival	Near total	1-stage EEA	Septic shock; pneumonia
		63/F	Headache, cognitive impairment	Clival with retrosellar involvement	Subtotal	1-stage EEA	Hypopituitarism

Abbreviations: FOZ, Fronto-orbito-zygomatic; NA, not available.

Data from Refs.[14–21]

pneumocephalus that can cause mass effect symptoms. Bleeding is a risk in any surgical procedure, but seldom are so many important vessels susceptible to injury. The transnasal transclival approach outlined previously visualizes and puts at risk the following vessels:

- Sphenopalatine and maxillary arteries and their branches
- Internal carotid artery
- Basilar and vertebral arteries and their branches
- Small brainstem perforator arteries
- Venous sinuses of the skull base (basilar venous plexus, cavernous sinus)

Immediate complications occur during surgery. The most frequent of these are CSF leakage, intraoperative bleeding, and injuries to the brain and CNs. Delayed complications include meningitis, bleeding, synechia, and infection.

POSTOPERATIVE CARE

A satisfactory postoperative result depends on both appropriate operative technique and meticulous postoperative care. Wide-spectrum antibiotics are given during the operation and for 10 days postoperatively or until removal of the nasal packing. Adequate postoperative care of the operative site requires appropriate instrumentation, including 4-mm 0° and 45° endoscopes, straight and curved atraumatic aspirators, and straight and curved microforceps, for debridement and follow-up of outpatients.

- The anterior pack is removed in 5 to 7 days.
- The ribbon gauze is removed after 10 to 14 days.
- Vigilance is required in the postoperative period for CSF leaks and the risk of infections.
- After removal of the packing, the operative cavity is carefully suctioned and any residual bony fragments are removed.
- The patient is instructed to perform frequent nasal irrigations with buffered 0.9% saline solution.

OUTCOMES
Illustrative Cases

Case 1
A 50-year-old woman was referred for neurosurgical evaluation of a mass discovered on MRI. She had experienced 3 to 4 months of persistent headaches. On physical examination, including a detailed visual examination, no gross neurologic deficits were noted. MRI and CT were performed, demonstrating an intradurally located, contrast-enhancing dural-based lesion at the midclival region; significant mass effect on the ventral surface of the brainstem; and mild ventricular dilation (**Fig. 3**).

A 1-stage endoscopic transclival approach and skull base reconstruction was performed as described previously (**Fig. 4**). The authors decided not to install an intraoperative or postoperative CSF shunt system. There was significant intraoperative manipulation of the left CN VI, which was encased by the tumor. A near-total resection was achieved, with a residual tumor left on the inferolateral left side. The patient evolved left CN VI palsy and CSF leak, requiring 2 other procedures for skull base reconstruction and vetriculoperitoneal shunt placement.

Case 2
A 60-year-old woman presented with 3 months of ataxia. On radiologic investigation, a mass lesion on the posterior fossa was discovered. On physical examination, including a detailed visual examination, no gross neurologic deficits were noted. MRI and CT were performed, demonstrating an intradurally located, contrast-enhancing dural-based lesion at the midclival region; significant mass effect on the ventral surface of the brainstem; and mild ventricular dilation (**Fig. 5**).

A 1-stage endoscopic transclival approach and skull base reconstruction was performed as described previously. A near-total resection was achieved uneventfully, with a residual tumor left on the inferior region. There were no postoperative deficits. However, the patient died 2 weeks after the surgery owing to septic shock secondary to pneumonia.

Case 3
A 63-year-old woman presented with 1 year of intermittent headache and mild cognitive impairment. She was referred for neurosurgical evaluation after radiologic investigation. The physical examination showed no abnormalities. MRI and CT were performed, demonstrating an intradurally located, contrast-enhancing dural-based lesion at the upper and midclival region with a retrosellar component and significant mass effect on the ventral surface of the brainstem (**Fig. 6**).

A 1-stage endoscopic transclival approach and skull base reconstruction was performed as described previously. In addition, an intradural pituitary transposition was done to maximize the resection of the retrosellar component of the tumor (see **Fig. 6**). A subtotal resection was achieved uneventfully with a residual tumor left on the superior region. There were no postoperative neurologic deficits. However, the patient developed permanent hypopituitarism, requiring hormonal replacement.

Advantages and Limitations of the Endoscopic Endonasal Approach

The main advantages of approaching the ventral posterior fossa through an endoscopic transclival approach include the ability to avoid any cerebral retraction and decrease the incidence of injury to the CNs. It enables tumor resection without crossing the CN plane (see **Fig. 1**).[12,15,36–38] In addition, the approach uses a natural corridor providing direct and quick access to the tumor. Early access to the meningioma vascular supply (cranial base dura) can greatly reduce intraoperative blood loss and facilitate removal. Further advantage of this approach includes removal of involved bone and dura as a part of the approach, which allows a Simpson grade I resection.

Even though endoscopes do not allow a 3-dimensional perspective, they do provide a close and wide view of the operative field from different angles. However, endoscopes allow only for a narrow operative field, which is surrounded by critical neurovascular structures, making the risks of major intradural bleeding, CSF leakage, and neural damage still possible.[17]

The main disadvantages of EEA are related to the resection of lateral extension of tumors and the reconstruction of large dural and bone defects of the posterior fossa, with high CSF leak rates (ranging between 4% and 33.3%).[15,36,39]

Literature Review

The current literature on endoscopic management of posterior fossa meningiomas is scarce. The authors, including their series, found 17 cases reported of meningiomas operated through an EEA (**Table 1**).[14–21]

Most of them are part of series addressing the transclival approach or skull base reconstruction, rather than specifically addressing the surgical management of meningiomas. Thus, not all cases have complete information regarding patient characteristics, procedure, and complications.

The difficulty in resecting clival, petroclival, jugular tubercle/foramen and foramen magnum meningiomas is beyond the surgical approach. The literature review on the endoscopic removal of these tumors reinforces the associated morbidities (eg, CN palsies, CSF leak) seen on the posterior surgical routes.[8] The expanded EEA, in its current form, is not a substitute for the posterior skull base approaches in the treatment of ventral posterior fossa meningiomas. It is a safe alternative for the rare cases of meningiomas with most part of the dural base at the midline clival region, and it may be used solely or in combination with other approaches. Thus, appropriate case selection may optimize the advantages of the approach and reduce morbidity of this complex pathologic condition.

SUMMARY

- Clival, petroclival, and foramen magnum meningiomas are challenging lesions to manage independently of the selected surgical approach.
- The current literature involving the endoscopic management of ventral posterior fossa meningioma is scant mainly because of the rarity of the pathologic condition, limited indications, and technical difficulties in tumor resection and skull base reconstruction.
- The main challenge in the management of ventral posterior fossa meningioma is the surgical approach selection.
- Careful anatomoradiologic evaluation, patient's clinical condition, and surgical team's expertise must guide the surgical route selection.
- Nuances of the endoscopic transclival approach and skull base reconstruction are highlighted.

ACKNOWLEDGMENTS

The authors acknowledge Luiz Felipe Ulrich de Alencastro (MD) for his contribution with the anatomic image in **Fig. 1**.

REFERENCES

1. Cushing H. Meningiomas: their classification, regional behaviour, life history, and surgical end results. Baltimore (MD): Thomas; 1938.
2. Arnautović KI, Al-Mefty O, Husain M. Ventral foramen magnum meningiomas. J Neurosurg 2000;92:71–80.
3. Maclean J, Fersht N, Short S. Controversies in radiotherapy for meningioma. Clin Oncol (R Coll Radiol) 2014;26:51–64.
4. Rogers L, Barani I, Chamberlain M, et al. Meningiomas: knowledge base, treatment outcomes, and uncertainties. A RANO review. J Neurosurg 2014;24:1–20.
5. Campbell E, Whitfield RD. Posterior fossa meningiomas. J Neurosurg 1948;5:131–53.
6. Bricolo AP, Turazzi S, Talacchi A, et al. Microsurgical removal of petroclival meningiomas: a report of 33 patients. Neurosurgery 1992;31:813–28.
7. Natarajan SK, Sekhar LN, Schessel D, et al. Petroclival meningiomas: multimodality treatment and outcomes at long-term follow-up. Neurosurgery 2007;60:965–79.

8. Almefty R, Dunn IF, Pravdenkova S, et al. True petro-clival meningiomas: results of surgical management. J Neurosurg 2014;120:40–51.

9. Jho HD, Carrau RL. Endoscopic endonasal trans-sphenoidal surgery: Experience with 50 patients. J Neurosurg 1997;87:44–51.

10. Cavallo LM, Messina A, Cappabianca P, et al. Endo-scopic endonasal surgery of the midline skull base: anatomical study and clinical considerations. Neuro-surg Focus 2005;19:E2.

11. Kassam A, Snyderman CH, Mintz A, et al. Expanded endonasal approach: the rostrocaudal axis. Part I. Crista galli to the sella turcica. Neurosurg Focus 2005;19:E3.

12. Kassam A, Snyderman CH, Mintz A, et al. Expanded endonasal approach: the rostrocaudal axis. Part II. Posterior clinoids to the foramen magnum. Neuro-surg Focus 2005;19:E4.

13. Beer-Furlan A, Evins AI, Rigante L, et al. Dual-Port 2D and 3D endoscopy: expanding the limits of the endonasal approaches to midline skull base lesions with lateral extension. J Neurol Surg B Skull Base 2014;75:187–97.

14. Gardner PA, Kassam AB, Thomas A, et al. Endo-scopic endonasal resection of anterior cranial base meningiomas. Neurosurgery 2008;63:36–52.

15. Fraser JF, Nyquist GG, Moore N, et al. Endoscopic endonasal minimal access approach to the clivus: case series and technical nuances. Neurosurgery 2010;67:ons150–8.

16. Alexander H, Robinson S, Wickremesekera A, et al. Endoscopic transsphenoidal resection of a midclival meningioma. J Clin Neurosci 2010;17:374–6.

17. Prosser JD, Vender JR, Alleyne CH, et al. Expanded endoscopic endonasal approaches to skull base meningiomas. J Neurol Surg B Skull Base 2012;73: 147–56.

18. Fernandez-Miranda JC, Morera VA, Snyderman CH, et al. Endoscopic endonasal transclival approach to the jugular tubercle. Neurosurgery 2012;71:146–58.

19. Fernandez-Miranda JC, Gardner PA, Rastelli MM Jr, et al. Endoscopic endonasal transcavernous poste-rior clinoidectomy with interdural pituitary transposi-tion. J Neurosurg 2014;121:91–9.

20. Simal Julian JA, Sanromán Álvarez P, Miranda Lloret P, et al. Full endoscopic endonasal transclival approach: Meningioma attached to the ventral surface of the brainstem. Neurocirugia (Astur) 2014;25:140–4.

21. Iacoangeli M, Di Rienzo A, di Somma LG, et al. Improving the endoscopic endonasal transclival approach: the importance of a precise layer by layer reconstruction. Br J Neurosurg 2014;28:241–6.

22. Buetow MP, Buetow PC, Smirniotopoulos JG. Typical, atypical, and misleading features in menin-gioma. RadioGraphics 1991;11:1087–106.

23. Osborn AG, Salzman KL, Barkovich AJ. Meningioma and atypical and malignant meningioma. In:

Osborn AG, editor. Diagnostic imaging: brain. 2nd edition. Salt Lake City (UT): Lippincott Williams & Wilkins/Amirys; 2009. p. 72–81.

24. Ojemann RJ. Management of cranial and spinal me-ningiomas. Clin Neurosurg 1993;40:321–83.

25. Hallinan JT, Hegde AN, Lim WE. Dilemmas and diagnostic difficulties in meningioma. Clin Radiol 2013;68:837–44.

26. Castellano F, Ruggiero G. Meningiomas of the pos-terior fossa. Acta Radiol Suppl 1953;104:1–177.

27. Sekhar LN, Wright DC, Richardson R, et al. Petroclival and foramen magnum meningiomas: surgical ap-proaches and pitfalls. J Neurooncol 1996;29:249–59.

28. Al-Mefty O. Preface. In: Al-Mefty O, editor. Meningi-omas. New York: Raven Press; 1991. p. vii.

29. Farb RI, Scott JN, Willinsky RA, et al. Intracranial venous system: gadolinium-enhanced three-dimen-sional MR venography with auto-triggered elliptic centric-ordered sequence—initial experience. Radi-ology 2003;226:203–9.

30. Schmitz B, Hagen T, Reith W. Three-dimensional true FISP for high-resolution imaging of the whole brain. Eur Radiol 2003;13:1577–82.

31. Mikami T, Minamida Y, Yamaki T, et al. Cranial nerve assessment in posterior fossa tumors with fast imag-ing employing steady-state acquisition (FIESTA). Neurosurg Rev 2005;28:261–6.

32. Stamm AC, Pignatari SS. Transnasal endoscopic-assisted surgery of the skull base. In: Cummings CW, Flint PW, Harker LA, editors. Otolar-yngology head neck surgery. 4th edition. Philadel-phia: Elsevier Mosby; 2005. p. 3855–76.

33. Stamm AC, Pignatari S, Vellutini E, et al. A novel approach allowing binostril work to the sphenoid si-nus. Otolaryngol Head Neck Surg 2008;138:531–2.

34. Hadad G, Bassagasteguy L, Carrau RL, et al. A novel reconstructive technique after endoscopic expanded endonasal approaches: vascular pedicle nasoseptal flap. Laryngoscope 2006;116:1882–6.

35. Stamm AC, Pignatari SS, Vellutini E. Transnasal endoscopic surgical approaches to the clivus. Oto-laryngol Clin North Am 2006;39:639–56.

36. Dehdashti AR, Karabatsou K, Ganna A, et al. Expanded endoscopic endonasal approach for treatment of clival chordomas: early results in 12 patients. Neurosurgery 2008;63:299–307.

37. Frank G, Sciarretta V, Calbucci F, et al. The endoscopic transnasal transsphenoidal approach for the treatment of cranial base chordomas and chondrosarcomas. Neurosurgery 2006;59:ons50–7.

38. Stippler M, Gardner PA, Snyderman CH, et al. Endo-scopic endonasal approach for clival chordomas. Neurosurgery 2009;64:268–78.

39. Shiley SG, Limonadi F, Delashaw JB, et al. Inci-dence, etiology, and management of cerebrospinal fluid leak following trans-sphenoidal surgery. Laryngoscope 2003;113:1283–8.

Endoscopic Endonasal Odontoidectomy

Matteo Zoli, MD[a],*, Diego Mazzatenta, MD[a], Adelaide Valluzzi, MD[a], Carmelo Mascari, MD[a], Ernesto Pasquini, MD[b], Giorgio Frank, MD[a]

KEYWORDS

- Endoscopic endonasal surgery • Craniovertebral junction • Odontoidectomy • Basilar invagination
- Occipital-cervical degenerative disease

KEY POINTS

- Odontoidectomy is the treatment of choice for irreducible ventral compression of the brainstem.
- Endoscopic endonasal odontoidectomy is well tolerated by patients, allows an immediate restoring of the spontaneous breathing, and permits a rapid resumption of oral feeding.
- Endoscopic endonasal odontoidectomy is a technical demanding procedure, due to the narrow and deep surgical corridor and it should be reserved to neurosurgeons well trained in endoscopic techniques.
- The endoscopic endonasal technique is a straightforward, panoramic, and direct approach to the odontoid even in cases with severe platybasia and high position of dens.
- All approaches to odontoidectomy present advantages and limits. The surgeon should select the approach that maximizes the advantages and minimizes the disadvantages in each case and should consider the peculiar anatomic and clinical conditions.

INTRODUCTION

The goal of the endoscopic endonasal odontoidectomy for craniovertebral junction degenerative disease is cervicomedullary decompression when irreducible ventral bony, ligamentous, or other disease compresses the brainstem. The standard approach for odontoidectomy is represented by transoral or transcervical approaches with microsurgical support. In 2005, Kassam and colleagues[1] proposed the endoscopic endonasal route as a less invasive approach to avoid splitting the soft or hard palate, retraction of the tongue, or the need for glossotomy or mandibulotomy with the

related sequelae and possible complications for the patients. This approach provided a more direct, panoramic, and straightforward route to the odontoid process. Since this pioneering report, many series have documented the safety and feasibility of this approach and demonstrated high patient tolerance. It also provides quick recovery time due to immediate airway reestablishment without the need for tracheostomy or prolonged orotracheal intubation. There is also rapid resumption of oral feeding, avoiding the risk of postoperative dysphagia or swallowing impairment.[2–13] However, some questions still remain open. In particular, the identification of proper and accurate

The authors state that the content of the submitted article, in part or in full, has not been published previously and has not been submitted elsewhere for review. There is no financial support received in conjunction with the generation of this submission and no conflict of interest. The authors certify that this article is a unique submission and is not being considered for publication with any other source in any medium. The authors have nothing to declare and nothing to disclose.

[a] Department of Neurosurgery, Center of Pituitary Tumors and Endoscopic Skull Base Surgery, IRCCS Scienze Neurologiche, via Altura, 3, Bologna 40139, Italy; [b] ENT Department, Azienda USL, via Altura, 3, Bologna 40139, Italy

* Corresponding author.

E-mail address: matteozeta@libero.it

surgical indications to maximize the advantages and minimize the limits of this approach. Furthermore, some technical points, such as whether to open the anterior arch of cervical vertebrae (C) 1 and management of the rhinopharyngeal mucosa (midline incision, direct skeletonization, or flap), are still debated. This article reviews the authors' surgical experience and the current literature with the aim to identify in which conditions this approach is indicated. A variant of the surgical technique for the cases of craniovertebral malformation with platybasia and high position of the dens, which can provide a more direct access to the odontoid for such patients, is discussed.

ENDOSCOPIC ENDONASAL ANATOMY OF CRANIOVERTEBRAL JUNCTION

The craniovertebral junction comprises the occipital bone and C1 and C2. It envelops and protects the brainstem, the upper spinal cord, the last cranial and the first spinal nerves, and the vertebral arteries. From the endoscopic endonasal perspective, this region represents the more caudal midline extension of this approach. Indeed, the inferior limit of the endoscopic endonasal

approach is represented by a line passing through the anterior nasal spine and the posterior border of hard palate.[14] Thus, normally, the endoscopic endonasal approach allows the surgeon to reach the body of C2, giving excellent exposure of the craniovertebral junction (**Fig. 1A**).[14,15] The superior part of the craniovertebral junction is formed by the occipital bone, which constitutes the foramen magnum, where the medulla passes to the spinal canal and the atlas articulates with the skull base. Thus, from the endoscopic endonasal view, the dissection of the inferior third of the clivus permits reaching and exposing the foramen magnum at the midline (see **Fig. 1B**). Laterally, this exposure is hampered by the presence of the 2 occipital condyles, where the first cervical vertebra connects with the skull and the hypoglossal canals are contained. To approach the dens, a strictly midline approach is sufficient because occipital condyles do not limit the view (see **Fig. 1B**). Furthermore, their preservation prevents injuries to cranial nerve XII, passes the hypoglossal canal, and reduces postoperative instability. The posterior surface of anterior arch of the C1 arch joins with the odontoid process of C2 (see **Fig. 1B**). Indeed, the axis has a typical shape, with this

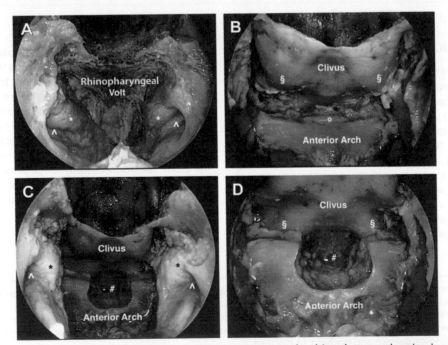

Fig. 1. Cadaveric dissection, 0° scope. (*A*) After posterior septostomy, the rhinopharyngeal region is exposed. The craniovertebral junction is in the midline by the inferior third of the clivus and the first cervical spine segments. This area is covered by the rhinopharyngeal mucosa and muscles. (*B*) After removal of the rhinopharyngeal mucosa and muscles, the occipital bone and the anterior arch of C1 are completely exposed. In normal conditions, the odontoid is covered for the most of its extension by this arch. (*C, D*) After opening of the anterior arch of C1, the dens can be exposed and resected, showing the dura behind the odontoid process. *, eustachian tubes; ^, Rosenmüller fossae; §, occipital condyles; °, odontoid process; #, cervical spine dura.

upward process, deriving from its body, which is completely visible, from an endoscopic endonasal point of view after the removing of the anterior arch of the atlas (see **Fig. 1**C, D). Occipital bones, C1 and C2, are also connected by multiple ligaments. The anterior longitudinal ligament must be opened to access to the craniovertebral junction from a ventral route. It covers the atlantooccipital membrane, a broad and dense fibrous tissue that extends from the inferior border of the foramen magnum to the superior edge of C1. Its incision allows access to the bony structures of the region. When exposed, the dens is surrounded by a complex ligamentous system, formed by the alar, the apical, and the cruciform ligaments. The alar ligaments are thick fibrous structures that connect the dens to the occipital condyles. The apical is a midline structure that rises from the tip of odontoid to the foramen magnum. All of these ligaments should be sectioned to free the odontoid process and allow its removal.

INDICATIONS AND PREOPERATIVE MANAGEMENT

Odontoidectomy is indicated in craniovertebral junction abnormalities of any origin (congenital, inflammatory, developmental, or traumatic) when there is a pure ventral irreducible cervicomedullary compression.[1–7] When the abnormality is reducible, such as in some atlantoaxial subluxations, its realignment, followed by immobilization and/or posterior arthrodesis, is the treatment of choice. When the abnormality is irreducible, decompression is necessary and the surgery should be tailored based on the origin of the brainstem compression. For instance, in a case of dorsal compression, such as Arnold-Chiari malformation, a posterior decompression is indicated. Conversely, in a case of ventral compression, such as odontoid invagination, a ventral decompression (ie, odontoidectomy) is indicated.[1–13] As a first step, the stability of the craniovertebral junction should be assessed. Radiographic studies in a flexion-extension position are the gold standard for this evaluation. If an unstable craniovertebral junction condition is observed, a posterior fusion (or a revision, if already performed) should be the first line of treatment.[13,16,17] This is because, in multiple degenerative diseases of this region, such as rheumatoid arthritis, instability plays a key role in the development of the an inflammatory pannus around the odontoid, which exerts compression on the brainstem.[18,19] For these cases, a simple posterior arthrodesis, resolving the first element of the pathogenesis of the disease, can be curative and favors the regression of the ventral reactive pannus through the immobilization

of the junction.[19] Thus, only for cases of ventral irreducible compression, the odontoidectomy is properly indicated. These cases are extremely rare, which justifies the low number of series and cases reported in literature.[1–13] The indication for an endoscopic endonasal approach should be evaluated case by case. Two main elements should be considered: the radiological features of the brainstem compression and patient-related peculiarities, such as the presence of relative or absolute contraindications to the transoral approach. Crockard[20] observed that, in cases of oral sepsis, reduced oral opening, or fixed flexion deformity of the head on the neck that does not allow sufficient opening of the mouth, the transoral approach should be discouraged. Macroglossia is another complication for the surgeon because it reduces the surgical field and increases the risk of postoperative ventilatory impairment. For these cases, the authors advise the endoscopic endonasal approach as an alternative to the transoral because the reduced oral surgical field does not impair it. CT scan and MRI give different information that should be considered in the preoperative surgical planning. In particular, the presence of cranial-vertebral junction malformations, especially platybasia and high position of the dens that causes brainstem compression, are relevant features for the surgical planning.[21–23] Indeed, in these cases, the transoral approach is complicated by the vertical direction of work and the long route, whereas the endoscopic endonasal approach allows a direct and short path to the odontoid, thus it can be advantageously chosen.[22,23]

ENDOSCOPIC ENDONASAL TECHNIQUE
Patient Position

The patient is placed in a semisitting position with orotracheal intubation and packing of the oropharynx to prevent blood leakage into the stomach. At the beginning of the procedure, the authors retract the soft palate and widen the exposure of the rhinopharynx with 2 thin rubber nasogastric probes inserted through the nose and extracted through the mouth (**Fig. 2**A, B). A controlled arterial hypotension is required in the nasal phase.

Instrumentation

Because endoscopic endonasal odontoidectomy is a strictly midline approach, angled optic scopes are not required. A high-speed diamond drill is necessary, as well as Kerrison rongeurs. A diode laser can be useful to speed the dissection of the rhinopharynx muscles and to avoid blood loss in this phase. The laser is extremely useful because the bony attachments of the rhinopharynx muscles are extremely tenacious. The neuronavigation

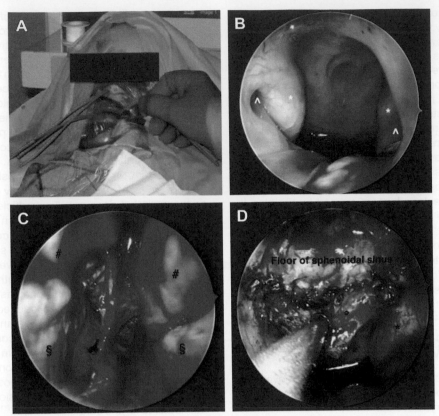

Fig. 2. Intraoperative images. 0° scope. (*A*, *B*) The insertion of 2 rubber nasogastric probes in the nasal fossa and extracted from the mouth allows restriction of the soft palate and improved working room. (*C*) The posterior septostomy allows creation of a single surgical cavity and use of the 2 nostrils–4 hands technique. (*D*) Through the diode laser, the rhinopharyngeal volt is progressively detached from the floor of sphenoidal sinus and the middle and inferior clivus, creating an inverted U-shaped flap that can be retracted through a suture. *, eustachian tubes; ̂, Rosenmüller fossae; §, inferior turbinates; #, middle turbinates; °, rhinopharyngeal flap.

system is strongly recommended because it allows orientation in all 3 planes (not only in the sagittal plan as with the fluoroscope). Before surgery, we perform a CT angiogram (CTA) for neuronavigation purposes. The aim is to consider the bony nasal anatomy of the patient, as well as the course of the vertebral arteries laterally and the carotid arteries, which can rarely present some midline loops in its pharyngeal tract. Micro-Doppler (16 MHz) can be also useful to intraoperatively confirm the course of the main vessels and, in particular, of the carotid artery, which can be identified by the neuronavigation system. The microdebrider has proven very useful to complete the skeletonization of the clivus and, in cases of a fibrous pannus around the dens, to improve the cervicomedullary decompression.

Approach Phase

A binostril approach is performed. The middle and inferior turbinates are displaced laterally. Usually,

their resection is not required but, when necessary, the posterior tail of inferior turbinate can be removed to widen the surgical corridor. The vomer is detached from its insertion and it is resected together with the posterior quarter of the septum, creating a single surgical cavity accessible through both nostrils (see **Fig. 2**C). This surgical field is basically the choana comprised of the floor of the sphenoidal sinus superiorly, the upper part of oropharynx inferiorly, and in between the eustachian tubes and Rosenmüller fossae laterally (see **Figs. 1**A and **2**C). We create an inverted U-shaped flap on the rhinopharyngeal volt using laser to incise the mucosal and the muscular layers from immediately behind the eustachian tube to the other, connecting both Rosenmüller fossae (see **Fig. 2**D). The eustachian tube is the main landmark of the parapharyngeal carotid artery, which runs posterolaterally. Therefore, the incision should be medial to the tube to avoid to injury the carotid. The preoperative CTA has a crucial role in this phase, especially if a median loop of internal carotid artery is present. Some investigators prefer a midline incision of the rhinopharynx volt, followed by direct skeletonization of the clivus and the craniovertebral junction.[1] The authors prefer the rhinopharyngeal flap, although it is a moderately bloody and time-consuming procedure, because it allows an effective plastic reconstruction in case of cerebrospinal fluid (CSF) leak. At this point, 2 routes can be taken to reach the odontoid process, depending on the craniovertebral junction anatomic abnormalities.

Endosinusal Route

In cases of marked platybasia, with horizontal direction of the clivus and, especially, with high positioning of the dens, the authors prefer a route passing through the sphenoid sinus (**Fig. 3**). For these cases, this is the more direct corridor and it allows a more extensive and straightforward view of the odontoid process. This route requires, after the skeletonization of the floor of the sphenoid sinus and clivus, an anterior sphenoidotomy and complete drilling of the floor of the sphenoid sinus so that it may be used as part of the surgical corridor (see **Fig. 3**A). It is possible to start drilling the clivus just below the sellar bulge (see **Fig. 3**B), allowing creation of a funnel-shape canal along the

clivus up to the odontoid process (see **Fig. 3**C–E). The last third of clivus can be completely resected to fully expose the craniovertebral junction.

Extrasinusal Route

For all other cases, the authors perform a complete extrasinusal route, not opening the sphenoidal sinus (**Fig. 4**). After the complete skeletonization of the clivus, its inferior third or less, depending on the height of the dens, is drilled out without opening the sphenoidal sinus (see **Fig. 4**A). Thus, the foramen magnum is ventrally opened and the anterior arch of C1, followed by the odontoid process, is posteriorly exposed (see **Fig. 4**B–D).

Odontoidectomy

To skeletonize the atlantoaxial articulation, it is necessary to resect the anterior longitudinal ligament. In the first case, described by Kassam and colleagues,[1] the C1 anterior arch was resected to widely expose the odontoid process. Other investigators propose preservation of the anterior C1 arch to reduce the risk of craniocervical instability.[17,24,25] The authors agree that it is preferable to preserve the anterior arch because its integrity is an important element of craniocervical stability. Thus, in cases with a sufficient exposure of the

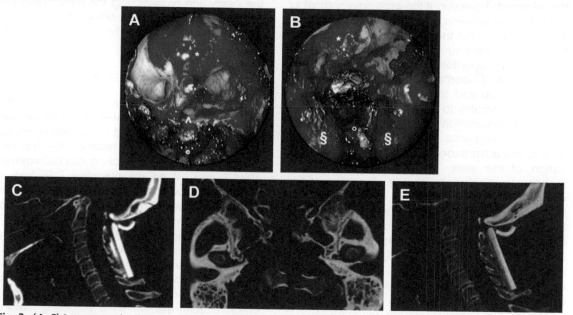

Fig. 3. (*A, B*) Intraoperative images. 0° scope. (*C–E*) CT scan with no enhancement. (*A*) In the endosinusal route, the floor of the sphenoidal sinus is resected and the sinus is entirely opened. (*B*) The clivus is drilled just behind the sellar bulge in a direction that depends on the degree of platybasia and on the location of the dens. (*C*) Preoperative sagittal CT scan of the neuroradiological features (platybasia and high position of the dens) that make the endosinusal route direct and straightforward to the dens. (*D*) Axial early postoperative CT scan of the funnel-shaped path in the clivus to reach the dens, which the endosinusal route allows. (*E*) Sagittal early postoperative CT scan of the corridor of the endosinusal route to reach the odontoid and the degree of resection. *, sellar bulges; ˄, floor of sphenoidal sinus; °, rhinopharyngeal flaps; §, eustachian tubes.

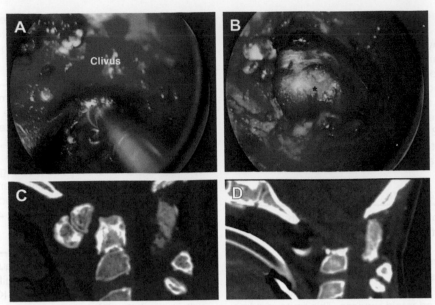

Fig. 4. (*A, B*) Intraoperative images. 0° scope. (*C, D*) CT scan with no enhancement. (*A*) In the extrasinual route, the floor of the sphenoidal sinus is spared; the sinus is not opened; and, after its skeletonization, the inferior third of the clivus is drilled out. (*B*) The craniovertebral junction is accessed and exposed. (*C*) Preoperative sagittal CT scan of an atlantoaxial subluxation and os odontoideum. (*D*) Sagittal early postoperative CT scan of the corridor of the extrasinual route to reach the odontoid and the degree of resection. *, os odontoideum.

dens, without resection of C1, we prefer to spare this element; however, if the arch covers most of the odontoid process, its removal is unavoidable. We prefer to resect the anterior arch with the Kerrison punch instead of the drill. After it is fully exposed, the odontoid process can be removed. The amount of odontoid to be resected (only the top or the top and the caudal portion) depends on the abnormality to be treated. For example, in odontoid invagination it is the entity of the invagination that suggests the amount of odontoid to resect; the advantage represented by the preservation of the atlas, leaving the craniovertebral stability unaffected, is intuitive. The core of the odontoid is drilled out with a diamond drill and the residual shell of the odontoid is removed before cutting the surrounding fibrous pathologic tissue, if present, or sectioning of apical, alar, and cruciate ligaments (**Fig. 5**). In patients with rheumatoid arthritis or other inflammatory diseases, the thickening of ligaments and surrounding tissue is a crucial part of the compression. Obtaining a satisfactory ventral decompression is necessary to remove the granulomatous tissue and the hypertrophied ligaments.

Closure

In cases of CSF leak, an adequate repair is mandatory (**Fig. 6**A). The authors perform the reconstruction by introducing abdominal fat into the cavity and repositioning the rhinopharyngeal flap with a suture (see **Fig. 6**B, C). A single 8-cm Merocel (Merocel Corp., Mystic, CT) is useful to maintain placement.

POSTOPERATIVE MANAGEMENT

This technique allows awaking the patient at the end of procedure, immediately removing the orotracheal tube, and restoring spontaneous ventilation. Oral feeding can be resumed the first day after surgery and nasal packing can be removed after 2 days. If no intraoperative CSF leak is observed, the patient can stand up about the first day after surgery. Otherwise, 3 days of bed rest are required. In the first days after surgery, a CT scan is advised to confirm odontoid resection and rule out early complications. A Philadelphia neck brace can be adopted to avoid dramatic postoperative consequences and a tomogram in the flexion-extension position is advised to assess craniovertebral stability while resuming motility. The patient can be discharged few days after surgery. The first endoscopic nasal debridement is suggested in the first month after surgery and an MRI control after 3 months. The postoperative rehabilitation can be started as soon as possible after surgery, depending on the clinical condition of the patient.

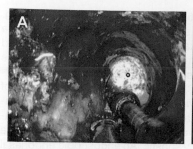 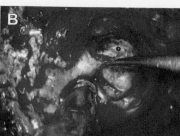 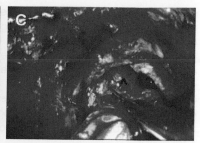

Fig. 5. Intraoperative images. 0° scope. (*A*) The core of odontoid process is progressively drilled. (*B*) The shell of dens is detached by surrounding tissues. (*C*) The fibrous tissue, when present as in rheumatoid arthritis, is resected to complete the cervicomedullary decompression. °, odontoid processes; ̂, fibrous pannus.

ADVANTAGES AND LIMITS OF ENDOSCOPIC ENDONASAL ODONTOIDECTOMY

The transoral route is a more common approach and it still is the gold standard access for odontoidectomy.[1] Recently, the endonasal endoscopic approach has been proposed because it presents some advantages in respect to the more traditional approaches.[1] This approach is well tolerated by patients for several reasons.[2–13] It avoids soft or hard palate cut or glossotomy or, in general, tongue manipulation because the soft palate is simply retracted. This reduces the risk of the frequent complications related to its defective repair, such as nasal voice or incontinence of the soft palate with regurgitation of liquids and solids through the nose. Tongue compression for a long period is not required. It also avoids complications such as tongue base edema, necrosis, and respiratory impairment. This allows prompt and safe orotracheal extubation after surgery.[2–13] As elegantly demonstrated by Van Abel and colleagues,[26] this approach reduces the risk of dysphagia because it limits the incision of the rhinopharynx muscle above the palatal line, which lowers the risk of damaging the high-density neural plexus found in the oropharyngeal wall and allows a prompt resumption of oral feeding. Another advantage is the reduced infection risk that is one of the more dramatic complications of the transoral approach due to the contamination of the surgical field by saliva and oral bacterial flora. Conversely, with the risk of postoperative meningitis is low, observed in rare cases in the literature.[1–13] The authors believe that with this approach, especially if a rhinopharyngeal flap is performed in the approach phase, the intraoperative CSF leak can be effectively repaired, reducing the risk of CSF bacterial contamination. Furthermore, one of the main advantages of the endoscopic endonasal approach is the angle of attack of the odontoid. The odontoid process is approached in a caudocranial direction and resection of the anterior arch of C1 to expose the odontoid is often necessary. Endonasal endoscopic approaches, through either an extrasinusal or an endosinusal route, allow the surgeon to reach the odontoid process ventrally or in a craniocaudal direction, permitting resection of the odontoid, preserving, in certain cases, the arch of the atlas. Moreover, the endosinusal endoscopic endonasal route allows the surgeon to reach ventrally with a direct angle of approach even in demanding cases with a severe platybasia and high position of the dens. However, the

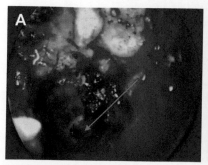 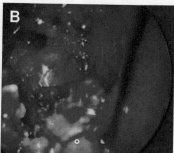 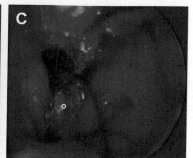

Fig. 6. Intraoperative images. 0° scope. (*A*) After the odontoid resection, a CSF leak is evident through a dura defect (*arrow*). (*B*) Plastic repair is performed with abdominal fat, which is put in place to fill the surgical cavity, and the U-shaped rhinopharyngeal flap. (*C*) The flap is repositioned with a suture to complete the reconstruction phase. °, rhinopharyngeal flaps.

odontoidectomy, regardless of the approach, still remains a challenging neurosurgical procedure due to the deepness of the target, the narrowness of the corridor, and the risk of potentially dramatic neurologic sequelae related to the close relationship with the brainstem-spinal cord passage. Specifically, the endonasal endoscopic odontoidectomy is technically demanding and it should be reserved for well-trained surgeons.

EXPLICATIVE CASES

Two illustrative cases from previously published series describe the management, outcome, and surgical technique adopted for these cases.[6,24]

First Case

A 34-year-old man, affected by Down syndrome, came to our attention for progressive tetraparesis, confirmed by motor evoked potentials (MEPs) and sensitive evoked potentials (SEPs). Four years earlier, he had undergone an occipitocervical fixation for an atlantoaxial subluxation but the

neurologic deficits were progressively worsening. The CT scan showed a basilar invagination due to the subluxation and the MRI demonstrated brainstem compression with a new spontaneous hyperintense signal in a T2-weighted image (T2-WI) (**Fig. 7**A, C). Flexion-extension radiography of the craniocervical junction demonstrated the stability of the fixation system. At admission, the patient was still able to walk with support and the gait was frankly spastic. An endoscopic endonasal odontoidectomy through an extrasinusal route was performed. No intraoperative CSF leak was observed. The postoperative course was unremarkable and the patient was discharged and had no additional neurologic deficits after 4 days with a home rehabilitation program. Postoperative CT scan and MRI showed the complete resection of the odontoid process and the relief of the brainstem compression (see **Fig. 7**B, D). Three years later, the clinical worsening progression is arrested, the neurologic condition is stable, and the patient can walk autonomously without support after the rehabilitation program.

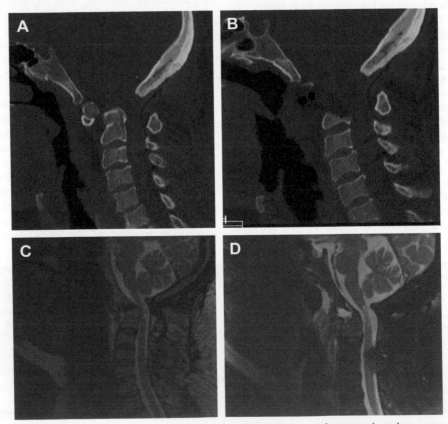

Fig. 7. (*A, B*) Sagittal CT scans. (*C, D*) T2WI sagittal MRIs. (*A, C*) Preoperative neuroimaging assessments of an atlantoaxial subluxation with consequent brainstem compression. (*B, D*) Postoperative neuroimaging assessments demonstrating the satisfactory odontoidectomy and the decompression of cervicomedullary junction obtained through an endoscopic endonasal extrasinusal approach.

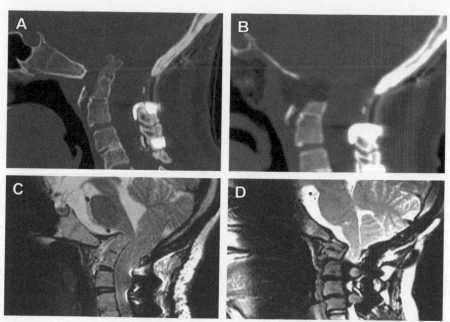

Fig. 8. (*A, B*) Sagittal CT scans. (*C, D*) T2WI sagittal MRIs. (*A, C*) Preoperative neuroimaging assessments of a basilar invagination, platybasia, and inflammatory pannus around the dens. (*B, D*) Postoperative neuroimaging assessments demonstrating the odontoidectomy and the decompression of neural structures, obtained through an endoscopic endonasal endosinusal approach.

Second Case

A 29-year-old woman, affected by rheumatoid arthritis, came to our attention presenting progressively worsening mild tetraparesis, confirmed by MEPs and SEPs. Three years earlier, the patient had undergone an occipitocervical fixation for a basilar invagination. The CT scan and the MRI showed a complex malformation of the craniovertebral junction with platybasia, high position of the odontoid process surrounded with rheumatoid pannus, and compression of the brainstem (**Fig. 8**A, C) A flexion-extension radiography of the craniocervical junction was performed to demonstrate the stability of the fixation system. Endoscopic endonasal odontoidectomy through an endosinusal route was performed. An intraoperative CSF leak was repaired with fat and with the rhinopharyngeal flap. The patient was discharged in excellent clinical condition after 3 days. The postoperative neuroimaging examinations showed the removal of the odontoid and brainstem decompression (see **Fig. 8**B, D). Two years later, the patient is in good clinical condition and an early improvement in superior limbs strength is observed.

SUMMARY

Odontoidectomy is indicated in selected cases of ventral irreducible compression of the cervicomedullary junction. It is complementary and not alternative to other surgical techniques, such as the transoral or the transcervical, because it can be performed for cases with contraindication to the other approaches or in situations in which it could be particularly demanding with traditional routes. The main advantages compared with other techniques are improved patient tolerance, prompt oral feeding, and restoration of spontaneous ventilation. Technically, it allows a tailored odontoidectomy (removing only the amount of odontoid or fibrous tissue necessary) and gives the surgeon a frontal and direct angle of attack, even in cases with a marked platybasia and high position of the dens, especially if an endosinusal route is adopted. The authors strongly believe that there is not a single ideal procedure for the treatment of craniovertebral abnormalities and endoscopic endonasal odontoidectomy is one of several surgical procedures that should be selected case by case to give to each patient the best possible treatment.

ACKNOWLEDGMENTS

Fig. 1 was taken by one of the Author of this article at the ALT-vision at Wexner Medical Center, The Ohio State University, Columbus, Ohio, USA. We thank Dr D. Prevedello, Dr R. Carrau, and Dr B. Otto, directors of laboratory, for the permission to use these pictures.

REFERENCES

1. Kassam AB, Snyderman C, Gardner P, et al. The expanded endonasal approach: a fully endoscopic transnasal approach and resection of the odontoid process: technical case report. Neurosurgery 2005;57(Suppl 1):E213.

2. Duntze J, Eap C, Kleiber JC, et al. Advantages and limitations of endoscopic endonasal odontoidectomy. A series of nine cases. Orthop Traumatol Surg Res 2014;100(7):775–8.

3. Ponce-Gómez JA, Ortega-Porcayo LA, Soriano-Barón HE, et al. Evolution from microscopic transoral to endoscopic endonasal odontoidectomy. Neurosurg Focus 2014;37(4):E15.

4. Choudhri O, Mindea SA, Feroze A, et al. Experience with intraoperative navigation and imaging during endoscopic transnasal spinal approaches to the foramen magnum and odontoid. Neurosurg Focus 2014;36(3):E4.

5. Iacoangeli M, Gladi M, Alvaro L, et al. Endoscopic endonasal odontoidectomy with anterior C1 arch preservation in elderly patients affected by rheumatoid arthritis. Spine J 2013;13(5):542–8.

6. Mazzatenta D, Zoli M, Mascari C, et al. Endoscopic endonasal odontoidectomy: clinical series. Spine (Phila Pa 1976) 2014;39(10):846–53.

7. Goldschlager T, Härtl R, Greenfield JP, et al. The endoscopic endonasal approach to the odontoid and its impact on early extubation and feeding. J Neurosurg 2014;31:1–8.

8. Wu JC, Mummaneni PV, El-Sayed IH. Diseases of the odontoid and craniovertebral junction with management by endoscopic approaches. Otolaryngol Clin North Am 2011;44:1029–42.

9. Wu JC, Huang WC, Cheng H, et al. Endoscopic transnasal transclival odontoidectomy: a new approach to decompression: technical case report. Neurosurgery 2008;63(Suppl 1):ONSE92–4.

10. Gempt J, Lehmberg J, Meyer B, et al. Endoscopic transnasal resection of the odontoid in a patient with severe brainstem compression. Acta Neurochir (Wien) 2010;152:559–60.

11. Gempt J, Lehmberg J, Grams AE, et al. Endoscopic transnasal resection of the odontoid: case series and clinical course. Eur Spine J 2011;20:661–6.

12. Leng LZ, Anand VK, Hartl R, et al. Endonasal endoscopic resection of an os odontoideum to decompress the cervicomedullary junction: a minimal access surgical technique. Spine 2009;34:E139–43.

13. Cornelius JF, Kania R, Bostelmann R, et al. Transnasal endoscopic odontoidectomy after occipitocervical fusion during the same operative setting technical note. Neurosurg Rev 2011;34:115–21.

14. de Almeida JR, Zanation AM, Snyderman CH, et al. Defining the nasopalatine line: the limit for endonasal surgery of the spine. Laryngoscope 2009;119(2):239–44.

15. Kassam A, Snyderman CH, Mintz A, et al. Expanded endonasal approach: the rostrocaudal axis. Part II. Posterior clinoids to the foramen magnum. Neurosurg Focus 2005;19(1):E4.

16. Goel A, Bhatjiwale M, Desai K. Basilar invagination: a study based on 190 surgically treated patients. J Neurosurg 1998;88:962–8.

17. Shetty A, Kumar A, Chacko A, et al. Reduction techniques in the management of atlantoaxial subluxation. Indian J Orthop 2013;47:333–9.

18. Schreiber AL. Manifestations of rheumatoid arthritis: epidural pannus and atlantoaxial subluxation resulting in basilar invagination. PM R 2012;4(1):78–80.

19. Young RM, Sherman JH, Wind JJ, et al. Treatment of craniocervical instability using a posterior-only approach: report of 3 cases. J Neurosurg Spine 2014;21(2):239–48.

20. Crockard HA. Transoral surgery: some lessons learned. Br J Neurosurg 1995;9(3):283–93.

21. Burke K, Benet A, Aghi MK, et al. Impact of platybasia and anatomic variance on surgical approaches to the craniovertebral junction. Laryngoscope 2014;124(8):1760–6.

22. Seker A, Inoue K, Osawa S, et al. Comparison of endoscopic transnasal and transoral approaches to the craniovertebral junction. World Neurosurg 2010;74:583–602.

23. Baird CJ, Conway JE, Sciubba DM, et al. Radiographic and anatomic basis of endoscopic anterior craniocervical decompression: a comparison of endonasal, transoral, and transcervical approaches. Neurosurgery 2009;65(Suppl 6):158–63.

24. Magrini S, Pasquini E, Mazzatenta D, et al. Endoscopic endonasal odontoidectomy in a patient affected by Down syndrome: technical case report. Neurosurgery 2008;63:E373–4.

25. El-Sayed IH, Wu JC, Dhillon N, et al. The importance of platybasia and the palatine line in patient selection for endonasal surgery of the craniocervical junction: a radiographic study of 12 patients. World Neurosurg 2011;76:183–8.

26. Van Abel KM, Mallory GW, Kasperbauer JL, et al. Transnasal odontoid resection: is there an anatomic explanation for differing swallowing outcomes? Neurosurg Focus 2014;37(4):E16.

Chordomas: A Review

Bernard George, MD[a], Damien Bresson, MD[a], Philippe Herman, MD[b],
Sébastien Froelich, MD[a],*

KEYWORDS

- Chordomas • Endonasal approach • Proton beam therapy

KEY POINTS

- There has been progress in the understanding of chordomas (CHs), but it remains a challenging lesion to treat and a deadly tumor.
- Positive diagnosis is no more an issue with the use of immunohistology markers such as brachyury.
- A marker of the biological behavior of each CH is still needed in order to be able to adjust the treatment strategy to the aggressiveness of the tumor.
- Radical resection at first presentation should be applied on all CHs because the extent of resection is the best prognostic factor.
- Complementary proton therapy irrespective of the quality of resection is now routinely proposed even if its efficacy is not clearly demonstrated in every case, especially in case of incomplete resection.
- The future of CH treatment is certainly related to a better understanding of the molecular biology and oncogenesis of CHs and consequently to the development of efficient targeted chemotherapies.

INTRODUCTION

CHs are tumors that have a benign histopathology but exhibit aggressive clinical behavior with invasive and metastatic potential. CHs are challenging tumors to treat, and there are still many questions especially about their optimum treatment. In the best cases, recurrence is delayed, but it is inevitable after 10 or 20 years. However, important improvements have been made over the past decade. First, with the advances of new techniques such as endoscopic endonasal approach (EEA) of skull base (SB) CH, the extent of surgical resection has improved, which has tremendous importance because complete tumor removal is still the most important prognostic factor. Second, complementary targeted chemotherapy is being developed based on a better knowledge of the

signaling pathways involved in the oncogenesis of CHs.

DEFINITION

CHs are gelatinous (jellylike), grayish, and more or less encapsulated and infiltrative tumors originating from extradural vestiges of the notochord (NC). The NC is the primary axis of the embryo along which are organized the neuraxis, the spinal axis, and the SB up to the dorsum sellae.[1] The NC runs from the sacrum (S) all along the spine, across the vertebral bodies up to the odontoid process and the lower clivus where it crosses the bone (mediobasal canal) to reach the pharynx; it then runs into the pharyngeal soft tissues, in front of the clivus to its upper limit where it crosses again the bone and ends its course at the top of the

[a] Department of Neurosurgery, Hôpital LARIBOISIERE, Assistance Publique – Hôpitaux de Paris, Université Paris Diderot, 2 rue Ambroise Paré, Paris 75475, France; [b] ENT Department, Hôpital LARIBOISIERE, Assistance Publique – Hôpitaux de Paris, Université Paris Diderot, 2 rue Ambroise Paré, Paris 75475, France
* Corresponding author.
E-mail address: sebastien.froelich@lrb.aphp.fr

Neurosurg Clin N Am 26 (2015) 437–452
http://dx.doi.org/10.1016/j.nec.2015.03.012
1042-3680/15/$ – see front matter © 2015 Elsevier Inc. All rights reserved.

dorsum sellae (**Fig. 1**). The NC starts to regress on the sixth or seventh week and completely disappears during the first years of life. The last remnant of the NC is the nucleus pulposus of the intervertebral disks, but it cannot be considered as a possible origin of CHs. In fact, intervertebral disks are never involved in CHs even in the case of multiple vertebrae invasion. Moreover, CHs are found in structures without disks such as the clivus or the S. Therefore the last remnants must be distinguished from the vestiges of NC, the latter being the only true origin of CHs. One of these vestiges is well known and was discovered by Luschka[2] (1856) and Virchow[3] (1857); it first was erroneously called ecchondrosis physaliphora because it was supposed to be of cartilaginous origin. The origin of this vestige from the NC was established by Muller[4] in 1858 and linked to CHs only in 1895 by Ribbert.[5] Since then, it is named ecchordosis physaliphora (EP). The EP is a small (<1 cm) round mass located behind the clivus (sometimes connected to it by a pedicle) in the prepontine area and observed in 0.4% to 2% of the cases at autopsy[6,7] or on MRI (**Fig. 2**).[8] Another likely vestige is called benign notochord cell tumor (BNCT); it is most commonly described in vertebral bodies and sometimes in association with true CHs.[9,10] Yamaguchi and colleagues[11] found 20 BNCTs in different locations from 100 autopsies. BNCTs present on MRI as noninvasive and nondestructive nodular lesions with signal similar to that of CHs on T1 and T2 sequences but without contrast enhancement. EP and BNCT are generally asymptomatic or only associated with local pain (**Table 1**).

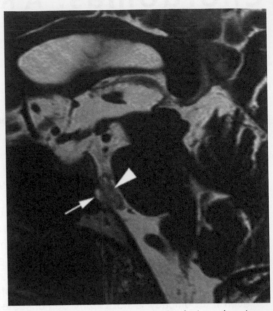

Fig. 2. T2 MRI sequence in sagittal view showing a prepontine EP connected to the clivus. *Arrow* indicates the part of the lesion into the clivus. *Arrowhead* indicates prepontine EP.

POSITIVE DIAGNOSIS

CHs exhibit particular but not specific features on computed tomography and MRI (**Figs. 3 and 4**)[12,13]: essentially destructive and invasive aspects with hyposignal in T1 sequences, hypersignal in T2 sequences, and contrast enhancement. Rather than calcifications, bony remnants can be seen inside the tumors (**Fig. 5**).

Histology is also particular with largely vacuolated cells called physaliphora cells surrounded by a myxoid matrix. There are 3 histologic types of CHs: classical, chondroid with a partially chondroid matrix, and dedifferentiated (or sarcomatous). In the dedifferentiated type, there are areas with classic features of CHs and other parts with features of sarcomas.

CHs are mainly confused with chondrosarcomas on radiologic diagnosis, which have similar radiological features but harbor more frequently true calcifications. Histologic aspects may also be confusing, but nowadays, immunohistology allows a clear differentiation. The most specific and sensitive markers are cytokeratins and brachyury. Brachyury is a protein linked with a specific gene locus (6q27) and is an intranuclear transcription factor without which the development of the NC is abnormal.[14] Brachyury is always found in any tissue or lesion that is derived from the NC including CHs, EP, and BNCTs, as well as in the

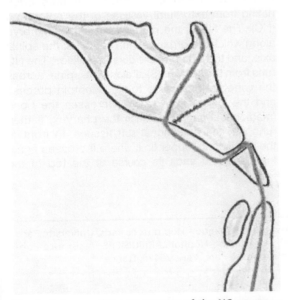

Fig. 1. Scheme of the upper part of the NC course.

Table 1
Main characteristics of notochordal entities

Entity	Localization	Most Frequent Symptoms	Size	IRM TDM	Histo	Evolution
EP	Intradural prepontine	None	<1 cm	Contrast = 0	Matrix myxoid = 0 Brachyury +	None
CH ID	Prepontine (56%)	Focal (localization)	>1 cm	Contrast = +	Matrix myxoid = + Brachyury +	Little
BNCT	Intra osseous	None	Small	Contrast = 0 Bone lysis = 0	Matrix myxoid = 0 Brachyury +	Little or none
CH extra-axial	Bone + soft tissue	Mass + Pain	Various	Contrast = +	Matrix myxoid= + Brachyury +	Little
Parachordoma	Bone + soft tissue	Mass + Pain	Various	Contrast = +	Brachyury 0	Little
CH	Bone + extraosseous	Focal (localization)	>5 cm	Contrast = + Bone lysis = +	Matrix myxoid = + Brachyury +	Recurrences and metastases

NC itself. However, it is not found in the nucleus pulposus. This protein is also present in hemangioblastomas and in few testicular tumors. Brachyury may also be present in some tumors called parachordomas, that are very similar to CHs but located outside of the NC axis, most commonly in the limbs. In the last literature review by Clabeaux and colleagues[15] (2008), 45 cases were reported located in any part of the body. However, Tirabosco and colleagues[16] (2008) found only 10 cases positive for brachyury and suggested to call them extra-axial CHs. Only brachyury-negative tumors should be named parachordomas; they have been included by the World Health Organization in the group of mixed tumors and myoepitheliomas.[17]

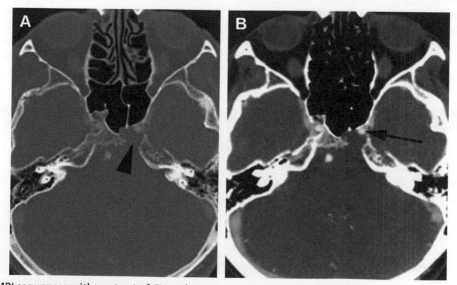

Fig. 3. T1 MRI sequences with contrast of CH at the craniocervical junction (*A*) and at the upper clivus (*B*). *Arrow* indicates the part of the lesion into the clivus. *Arrowhead* indicates prepontine EP.

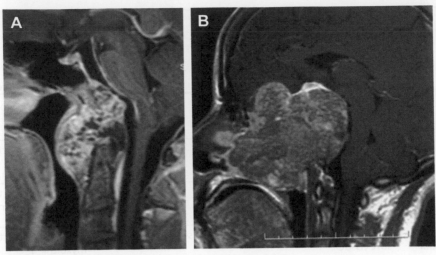

Fig. 4. (*A, B*) Computed tomographic axial views of a small clival CH.

Tests for brachyury yield positive results homogeneously in every part of a CH, except in the sarcomatous part of the dedifferentiated CHs.

EPIDEMIOLOGY

CHs account for 1.4% of all primary malignant bone tumors, 0.4% of all intracranial tumors,[18,19] 0.2% of SB tumors,[20] and 17% of primary bone tumors of the spine, most commonly at the C1-C2 level.[21]

In an American register (McMaster and colleagues[22]) collecting 400 cases over 22 years, CHs were observed in 0.8 of 1,000,000 people and were equally distributed between the three most frequent location of chordomas: 29.2% in the S, 32% in the SB, and 32.8% in the mobile spine (MS) (**Figs. 6** and **7**); SB location is more frequent in females (39%). CH occurs predominantly in males (60%), and the median age is

58.5 years. Patients with SB CHs are younger than those with S and MS CHs (49 vs 69 years).

PARTICULAR FORMS

The course of the NC explains that CHs can be observed in the pharynx without any bone involvement. On the contrary, location away from the midline can only be explained by an NC forking[1]; jugular foramen location has been reported in 9 cases and location in Meckel cave has been reported in 5.[23]

Most CHs are located extradurally at least at the beginning of their evolution (**Fig. 8**); after some time, they may rupture the dura and extend into the intradural (ID) space (**Fig. 9**); ID CHs often remain subdural, and true subarachnoid extension and even pia mater infiltration are rare and occur more frequently at the time of recurrence. Some rare CHs are initially located in the ID space mostly

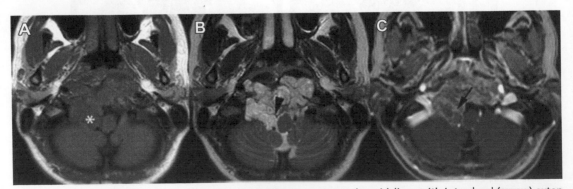

Fig. 5. Axial T1 (*A*), T2 (*B*), and T1 with contrast (*C*) MRI sequences at the midclivus with intradural (*arrow*) extension, Hyposignal T1 zone (*asterik*), Hyposignal septa (*arrowhead*).

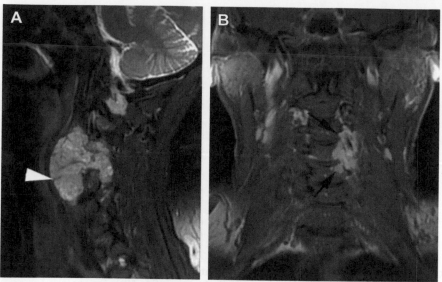

Fig. 6. Sagittal (*A*) and coronal (*B*) T1 (*A*) and T2 (*B*) MRI sequences of a cervical spine CH. *Arrows* indicate the part of the lesion into the clivus. *Arrowhead* indicates prepontine EP.

in the prepontine area but this is not the only location. In the literature, 34 ID cases were reported: 19 prepontine, 6 in the sellar region, 2 in the foramen magnum, 1 in the cerebellopontine angle, 1 in the Meckel cave, 4 cervical, and 1 thoracic.[23] When they are small, these ID CHs may be confused with EP; like any proliferative CH, ID CHs show contrast enhancement on MRI and have a myxoid matrix, whereas EP do not (as well as BNCTs). However, both yield positive results for brachyury (see **Table 1**).

CHs located inside the brain parenchyma were also observed in 4 cases, 1 hypothalamic, 1 cerebellar, 1 pineal, and 1 on both sides of the tentorium.[23] However, in these old reports, there is no immunohistological study.

FAMILIAL FORMS AND ASSOCIATIONS

Eleven families presenting with at least 2 CHs in the family (46 cases) have been reported.[24] CHs were most commonly located in the SB. Several

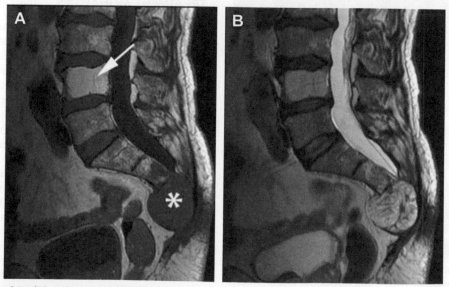

Fig. 7. Sagittal T1 (*A*) and T2 (*B*) MRI sequences of a sacral CH. Hyposignal T1 zone (*Asterik*), Hyposignal septa (*arrow*).

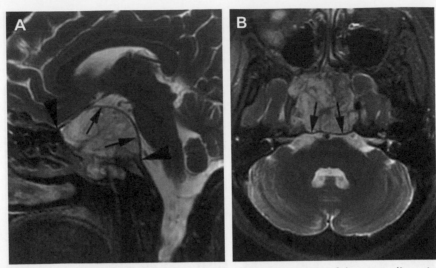

Fig. 8. Sagittal (*A*) and axial (*B*) T2 MRI sequences of an entirely extradural CH of the upper clivus. *Arrows* indicate the part of the lesion into the clivus. *Arrowheads* indicate prepontine EP.

studies showed mutations in different genes; the most convincing study found an alteration of the locus 6q27 (the brachyury locus) with the same modification being observed in all affected members in 4 of 7 families.[25,26]

Several associations of CHs with another pathologic condition have been described. Tuberous Sclerosis Complex (TSC) is the most interesting

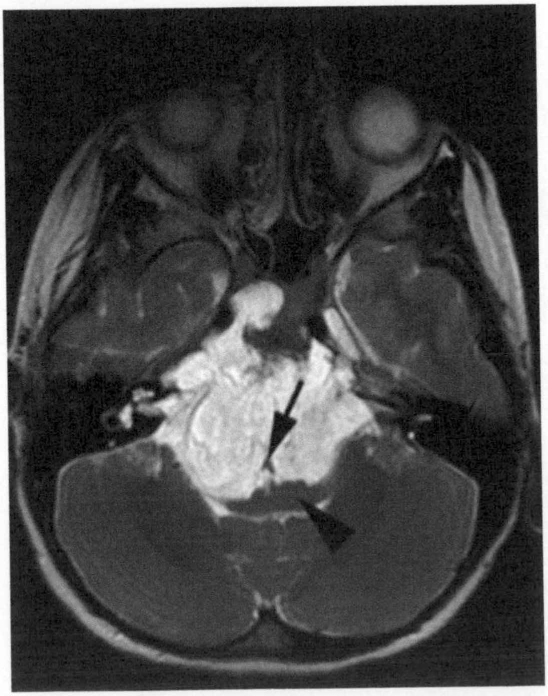

Fig. 9. Axial T2 MRI sequence of a clival CH with intradural extension (*arrowhead*); notice the displacement and the encasement of the basilar trunk. Basilar artery embedded into the tumor (*arrow*).

because this disease is due to inactivation of a suppressor gene that induces activation of mammalian target of rapamycin (mTOR) (transduction factor) and so stimulates tumor growth and proliferation.[27] In the 10 published cases,[28] the mean age was very less (6.2 months), there were 4 sacral CHs, and the prognosis was rather good (83% survival at 5 years).

Associations with Ollier disease, Maffucci syndrome,[29,30] and Crohn disease[31] suggest a gene modification but only a few cases have been published. Association with sellar pathologies (Rathke cleft cyst and Cushing syndrome)[32,33] may be explained by the course of NC that ends at this level.

TREATMENT MODALITIES

Surgery is the most efficient treatment because complete resection remains the most important prognostic factor. Considering the midline location of CH and the initial bone and extradural location, anterior approaches that do not cross the cranial nerves (CNs) and vessels are the most logical and should be favored. For long, transoral, transsphenoidal, and transfacial routes were used. Nowadays, EEAs are supplanting all of them.[34,35] Using the endoscope, it is possible to reach any part of the clivus from the dorsum sellae (with pituitary transposition) to its lower tip and even the craniocervical junction (CCJ). Lateral limits of the approach are venous structures (cavernous sinus and jugular bulb), CNs and arteries (carotid and vertebral arteries). However, it is now possible for experienced teams to reach the lateral SB and to control and work around these vessels and CNs with an acceptable risk. Micro-Doppler and neuronavigation are mandatory in those situations as well as in recurrent CHs. Monitoring of the CNs, especially the sixth and twelfth, also brings safety in the surgical resection. Balloon occlusion tests (BOTs) may also be a safe preoperative option, leading occasionally to a preoperative or intraoperative occlusion. In the authors' experience,[23] BOT was performed in 40 cases (33%) and the carotid and vertebral arteries were occluded, respectively, in 5 and 11 cases without complications (**Table 2**). One of the main issue with endoscopic techniques is the dural closure in case of ID extension (more than 50% of the authors' 128 cases). Recurrent cases are even more challenging to close because the nasoseptal flap that is the keystone of a successful closure may not be available anymore. In these recurrences, previous radiation therapy also increases the risk of cerebrospinal fluid (CSF) leak. If no other option for closure is available, the temporoparietal fascia flap can be a life-saving option for the patient. Despite recent improvements in closure techniques, the rate of postoperative CSF leak is still around 10%.

In case of lateral extension, EEA can be combined during the same or in a separate stage with transcranial approaches (**Figs. 10** and **11**) such as Dolenc transcavernous approach, subtemporal approach, anterior and/or posterior transpetrosal approaches, and CCJ anterolateral or posterolateral approaches (far and extreme lateral). Combination of 2 or more surgical approaches was used in 29.5% of the authors' cases (see **Table 2**). In addition to the surgical resection, a craniocervical fixation may be needed (28 of 47 CCJ CHs).[23] Whether the surgical strategy is with 1 or several approaches or in 1 or 2 stages, it is often a severe burden for the patient. In the authors' series, there was no mortality and a significant improvement of CN deficits, essentially oculomotor (54 preoperative vs 11 postoperative) and visual deficits (15 vs 6), was

observed. At the level of the CCJ, 17 patients had a preoperative lower CN palsy (14, 11, and 10 CNs IX, X, and XI palsies, respectively) and 28 had a CN XII palsy. Postoperatively, 15 patients had a lower CN palsy (15, 15, and 1 CNs IX, X, and XI palsies, respectively) and 6 had a permanent CN XII palsy. These lower CN deficits needed 14 tracheostomies and 7 gastrostomies. Besides these CN deficits, which improved with time in most cases, other complications were observed including 2 cases of stroke (perforating artery occlusions), 5 cases of permanent motor deficits, 5 cases of new Horner syndrome, and 16 cases of meningitis.[23]

The surgical strategy in CH must be as radical a resection as possible at first presentation.[36] However, in every series there are a large number of secondary patients (referred after recurrence or after an incomplete resection).[37,38] In secondary patients, who account for 36% of the authors' patients[23] (see **Table 2**), surgery is more difficult, associated with a higher morbidity and a higher rate of incomplete resection.

Complementary treatments include radiotherapy and chemotherapy.

A variety of radiation modalities have been used for CHs: fractionated radiotherapy, gamma knife, cyberknife, and hadrontherapy (proton and carbon ion). Their roles and efficiencies are discussed later in the article.

Targeted chemotherapy is an upcoming treatment modality based on the recent advances in the understanding of the molecular event involved in the oncogenesis of CHs.[39,40] Transformation into a tumoral cell is because of the activation of a cascade of factors from the cell surface into it (transduction) and then into the nucleus (transcription). The most important factors at the cell surface are the tyrosine kinase receptors (RTKs). To date 58 RTKs have been identified. RTKs are activated by different ligands, mostly growth factors; the

Table 2
Lariboisière series

	Total	Clivus	CCJ	Cervical Spine
Number	128	58	47	23
Age (y)	43	46	36	44
ID/ED (%)	53	65	49	27
Secondary patients (%)	36	23	45	57
Combined approaches (%)	29.5	32.5	25.5	26
BOT (occlusion)	40 (16)	18 (5 ICA)	18 (6 VA)	4 (5 VA)
RxTT (Proton), %	81 (79)	79 (93)	86 (68.5)	79 (60)

Abbreviations: ED, Extradural; ICA, Internal carotid artery; ID, Intradural; (Proton), N proton/N Radiotherapy; RxTT, radiotherapy; VA, Vertebral artery.

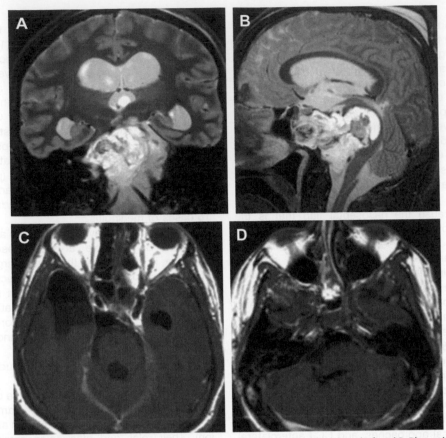

Fig. 10. CH of the upper clivus with ID and intrapontine extension before (*A, B*) and after (*C, D*) surgical resection through 3 approaches: (1) subtemporal approach, (2) posterolateral approach of the CCJ, and (3) endoscopic endonasal approach.

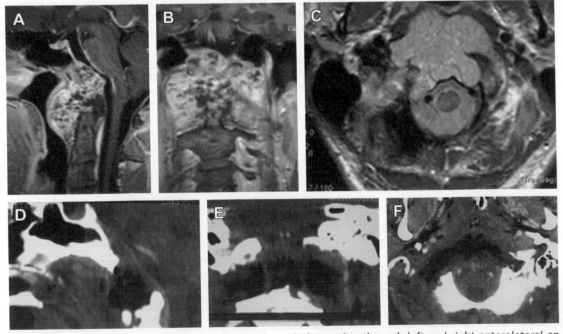

Fig. 11. CH of the CCJ before (*A–C*) and after (*D–F*) surgical resection through left and right anterolateral approaches followed by a posterior fixation.

most important are the platelet-derived growth factor (PDGF), the epidermal growth factor (EGF), and the transforming growth factor. These activated RTKs in turn activate different chains of transduction factors. Some of the most important are PI3K, ATK, and mTOR; the renin-angiotensin system; and the signal transducer and activator of transcription 3. All these chains of factors lead to activation of growth and proliferation; their disregulation may be caused by several mechanisms such as genetic mutation (eg, TSC genes), or overexpression of RTK ligands. At present, several inhibitors of these factors can be used against tumors and especially CHs. The most commonly used are inhibitors of the PDGF receptor (imatinib) or of the EGF receptor (cetuximab, gefitinib, erlotinib) and the inhibitor of mTOR (sirolimus). Several studies have been published, but they are mostly small series of CHs that recurred after other treatments (surgery and radiotherapy).[41–45] Until now, the benefit of such targeted therapies remains limited with at least 2 main explanations. One is the activation of other RTKs when one RTK is blocked by an inhibitor; another explanation in case of mTOR inhibition is a negative feedback with activation of the upstream factors and the deviation toward another chain of factors. Anyway, these studies raise a lot of hope in the treatment of CHs. Moreover, an inhibitor of brachyury has already been tested in vitro with good results. It is very likely that targeted chemotherapy will be used in the future as a complementary postoperative treatment or as a preoperative neoadjuvant treatment to reduce tumor size and to facilitate surgical resection.

Classical chemotherapy has almost no effect on CHs; however, repetitive direct intratumoral injections of chemotherapy were shown to slow down for some time the tumoral progression.[46,47]

PROGNOSIS

From the Surveillance, Epidemiology, and End Results program[22] in which 84% of the patients were treated by surgery with or without radiotherapy and 13% by radiotherapy only, the average length of survival is 6.29 years; it is longer, but not significantly, in females than in males (7.25 vs 5.93 years) and in SB than in MS location (6.94 vs 5.88 years). Overall survival (OS) is 67.6% at 5 years, 39.9% at 10 years, and 13.1% at 20 years.

In children, the prognosis is better[48–50] with an OS of 80% at 5 years and 60% at 10 years. However, in children younger than 5 years, the prognosis is much worse with 30% survival at 2 years because of a high number (65%) of atypical (more or less similar to dedifferentiated) forms in which survival is 0% at 6.6 months. In the Mayo Clinic series,[50] all the sacral CHs are atypical with a very short survival.

Metastases may occur but seem not to affect the length of survival. Metastases occur everywhere in the body but most commonly in the lungs, lymphatic nodes, bones, and subcutaneous tissues (Fig. 12). The delay of occurrence is 6 years on an average. Metastases are more frequently observed after a recurrence but may be found at the time of diagnosis or only at autopsy. CHs of the S are more likely to metastasize than those of the SB (73% vs 9%).[51,52]

There are 3 different types of seeding. The most frequent one (as much as 10%) is along the surgical pathways and especially during transphenoidal approach, transfacial approach, or EEA.[53,54]

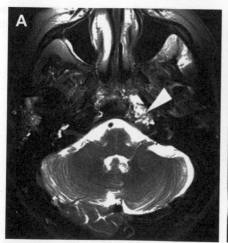 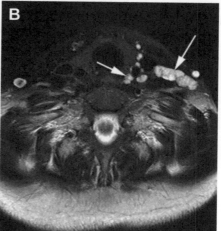

Fig. 12. (*A, B*) Small CH of the junction of the clivus and cerebellopontine angle with multiple lymph nodes metastases at the time of diagnosis. *Arrows* indicate the part of the lesion into the clivus. *Arrowhead* indicates prepontine EP.

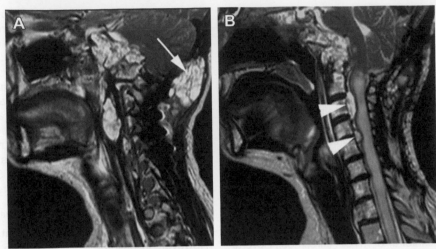

Fig. 13. (*A, B*) Second recurrence of a CH of the CCJ with surgical seeding in the upper neck (*arrow*) and 2 cervical localizations (*arrowheads*) away from the primary site.

Another way of seeding is along the subarachnoid spaces, obviously in cases of CHs with ID extension. Seeding is generally along the spinal cord, especially at the level of the conus and cauda equina (**Fig. 13**).[23] The last way of seeding is along a ventriculoperitoneal shunt; one case of pineal CH treated by radiotherapy and ventricular shunt was diagnosed after a seeding in the abdomen.[55]

FACTORS OF PROGNOSIS

In every published series including that of the authors (136 cases over 20 years: 58 clival, 47 CCJ, 28 cervical, and 8 sacral), it is striking to notice that some CHs recur and die in less than 2 years whatever be done and some others have a progression-free survival (PFS) of more than 10

or even 20 years. It seems that the biological behavior of each CH is quite different. This fact is quite clear in the authors' series, and 2 groups of patients can be distinguished: before 5 years, there is a sharp decline in the proportion of patients without disease progression and after 5 years the OS and PFS curves are almost horizontal (**Fig. 14**). Unfortunately, until now, no clinical, radiologic, or biological marker has been found to differentiate these 2 groups and hence it is not possible to adjust the aggressiveness of the treatment to the aggressiveness of each CH.

Analyzing all available publications, only 3 prognostic factors can be drawn: incomplete resection, secondary patients (after recurrence), and dedifferentiated forms.

Dedifferentiated forms that include sectors with sarcomatous features recur, metastasize, and

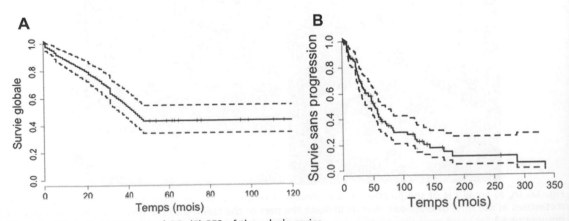

Fig. 14. (*A*) Actuarial curves of OS; (*B*) PFS of the whole series.

lead to the death of the patient in less than 1 year whatever is done.[56–58] These forms are observed at first presentation or more often secondarily after one or several recurrences.[59] It has been suggested that radiotherapy could induce these secondary transformations, but this has not been proven until now. Dedifferentiated forms have the same radiological aspects as classical CHs. However, it has been mentioned[60] that sarcomatous sectors may show hyposignal (instead of hypersignal) on T2 MRI sequences. It is worth noting that test for brachyury yields positive result in the typical CH feature sectors but negative result in the sarcomatous ones.

PFS of secondary patients referred after a recurrence is always shorter than the that of primary patients even if radical resection and complementary radiotherapy can be achieved. This fact is clearly established in all published series.[23,37,38] In the study by Di Maio and colleagues,[37] 95 patients were separated into 2 groups: group 1 with 56 patients treated between 1988 and 1999 and group 2 with 39 patients treated between 2000 and 2011. Best results were obtained in group 2. The investigators suggested that progresses in the surgical technique associated with radiotherapy in every patient and not only in those with incomplete resection explain these better results. However, they also mention a proportion of 66% of secondary patients in group 1 and only 39% in group 2. In the study by Wu and colleagues[38] (N = 79), the rate of recurrence at 5 years is 10% after complete resection and about 45% after partial or subtotal resection. In the authors' series (N = 136), the actuarial curve shows a highly significant statistical difference (P = .0001) of the PFS between primary and secondary patients (Fig. 15). In fact, all the largest series of CHs underline the same major problem in the analysis of the results obtained in the treatment of CHs: they are inhomogeneous,

including different locations of CH, primary and secondary patients, and different treatment modalities (surgery and radiotherapy). It is, therefore, difficult to draw valuable conclusions from such studies; dividing series in subgroups of patients seems to be a good work-around solution but leads to a very small number of cases. Therefore, meta-analysis seems to be the best way to obtain more or less useful conclusions. There are 2 main meta-analyses in the literature. Di Maio[61] collected 807 cases of CHs from 11 centers published between 1999 and 2009. Treatment was surgery followed by radiotherapy in case of incomplete resection. The rate of complete resection varied from 0% to 73%. Follow-up was 53.6 months on an average. OS at 5 and 10 years were, respectively, 70% and 63%, and rates of PFS were 54% and 26%, respectively. OS after complete resection was 95% versus 53% after partial resection. In case of incomplete resection, the 5-year rate of recurrence is multiplied by 3.83 and the 5-year rate of death by 5.85. Jian and colleagues[62,63] published 2 meta-analyses with contradictory results in 2010 and 2011. In the first study of 760 patients, they found a better prognosis of chondroid versus classical CHs (P = .0001) and of surgery combined with radiotherapy versus surgery alone (P = .0001). On the contrary, in their second study of 560 cases of CHs, no statistically significant difference was found between chondroid and classical CHs and between different types of treatment.

The extent of resection is in all studies is the main prognostic factor. In the series of sacral CHs, there is often a difference between total en bloc and marginal resection.[51,64,65] Ruggieri[64] gives a rate of 17% recurrence after en bloc resection and 71% to 81% after any other type of resection. Fuchs and colleagues[65] observed only 1 recurrence of 21 cases with radical resection and

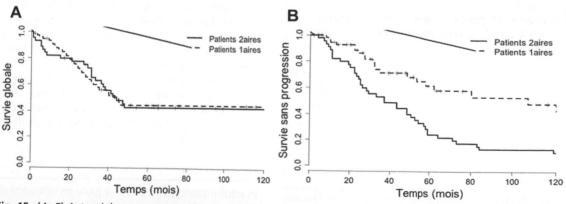

Fig. 15. (A, B) Actuarial curves comparing OS and PFS of primary and secondary patients.

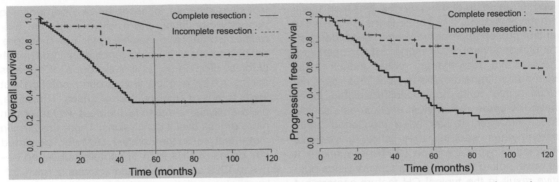

Fig. 16. Actuarial curves comparing OS and PFS in patients with complete and incomplete surgical resection.

22 of 31 with incomplete resection. These investigators do not carry out any complementary radiotherapy in case of en bloc resection. Obviously, these en bloc resections may have a higher cost in terms of sphincter disturbances. En bloc resection can also be achieved in some MS CHs involving only vertebral bodies.[66–68] However, series of MS CHs are very small or combine, for instance, cervical and CCJ locations.[69,70] At the level of the SB, en bloc resection cannot be achieved; piecemeal removal is the rule, with the goal of complete resection with no visible remnant on postoperative MRI. In the authors' series,[23] OS and PFS are clearly different between complete and incomplete resection (**Fig. 16**). With an average follow-up of 6.5 years in the authors' series of 136 cases, the rate of recurrence is 28%, 47.5%, and 75% and the rate of death is 20.5%, 52.5%, and 63%, respectively, after total, subtotal (>80%), and partial resection (**Table 3**).

Table 3
Lariboisière series; rate of partial, subtotal (>80%), and total resection and corresponding rate of recurrence and death

	%	Recurrence (%)	Death (%)
Partial resection	22	75	63
Subtotal resection	49	47.5	52.5
Total resection	28	28	20.5

Data from George B, Bresson D, Bouazza S, et al. Chordomas. Neurochirurgie 2014;60:1–140.

Complementary Treatment

There are some controversies about the usefulness of complementary radiotherapy. Some investigators use it only in case of postoperative remnant and some others in every case whatever be the extent of resection. Various types of radiotherapy have been used: fractionated radiotherapy, gamma knife, cyberknife, proton therapy, and carbon ion therapy. The last 2 types are generally considered as the most effective considering their powerful biological effect and the possibility of providing high treatment dose to the tumor even in close proximity to important sensitive structures. In the meta-analysis by Di Maio,[60] involving 517 patients treated by complementary radiotherapy, no statistical difference was observed in OS and PFS at 5 years between the different types of radiotherapy; at 10 years, there was a small difference in favor of carbon ion therapy. In the authors' series,[23] proton beam therapy was applied as often as possible (70% of the cases); on actuarial curves, for SB and CCJ CHs, surgery followed by proton beam therapy proved to be beneficial for OS and PFS ($P = .04$ and .03) but not for the whole series ($P = .05$ and .29) (**Fig. 17**). An important point was also found: combining complete resection and proton beam therapy seemed to significantly improve OS and PFS compared with incomplete resection with or without proton therapy ($P = .01$ and .003) (**Fig. 18**); at 6.5 years follow-up, the rate of recurrence is 26% versus 50% and the rate of death is 7% versus 50%.

Other Factors

In adult patients, age and sex have no influence on the results. In children, prognosis is better except

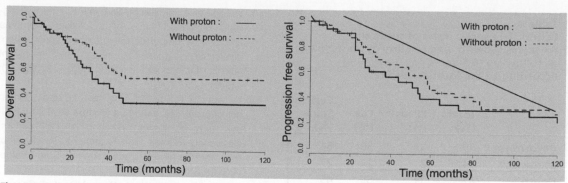

Fig. 17. Actuarial curves comparing OS and PFS in patients treated with and without proton. The axis indicates Global survival and time (month).

for children younger than 5 years in whom the prognosis is much worse.

Location seems to influence the prognosis. In the authors' series,[23,70] the delay before recurrence and death is much longer in SB CHs than in CCJ and cervical locations; the rates of recurrence, metastasis, and death are also lower in SB CHs (**Table 4**). Considering the SB, there is clearly a better prognosis in SB than in CCJ CHs, while the rates of total (25%), subtotal (50%), and partial (25%) resection are very similar.

SUMMARY

Progress has been made in understanding CHs, but they remain challenging lesions to treat and

deadly tumors. Positive diagnosis is no more an issue with the use of immunohistology markers such as brachyury. Location has some influence on the prognosis, and CCJ and cervical spine locations have a worse prognosis than the SB location. However, a marker of the biological behavior of each CH is still needed in order to be able to adjust the treatment strategy to the aggressiveness of the tumor. Radical resection at first presentation should be applied on all CHs because the extent of resection is the best prognostic factor. Complementary proton therapy irrespective of the quality of resection is now routinely proposed even if its efficacy is not clearly demonstrated in every case, especially in case of incomplete resection. The future of CH treatment is certainly related to a better understanding of

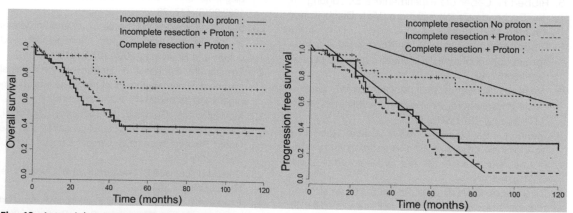

Fig. 18. Actuarial curves comparing OS and PFS in patients treated with complete resection and proton versus incomplete resection with or without proton.

Table 4
Lariboisière series; rates of recurrence, metastasis, death, and stability or no remnant at follow-up (6.5 years on an average) according to the locations of CHs

	Total (%)	Clivus (%)	CCJ (%)	Cervical Spine (%)
Recurrence	49.5	37	39	64
Metastasis	14	2	24	27
Death	47	39	59	45
Stable or no remnant	65	67	54.5	77

Data from George B, Bresson D, Bouazza S, et al. Chordomas. Neurochirurgie 2014;60:1–140.

the molecular biology and oncogenesis of CHs and consequently to the development of efficient targeted chemotherapies.

REFERENCES

1. Salisbury JR, Deverell MH, Cookson MJ, et al. Three dimensional reconstruction of human embryonic notochords: clue to the pathogenesis of chordoma. J Pathol 1993;171:59–62.
2. Luschka H. Die Altersveranderungen der Zwischenwirbelknorpel. Virchows Arch (Path Anat) 1856;9: 311–27.
3. Virchow R. Untersuchungen ueber die Entwicklung des Schaedelgrundes im gesunden und krankhaften Zustande und uber den Einfluss derselben auf Schadelform, Gesichtsbildung und Gehirnban. Berlin: G. Reimer 1857:47.
4. Muller H. Ueber das Vorkommen von Resten der Chorda dorsalis bei Menschen nach der Geburt und uber ihr Verhaltniss zu den Gallertgeschwulsten am Clivus. Zeitschrift fur ration. Medic 1858;2:202–29.
5. Ribbert H. Ueber die experimentelle Erzeugung einer Ecchondrosis physaliphora. Verh Dtsch Kongr Inn Med 1895;13:455–64.
6. Ribbert H, Steiner H. Uber die Ecchondrosis physaliphora sphenooccipitalis. Zentralbl Allg Pathol Anat 1894;5:457–61.
7. Wyatt RB, Schochet SS Jr, McCormick WF. Ecchordosis physaliphora. An electron microscopic study. J Neurosurg 1971;34(5):672–7.
8. Mehnert F, Beschorner R, Küker W, et al. Retroclival ecchordosis physaliphora: MR imaging and review of the literature. AJNR Am J Neuroradiol 2004; 25(10):1851–5.
9. Deshpande V, Nielsen GP, Rosenthal DI, et al. Intraosseous benign notochord cell tumors (BNCT): further evidence supporting a relationship to chordoma. Am J Surg Pathol 2007;31(10):1573–7.
10. Yamaguchi T, Yamato M, Saotome K. First histologically confirmed case of a classic chordoma arising in a precursor benign notochordal lesion: differential diagnosis of benign and malignant notochordal lesions. Skeletal Radiol 2002;31(7): 413–8.
11. Yamaguchi T, Suzuki S, Ishikawa H, et al. Benign notochordal cell tumors: a comparative histological study of benign notochordal cell tumors, classic chordomas, and notochordal vestiges of fetal intervertebral discs. Am J Surg Pathol 2004;28(6):756–61.
12. Meyers SP, Hirsch WL Jr, Curtin HD, et al. Chordomas of the skull base: MR features. AJNR Am J Neuroradiol 1992;13(6):1627–36.
13. Sze G, Uichanco LS 3rd, Brant-Zawadzki MN, et al. Chordomas: MR imaging. Radiology 1988;166(1 Pt 1):187–91.
14. Vujovic S, Henderson S, Presneau N, et al. Brachyury, a crucial regulator of notochordal development, is a novel biomarker for chordomas. J Pathol 2006;209(2):157–65.
15. Clabeaux J, Hojnowski L, Valente A. Case report: parachordoma of soft tissues of the arm. Clin Orthop Relat Res 2008;466(5):1251–6.
16. Tirabosco R, Mangham DC, Rosenberg AE, et al. Brachyury expression in extra-axial skeletal and soft tissue Chordomas: a marker that distinguishes chordoma from mixed tumor/Myoepithelioma/Parachordoma in soft tissue. Am J Surg Pathol 2008; 32(4):572–80.
17. Kilpatrick SE, Limon J. Mixed tumour/myoepithelium/parachordoma. In: Fischer CD, Unni KK, Mertens F, editors. World Health Organization classification of tumours: pathology and genetics of tumour of soft tissue and bone. Lyon (France): Iarc Press; 2002. p. 198–9.
18. Dahlin DC, Maccarty CS. Chordoma. Cancer 1952; 5(6):1170–8.
19. Healey JH, Lane JM. Chordoma: a critical review of diagnosis and treatment. Orthop Clin North Am 1989;20(3):417–26.
20. Samii A, Gerganov VM, Herold C, et al. Chordomas of the skull base: surgical management and outcome. J Neurosurg 2007;107(2):319–24.
21. Fuentes JM, Benezech J. Strategy of the surgical treatment of primary tumors of the spine. Neurochirurgie 1989;35(5):323–7, 352. [in French].
22. McMaster ML, Goldstein AM, Bromley CM, et al. Chordoma: incidence and survival patterns in the United States, 1973–1995. Cancer Causes Control 2001;12(1):1–11.
23. George B, Bresson D, Bouazza S, et al. Chordomas. Neurochirurgie 2014;60:1–140.
24. Bhadra AK, Casey AT. Familial chordoma. A report of two cases. J Bone Joint Surg Br 2006;88(5): 634–6.

25. Yang C, Schwab JH, Schoenfeld AJ, et al. A novel target for treatment of chordoma: signal transducers and activators of transcription 3. Mol Cancer Ther 2009;8(9):2597–605.

26. Yang XH, Ng D, Alcorta DA, et al. T (Brachyury) gene duplication confers major susceptibility to familial chordoma. Nat Genet 2009;41(11):1176–8.

27. Ma XM, Blenis J. Molecular mechanisms of mTOR-mediated translational control. Nat Rev Mol Cell Biol 2009;10:307–18.

28. McMaster ML, Goldstein AM, Parry DM. Clinical features distinguish childhood chordoma associated with tuberous sclerosis complex (TSC) from chordoma in the general paediatric population. J Med Genet 2011;48(7):444–9.

29. Ranger A, Szymczak A. Do intracranial neoplasms differ in Ollier disease and Maffucci syndrome? An in-depth analysis of the literature. Neurosurgery 2009;65(6):1106–13.

30. Liu J, Hudkins PG, Swee RG, et al. Bone sarcomas associated with Ollier's disease. Cancer 1987; 59(7):1376–85.

31. De Jesús-Monge WE, Torres EA, Báez VM, et al. Crohn's disease associated to chordoma: a case report. P R Health Sci J 2004;23(3):233–6.

32. Li ZS, Wei MQ, Fu X, et al. Chordoma coexisting with Rathke's cleft cyst: case report and literature review. Neuropathology 2011;31(1):66–70.

33. Arita-Melzer O, Medina H, Borsotto G, et al. An ectopic adrenocorticotropic hormone syndrome caused by a sacro-coccygeal chordoma: report of a case with a slow progression. Endocr Pract 1998;4(1):37–40.

34. Koutourousiou M, Gardner PA, Tormenti MJ, et al. Endoscopic endonasal approach for resection of cranial base chordomas: outcomes and learning curve. Neurosurgery 2012;71(3):614–24.

35. Tippler M, Gardner PA, Snyderman CH, et al. Endoscopic endonasal approach for clival chordomas. Neurosurgery 2009;64(2):268–77.

36. Carpentier A, Polivka M, Blanquet A, et al. Suboccipital and cervical chordomas: the value of aggressive treatment at first presentation of the disease. J Neurosurg 2002;97(5):1070–7.

37. Di Maio S, Rostomily R, Sekhar LN. Current surgical outcomes for cranial base chordomas: cohort study of 95 patients. Neurosurgery 2012;70(6):1355–60.

38. Wu Z, Zhang J, Zhang L, et al. Prognostic factors for long-term outcome of patients with surgical resection of skull base chordomas-106 cases review in one institution. Neurosurg Rev 2010;33(4):451–6.

39. Presneau N, Shalaby A, Idowu B, et al. Potential therapeutic targets for chordoma: PI3K/AKT/TSC1/TSC2/mTOR pathway. Br J Cancer 2009;100(9):1406–14, 6002.

40. Han S, Polizzano C, Nielsen GP, et al. Aberrant hyperactivation of AKT and mammalian target of rapamycin complex 1 signaling in sporadic chordomas. Clin Cancer Res 2009;15(6):1940–6.

41. Stacchiotti S, Marrari A, Tamborini E, et al. Response to imatinib plus sirolimus in advanced chordoma. Ann Oncol 2009;20(11):1886–94.

42. Casali PG, Messina A, Stacchiotti S, et al. Imatinib mesylate in chordoma. Cancer 2004;101(9):2086–97.

43. Casali PG, Stacchiotti S, Sangalli C, et al. Chordoma [review]. Curr Opin Oncol 2007;19(4):367–70.

44. Stacchiotti S, Longhi A, Ferraresi V, et al. Phase II study of imatinib in advanced chordoma. J Clin Oncol 2012;30(9):914–20.

45. Barry JJ, Jian BJ, Sughrue ME, et al. The next step: innovative molecular targeted therapies for treatment of intracranial chordoma patients. Neurosurgery 2011;68(1):231–40.

46. Guiu S, Guiu B, Feutray S, et al. Direct intratumoral chemotherapy with carboplatin and epinephrine in a recurrent cervical chordoma: case report. Neurosurgery 2009;65(3):E629–30.

47. Guan JY, He XF, Chen Y, et al. Percutaneous intratumoral injection with pingyangmycin lipiodol emulsion for the treatment of recurrent sacrococcygeal chordomas. J Vasc Interv Radiol 2011;22(8):1216–20.

48. Borba LA, Al-Mefty O, Mrak RE, et al. Cranial chordomas in children and adolescents [review]. J Neurosurg 1996;84(4):584–91.

49. Hoch BL, Nielsen GP, Liebsch NJ, et al. Base of skull chordomas in children and adolescents: a clinicopathologic study of 73 cases. Am J Surg Pathol 2006;30(7):811–8.

50. Ridenour RV 3rd, Ahrens WA, Folpe AL, et al. Clinical and histopathologic features of chordomas in children and young adults. Pediatr Dev Pathol 2010;13(1):9–17.

51. Bergh P, Kindblom LG, Gunterberg B, et al. 5 Prognostic factors in chordoma of the sacrum and mobile spine: a study of 39 patients. Cancer 2000;88(9):2122–34.

52. Chambers PW, Schwinn CP. Chordoma. A clinicopathologic study of metastasis. Am J Clin Pathol 1979;72(5):765–76.

53. Arnautovic KI, Al-Mefty O. Surgical seeding of chordomas. J Neurosurg 2001;95(5):798–803.

54. Fischbein NJ, Kaplan MJ, Holliday RA, et al. Recurrence of clival chordoma along the surgical pathway. AJNR Am J Neuroradiol 2000;21(3):578–83.

55. Figueiredo EG, Tavares WM, Welling L, et al. Ectopic pineal chordoma. Surg Neurol Int 2011;2:145.

56. Hanna SA, Tirabosco R, Amin A, et al. Dedifferentiated chordoma: a report of four cases arising 'de novo'. J Bone Joint Surg Br 2008;90(5):652–6.

57. Meis JM, Raymond AK, Evans HL, et al. "Dedifferentiated" chordoma. A clinicopathologic and immunohistochemical study of three cases. Am J Surg Pathol 1987;11(7):516–25.

58. Morimitsu Y, Aoki T, Yokoyama K, et al. Sarcomatoid chordoma: chordoma with a massive malignant spindle-cell component. Skeletal Radiol 2000; 29(12):721–5.

59. Ikeda H, Honjo J, Sakurai H, et al. Dedifferentiated chordoma arising in irradiated sacral chordoma. Radiat Med 1997;15(2):109–11.

60. Saifuddin A, Mann BS, Mahroof S, et al. Dedifferentiated chondrosarcoma: use of MRI to guide needle biopsy. Clin Radiol 2004;59:268–72.

61. Di Maio S, Temkin N, Ramanathan D, et al. Current comprehensive management of cranial base chordomas: 10-year meta-analysis of observational studies. J Neurosurg 2011;115(6):1094–105.

62. Jian BJ, Bloch OG, Yang I, et al. Adjuvant radiation therapy and chondroid chordoma subtype are associated with a lower tumor recurrence rate of cranial chordoma. J Neurooncol 2010;98(1):101–8.

63. Jian BJ, Bloch OG, Yang I, et al. A comprehensive analysis of intracranial chordoma and survival: a systematic review. Br J Neurosurg 2011;25(4):446–53.

64. Ruggieri P, Angelini A, Ussia G, et al. Surgical margins and local control in resection of sacral chordomas. Clin Orthop Relat Res 2010;468(11): 2939–47.

65. Fuchs B, Dickey ID, Yaszemski MJ, et al. Operative management of sacral chordoma. J Bone Joint Surg Am 2005;87(10):2211–6.

66. Cloyd JM, Chou D, Deviren V, et al. En bloc resection of primary tumors of the cervical spine: report of two cases and systematic review of the literature. Spine J 2009;9(11):928–35.

67. Boriani S, Bandiera S, Biagini R, et al. Chordoma of the mobile spine: fifty years of experience. Spine (Phila Pa 1976) 2006;31(4):493–503.

68. Chou D, Acosta F Jr, Cloyd JM, et al. Parasagittal osteotomy for en bloc resection of multilevel cervical chordomas. J Neurosurg Spine 2009;10(5):397–403.

69. Choi D, Melcher R, Harms J, et al. Outcome of 132operations in 97 patients with chordomas of the craniocervical junction and upper cervical spine. Neurosurgery 2010;66(1):59–65.

70. Carpentier A, Blanquet A, George B. Suboccipital and cervical chordomas: radical resection with vertebral artery control. Neurosurg Focus 2001; 10(3):E4.

The Endoscopic Endonasal Approach for Removal of Petroclival Chondrosarcomas

Leo F.S. Ditzel Filho, MD[a], Daniel M. Prevedello, MD[a,b],*,
Ricardo L. Dolci, MD[b], Ali O. Jamshidi, MD[a],
Edward E. Kerr, MD[a], Raewyn Campbell, MD[b],
Bradley A. Otto, MD[a,b], Ricardo L. Carrau, MD[a,b]

KEYWORDS

• Endonasal • Endoscopic • Chondrosarcoma • Petroclival • Skull base

KEY POINTS

- Skull base chondrosarcomas are locally aggressive and arise from the petroclival synchondrosis to involve multiple surrounding regions.
- Despite local aggressiveness, they often "respect" the dura, displacing rather than transgressing it like other skull base malignancies.
- Although the dura is often intact at the end of tumor resection, elevating a vascularized nasoseptal flap is still a key portion of the procedure to protect the exposed internal carotid artery (ICA).
- A standard wide transsphenoidal approach is coupled with other modules of the expanded endoscopic endonasal approaches, according to tumor characteristics.
- From its main component in the petroclival synchondrosis, the tumor may be "followed" into the cavernous sinus, Meckel's cave, the middle and posterior cranial fossae, and the craniovertebral junction.
- Removal of the posterior wall of the maxillary sinus grants access to the pterygopalatine fossa; locating the vidian nerve within it and tracing its path posteriorly will lead to the foramen lacerum and the transition between the petrous and paraclival portions of the ICA.

INTRODUCTION

Chondrosarcomas of the skull base are rare, locally invasive tumors that typically arise in the petroclival region, from degenerated chondroid cells located within the synchondrosis.[1–3] Given their usually slow growth rate, they are capable of reaching sizable dimensions, promoting bone erosion and significant displacement of neurovascular structures before causing symptomatology that will eventually lead to diagnosis; cranial neuropathies and headaches are common complaints. From the petroclival region, they may invade the upper clivus and cavernous sinus superiorly, Meckel's cave and the medial middle cranial fossa laterally, the posterior cranial fossa medially and posteriorly,[2] and the craniovertebral junction inferiorly. Moreover, chondrosarcomas have been shown to spill into the infratemporal fossa and the high cervical region, infiltrating the jugular foramen and even

---

[a] Department of Neurosurgery, Wexner Medical Center, The Ohio State University, 410 West 10th Avenue, Columbus, OH 43210, USA; [b] Department of Otolaryngology–Head & Neck Surgery, Wexner Medical Center, The Ohio State University, 410 West 10th Avenue, N-1049 Doan Hall, Columbus, OH 43210, USA
* Corresponding author. Department of Neurological Surgery, Wexner Medical Center, The Ohio State University, 410 West 10th Avenue, N-1049 Doan Hall, Columbus, OH 43210.
E-mail address: Daniel.Prevedello@osumc.edu

Neurosurg Clin N Am 26 (2015) 453–462
http://dx.doi.org/10.1016/j.nec.2015.03.008
1042-3680/15/$ – see front matter © 2015 Elsevier Inc. All rights reserved.

the jugular vein. Despite this local aggressiveness, these lesions often spare the dura, compressing and displacing rather than transgressing it. This behavior, coupled with their ability to affect multiple cranial compartments simultaneously, renders the ventral transnasal corridor particularly appealing for their surgical management. Due to their ventral trajectory, potential advantages of endoscopic endonasal approaches (EEAs) include the possibility of accessing multiple skull base compartments, even bilaterally, in a single procedure while avoiding retraction or manipulation of neurovascular structures; this is exceptionally displayed during endonasal resection of chondrosarcomas.[2,4–6]

Hence, herein the authors describe their indications, contraindications, surgical technique and anatomy, complication management, and perioperative care for the endoscopic endonasal resection of skull base chondrosarcomas. Nevertheless, one must be aware that this is a heterogeneous group that may present in a wide variety of scenarios; thus, we will focus on describing the rationale behind surgically addressing those lesions located mainly in the petroclival region with involvement of neighboring compartments.

INDICATIONS/CONTRAINDICATIONS

For indications and contraindications please refer to **Table 1**.

SURGICAL ANATOMY

The surgical anatomy of the petroclival region and its surroundings,[7–10] as well as of the related endonasal approaches,[11–17] has been described. The key landmarks and structures from a ventral perspective are illustrated in **Fig. 1**.

SURGICAL TECHNIQUE
Preoperative Planning

All patients undergoing endonasal resection of a petroclival chondrosarcoma are submitted to the following:

- Anesthesia evaluation with nasal swab and culture; all patients are treated on the morning of surgery with a single nasal application of a povidone-iodine solution at 5% (3M, St. Paul, MN); if positive for methicillin-resistant *Staphylococcus aureus* (MRSA), the patients also receive vancomycin during induction.
- Magnetic resonance imaging (MRI) of the brain and computed axial tomography (CT) scan, both thinly sliced (<3 mm) and fused for intraoperative navigation. Special attention is given to the relation of the tumor to the different segments of the internal carotid artery (ICA); this characteristic will ultimately dictate which EEA modules must be performed during tumor resection.
- Otolaryngology evaluation, to detect sinonasal abnormalities, especially signs of infection.
- Evaluation by the speech therapy/swallowing disorders team in case of jugular foramen involvement.
- Audiometry in case of involvement of the cerebellopontine angle, internal acoustic canal and/or cranial nerve VII/VIII complex.

Preparation and Patient Positioning

Preparation

- General anesthesia with orotracheal intubation.
- Prophylactic antibiotics: cefepime if MRSA negative, cefepime and vancomycin if positive.
- Urinary catheter placement.
- Copious nasal irrigation with oxymetazoline hydrochloride solution and facial/nasal decontamination with iodine solution; the abdomen and the right thigh are also prepped in case fat or muscle grafts are necessary, respectively.
- Insertion of intraoperative monitoring needles according to tumor characteristics (cavernous sinus/cerebellopontine angle/jugular foramen involvement).
- The navigation tower and at least 2 monitors are positioned according to the otolaryngologist's hand dominance (**Fig. 2**).

Table 1
Indications and contraindications

	Contraindications	
Indications	**Relative**	**Absolute**
• Petroclival chondrosarcoma with or without extension into adjacent compartments	• Presence of sinonasal infection[a]	• Clinical instability that prevents general anesthesia • Lack of appropriate personnel and/or equipment

[a] Treat for 3 weeks (if bacterial) or 6 weeks (if fungal) before proceeding with endonasal surgery.

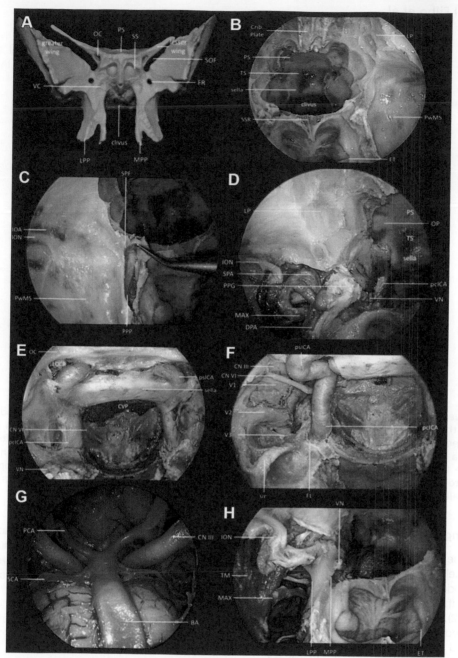

Fig. 1. Anatomic landmarks of the EEA to the petroclival region. (*A*) Anterior view of the sphenoid bone; observe the relation of the pterygoid process to the lower portion of the clivus. (*B*) Overview of the ventral skull base after a wide sphenoidotomy and left antrostomy. (*C*) Close-up view of the posterior wall of the maxillary sinus and sphenopalatine foramen; note that removal of this wall will grant access to the pterygopalatine fossa. (*D*) Exposure of the contents of the right pterygopalatine fossa and vidian canal; note that the nerve "points" to the ipsilateral ICA. (*E*) Dural landmarks after removal of the carotid canals and sellar and clival bones. (*F*) Exposure of the right medial middle cranial fossa and Meckel's cave. (*G*) View of the interpeduncular fossa and its contents after an upper clivectomy (angled endoscope pointing upward). (*H*) Initial exposure of the infratemporal fossa after removal of the pterygopalatine fossa contents. BA, basilar artery; CN III, oculomotor nerve; CN VI, abducens nerve; Crib. Plate, cribriform plate; CVP, clival venous plexus; DPA, descending palatine artery; ET, Eustachian tube; FL, foramen lacerum; FR, foramen rotundum; IOA, infraorbital artery; ION, infraorbital nerve; LOCR, lateral optic-carotid recess; LP, lamina papyracea; LPP, lateral pterygoid plate; MAX, internal maxillary artery; MPP, medial pterygoid plate; OC, optic canal; OP, optic nerve; PCA, posterior cerebral artery; pclICA, paraclival ICA; PPG, pterygopalatine ganglion; PPP, proximal pterygoid process; PS, planum sphenoidale; psICA, parasellar ICA; PwMS, posterior wall of maxillary sinus; SCA, superior cerebellar artery; SOF, superior orbital fissure; SPA, sphenopalatine artery; SPF, sphenopalatine foramen; SS, sphenoid sinus; SSR, sphenoid sinus rostrum; TM, temporalis muscle; TS, tuberculum sellae; V1, ophthalmic nerve; V2, maxillary nerve; V3, mandibular nerve; VC, vidian canal; VN, vidian nerve.

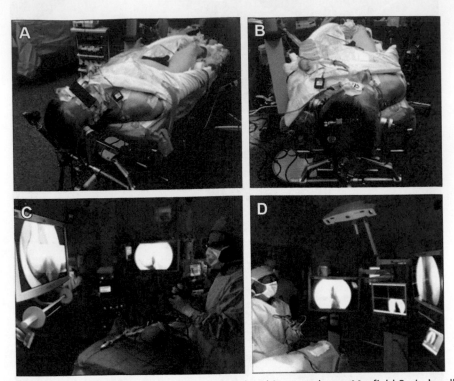

Fig. 2. Patient and room positioning. (*A*, *B*) The patient's head is secured on a Mayfield 3-pin headholder and turned to the right with slight neck extension; the body is secured with tape and protected with foam. Note the intraoperative monitoring needles; the abdomen and thigh are also prepped for possible grafts. (*C*) Room setup for a right-handed otolaryngologist; a monitor is positioned at the head of the patient and a second one at the feet, allowing both surgeons to stand to the right side of the patient. (*D*) Room setup for a left-handed otolaryngologist; 2 monitors are positioned at the head of the patient with the navigation tower between, allowing the surgeons to stand opposite each other on both sides of the patient.

Positioning

- Supine position, with the head fixed on the Mayfield 3-pin headholder. The neck is slightly extended and the head turned to the right, with the whole body tilted to the left (see **Fig. 2**). The right thigh is slightly flexed and rotated inward. The body is secured and protected with foam and tape; the navigation transmitter is attached to the headholder.

Surgical Approach

The surgical approach is composed of the following sequential steps (**Fig. 3**):

1. Right middle turbinectomy, performed with strong sinus scissors; extreme care is taken to avoid avulsing the turbinate from its insertion in the anterior cranial base and causing an early cerebrospinal fluid (CSF) leak.
2. Bilateral posterior ethmoidectomies, performed with microdebriders.
3. Elevation of the nasoseptal flap[18] on the contralateral side of the lesion (a transpterygoid

approach will ultimately dictate sacrificing the flap's blood supply). The flap is usually stored on the ipsilateral maxillary sinus to allow ample maneuvering within the lower clivus/craniovertebral junction regions.
4. Posterior septectomy.
5. Incision and rotation of the now-exposed contralateral septal mucosa to cover the denuded septum.[19]
6. Drilling of the sphenoid floor until flush with the clivus.
7. Removal of the posterior wall of the maxillary sinus on the tumor side, thus accessing the pterygopalatine fossa.
8. Identification of the pterygopalatine ganglion, infraorbital, and vidian nerves.
9. Progressive drilling of the vidian canal from anterior to posterior; depending on the amount of tumor lateral extension and the degree of pneumatization of the lateral sphenoid recess, the nerve may be spared or sacrificed during this step.[20]
10. The vidian nerve will ultimately lead the surgeon to the transition between the horizontal/petrous

and vertical/paraclival segments of the ICA, at the foramen lacerum.[21]

11. Drilling of the clivus (clival removal is dictated by the amount of tumor in the posterior fossa); during this step, the team must be prepared to encounter massive venous bleeding from invasion of the basilar plexus, which can be managed with direct infusion of various clot-inducing products.

12. Drilling of the petrous apex and skeletonization of the ICA.

Optional steps (according to tumor extension); these may be performed in different sequences in conjunction with the standard approach described previously:

1. Dissection of the ipsilateral torus tubarius and Eustachian tube; it may be removed or mobilized. The Eustachian cartilage is followed superiorly, continuing as the cartilage of the foramen lacerum; thus, use of the cautery while releasing the torus tubarius must be performed with caution.[22] This step is performed to grant access to tumor located inferior to the petrous apex.

2. Removal of the pterygoid processes[23] and musculature; this step grants access to the infratemporal fossa.

3. Drilling and removal of the lateral sphenoid recess; this step grants access to the anterior portion of the Meckel's cave[11] and the medial middle cranial fossa.

Note that the approach itself entails tumor resection; drilling and removal of the multiple bony structures mentioned is necessary to obtain complete resection in invasive tumors such as chondrosarcomas and chordomas.

Surgical Procedure

Actual tumor removal may not adhere to a rigid sequence of steps; it is determined by the location of the lesion's main component and the degree of surrounding involvement. In general, the following steps are taken (see **Fig. 3**):

1. Resection of tumor within the petrous apex (chondrosarcomas are usually soft and amenable to suction); however, very hard and calcified ones can be encountered.

2. Resection of tumor in the posterior fossa; if the dura has been transgressed, dissection is performed with a set of dissectors that enable direct stimulation with live feedback from the monitoring team to avoid damage to cranial nerves.

3. Lateralization of the now skeletonized ICA grants access to the petroclival synchondrosis and enables removal of tumor within it.

4. Once the main petroclival component has been resected, attention is given to the surrounding compartments, according to preoperative scans and intraoperative navigation. Typically, larger lesions will create a corridor from the petroclival synchondrosis to these regions, facilitating tumor removal. Dissection within the cavernous sinus, jugular foramen, infratemporal fossa, and high cervical region is also performed with stimulating dissectors to prevent cranial nerve injuries.

5. Once complete tumor resection, including removal of infiltrated bone, is achieved, copious irrigation of the operative field with warm saline takes place, promoting hemostasis and clearing debris.

6. Closure is performed based on the presence or absence of a CSF leak. When present, the dural defect is plugged with a partial inlay/onlay sheet of collagen matrix and covered with the nasoseptal flap elevated at the beginning of the procedure. If a leak is not found, the flap is then positioned over the skeletonized ICA for protection. Finally, the sphenoid sinus is obliterated with synthetic foam to preserve the flap in position.

COMPLICATIONS AND MANAGEMENT

- As with other pathologies addressed through an endoscopic endonasal technique, the main complication is postoperative CSF leakage,[24] which typically demands a second surgery for flap repositioning or bolstering with a fat graft.

- Meningitis is extremely rare,[25] even in the setting of a CSF leak. If present, it is managed with wide spectrum antibiotics aimed to cover the sinonasal flora.

- Sinonasal infection and scarring is uncommon and addressed as a typical sinus surgery postoperative recovery.

- Although uncommon, cranial neuropathies that are present preoperatively may be exacerbated because of manipulation during dissection; this phenomenon is usually transient and most patients experience recovery, even if partial, or maintenance of cranial nerve function. Steroids are routinely used intraoperatively and postoperatively. Permanent postoperative cranial nerve dysfunction is extremely rare.

- Vascular injuries also are rare; nonetheless, one must be aware that, among the pathologies treated with EEAs, chondroid tumors

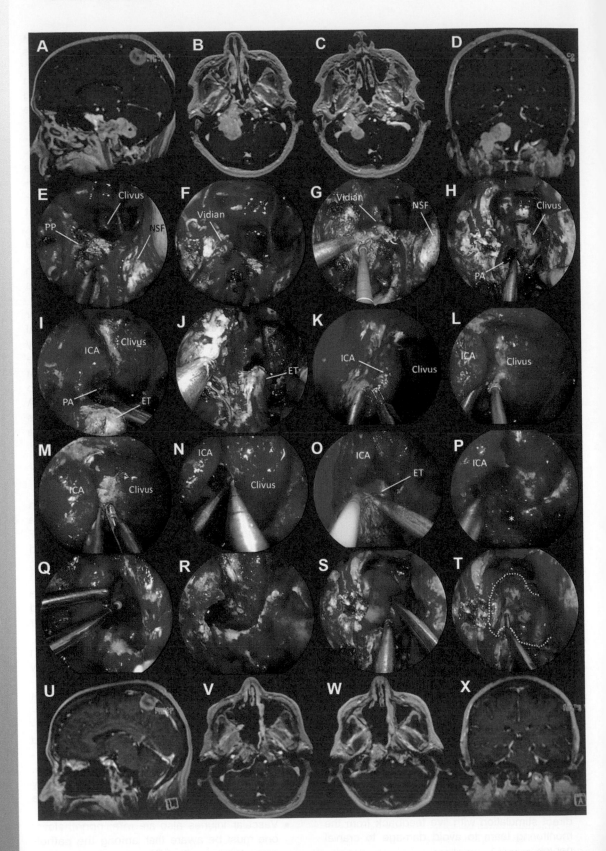

are the most frequently associated with carotid injuries.[26] In the event of an ICA rupture, intraoperative management is based on direct compression with a muscle graft from the thigh. Once the bleeding has been controlled, the patient is submitted to an angiography for potential definitive treatment of the vascular lesion. Repeat angiography must be performed within the following weeks to rule out pseudoaneurysm formation.

- Clinical complications (respiratory and urinary infections, deep vein thrombosis) must be addressed accordingly.

POSTOPERATIVE CARE

All patients submitted to endonasal resection of petroclival chondrosarcomas undergo the following:

- Postoperative care in the intensive care unit.
- Prophylactic antibiotics are given for 1 to 5 days after surgery; the same treatment initiated at the operating room (OR) is maintained through postoperative day 1 and replaced by sulfamethoxazole and trimethoprim or a third-generation cephalosporin after 24 hours. These are suspended when the nasal packing is removed, usually on postoperative day 5.
- A noncontrast head CT is performed as soon as feasible to rule out immediate complications and to determine the extent of bone removal. Within the first 24 hours, a brain MRI is also performed to determine the rate of resection and establish a postoperative baseline for future comparisons.

- General routine postoperative measures, such as pain management and deep vein thrombosis prophylaxis, are undertaken.
- To protect the skull base reconstruction until the flap heals, no cannulas, instruments, or catheters are permitted in the nasal cavity; straining is also avoided by the use of stool softeners and by orienting the patient to cough and sneeze with the mouth open. The use of incentive spirometry, bending, squatting, or lifting is also prohibited, especially within the first week after surgery. These measures are generally enforced for the first postoperative month.
- If a CSF leak was observed during surgery or is suspected during recovery, the patient is oriented to tilt the head forward to provoke fluid egress; if a leak is indeed present, this is usually in high volume. Clear nasal discharge in the first 24 hours after surgery may be saline solution trapped in the maxillary sinuses, which starts to exit through the nostrils once the patient begins to ambulate. A noncontrast head CT may aid in distinguishing between the 2 scenarios, as in a leak new or increased pneumocephalus will be present. Beta-2-transferrin test also may be used, although the somewhat long time required for its results and common false positives render it a less useful tool. If a CSF leak is suspected or obvious, the patient is returned to the OR for surgical exploration.
- If no complications occur, the patient is discharged at approximately postoperative day 2. The otolaryngology team removes the nasal packing on postoperative day 5; further

Fig. 3. Stepwise depiction of an endoscopic endonasal resection of a petroclival chondrosarcoma with extension into the right parapharyngeal space. Preoperative contrast-enhanced T1-weighted brain MRI sagittal (A), axial (B, C), and coronal (D) views demonstrate the presence of a large petroclival mass that arises from the right synchondrosis and extends into the parapharyngeal space, suggestive of a chondrosarcoma; a synchronous convexity meningioma is also seen. (E) The right middle turbinate is removed, a left nasoseptal flap (NSF) is raised (to allow right transpterygoid access), a wide sphenoidotomy is performed; the posterior wall of the maxillary sinus is also removed to expose the contents of the pterygopalatine fossa (PP). (F) Lateral displacement of the pterygopalatine ganglion exposes the vidian nerve entering its canal. (G) The vidian canal is progressively drilled from anterior to posterior until the ICA is reached at the foramen lacerum. (H) The petrous apex (PA) is reached; it has been eroded by tumor. (I) Tumor within the PA is aspirated; observe that the Eustachian tube (ET) prevents lateral and inferior dissection. (J) The cartilage of the ET continues superiorly and posteriorly as the cartilage of the foramen lacerum. (K) The paraclival portion of the ICA is drilled thin and elevated. (L) Once the carotid has been skeletonized, it is possible to displace it laterally to permit drilling of the petroclival synchondrosis and the lateral portion of the clivus. (M) The clivus is also drilled thin and elevated. (N) Tumor within the synchondrosis is removed; the posterior cranial fossa dura is displaced to facilitate its removal. (O) The ET is detached from the lacerum cartilage. (P) Removal of the ET exposes the tumor component located in the parapharyngeal space (asterisk), below the PA and the ICA. (Q) Angled endoscopes and instruments permit removal of the final, most lateral tumor components within the synchondrosis. (R) Hemostasis and irrigation of the surgical field demonstrate the exposure and resection. (S) A collagen matrix sheet is placed within the synchondrosis, despite the absence of a CSF leak, to reinforce reconstruction of the region. (T) The nasoseptal flap (dotted line) is placed covering the petroclival region and the exposed ICA. Postoperative contrast-enhanced T1-weighted sagittal (U), axial (V, W) and coronal (X) views confirm a thorough removal.

Table 2
Studies on endoscopic endonasal resection of skull base chondrosarcomas

Authors, Year	No. of Cases	Average Tumor Volume	Tumor Location	Rate of Resection	Complications
Frank et al,[4] 2006	2	Not available	Both with extension to clivus and cavernous sinus	2/2 (100%) GTR	1/2 (50%) with CSF leak
Zhang et al,[6] 2008	2	Not available	Not available	1/2 (50%) GTR 1/2 (50%) STR	Not available
Zanation et al,[27] 2009	3	Not available	Petrous apex	3/3 (100%) GTR	None
Ceylan et al,[28] 2009	1	Not available	Not available	1/1 (100%) STR	Not available
Fernandez-Miranda et al,[29] 2009	1	Not available	Clival, petroclival, with extension into right jugular tubercle	1/1 (100%) GTR	Middle ear effusion at 3-mo follow-up
Chivukula et al,[30] 2013	1	Not available	Not available	Not available	Not available
Battaglia et al,[31] 2014	1	Not available	Sinonasal cavity, extension into infratemporal fossa	1/1 (100%) GTR	None
Mesquita Filho et al,[2] 2014	5	Not available	Petrous apex, clivus and CPA (1) Petrous apex, clivus, jugular vein, high cervical region, CPA, cerebellum (1) Petrous apex, middle cranial fossa, clivus, CPA, jugular foramen, hypoglossal canal (1) Petrous apex, CPA, brainstem, parapharyngeal space (1) Petrous apex, clivus, CPA, jugular foramen, hypoglossal canal, brainstem, cerebellum (1)	2/5 (40%) GTR 3/5 (60%) NTR	None
Vellutini et al,[32] 2014	2	Not available	Clivus (2 in upper clivus, 1 with lateral extension)	1/2 (50%) GTR 1/2 (50%) STR	1/2 (50%) with abducens palsy
Moussazadeh et al,[5] 2015	8	9.8 cm^3	Petroclival	5/8 (62.5%) NTR 3/8 (37.5%) STR	1/8 (12.5%) with CSF leakage

Abbreviations: CPA, cerebellopontine angle; CSF, cerebrospinal fluid; GTR, gross total resection; NTR, near total resection; STR, subtotal resection.
Data from Refs.[2,4–6,27–32]

consults are dictated by the patient's response to surgery in terms of nasal healing and crusting. Within the first 30 days after surgery, the patient also visits the neurosurgery team and pathology results are reviewed; on confirmation of chondrosarcoma, most lesions are referred for adjuvant radiation, usually proton beam therapy. Follow-up is determined by pathology and rate of resection.

OUTCOMES

Given the rarity of skull base chondrosarcomas and the recent establishment of EEAs as a feasible technique for their surgical management, only a few reports can be found in the literature. Usually, these tumors are described along with chordomas, although the latter tend to occur more often in the midline and be significantly more aggressive. **Table 2** summarizes the *specific* results of the most recent series on endoscopic endonasal resection of skull base chondrosarcomas.

In brief, 26 patients were reported in 10 articles. Tumor dimensions were seldom provided; tumor location was mostly centered on the petrous apex and clivus/petroclival regions, with extensions into various surrounding compartments, including the cavernous sinus, jugular tubercle, cerebellopontine angle, jugular foramen and vein, middle cranial fossa, hypoglossal canal, brainstem, and cerebellum. Among the available data, gross total resection was possible in 11 (44%) of 25 cases, whereas near total and subtotal resection were possible in 8 (32%) of 25 cases and 6 (24%) of 25 cases, respectively. Complications were few; 2 patients (9%) presented with postoperative CSF leakage and 1 patient (4.5%) with an abducens nerve palsy. There were no surgery-related deaths or vascular injuries reported in these articles. These figures confirm the difficulty in achieving a complete resection of these invasive tumors, despite low complication rates.

SUMMARY

Endonasal endoscopic resection of petroclival chondrosarcomas appears to be a safe and feasible technique, capable of achieving total or near total removal in most cases, despite involvement of surrounding regions, with low complication rates. Nonetheless, further studies with a greater number of patients are necessary to confirm these initial impressions. The petrous apex and petroclival regions are their most common locations, with invasion of neighboring compartments frequently observed.

REFERENCES

1. Sekhar LN, Pranatartiharan R, Chanda A, et al. Chordomas and chondrosarcomas of the skull base: results and complications of surgical management. Neurosurg Focus 2001;10(3):E2.
2. Mesquita Filho PM, Ditzel Filho LF, Prevedello DM, et al. Endoscopic endonasal surgical management of chondrosarcomas with cerebellopontine angle extension. Neurosurg Focus 2014;37(4):E13.
3. Samii A, Gerganov V, Herold C, et al. Surgical treatment of skull base chondrosarcomas. Neurosurg Rev 2009;32(1):67–75 [discussion: 75].
4. Frank G, Sciarretta V, Calbucci F, et al. The endoscopic transnasal transsphenoidal approach for the treatment of cranial base chordomas and chondrosarcomas. Neurosurgery 2006;59:ONS50–7 [discussion: ONS50–7].
5. Moussazadeh N, Kulwin C, Anand VK, et al. Endoscopic endonasal resection of skull base chondrosarcomas: technique and early results. J Neurosurg 2015;122(4):735–42.
6. Zhang Q, Kong F, Yan B, et al. Endoscopic endonasal surgery for clival chordoma and chondrosarcoma. ORL J Otorhinolaryngol Relat Spec 2008;70(2):124–9.
7. Rhoton AL Jr, Tedeschi H. Lateral approaches to the cerebellopontine angle and petroclival region (honored guest lecture). Clin Neurosurg 1994;41:517–45.
8. Rhoton AL Jr. The sellar region. Neurosurgery 2002;51(Suppl 4):S335–74.
9. Rhoton AL Jr. The cavernous sinus, the cavernous venous plexus, and the carotid collar. Neurosurgery 2002;51(Suppl 4):S375–410.
10. Rhoton AL Jr. The cerebellopontine angle and posterior fossa cranial nerves by the retrosigmoid approach. Neurosurgery 2000;47(Suppl 3):S93–129.
11. Kassam AB, Prevedello DM, Carrau RL, et al. The front door to Meckel's cave: an anteromedial corridor via expanded endoscopic endonasal approach—technical considerations and clinical series. Neurosurgery 2009;64(Suppl 3):71–82 [discussion: 82–3].
12. Kassam AB, Vescan AD, Carrau RL, et al. Expanded endonasal approach: vidian canal as a landmark to the petrous internal carotid artery. J Neurosurg 2008;108(1):177–83.
13. Morera VA, Fernandez-Miranda JC, Prevedello DM, et al. "Far-medial" expanded endonasal approach to the inferior third of the clivus: the transcondylar and transjugular tubercle approaches. Neurosurgery 2010;66(6 Suppl Operative):211–9 [discussion: 219–220].
14. Benet A, Prevedello DM, Carrau RL, et al. Comparative analysis of the transcranial "far lateral" and endoscopic endonasal "far medial" approaches: surgical anatomy and clinical illustration. World Neurosurg 2014;81:385–96.

15. de Notaris M, Cavallo LM, Prats-Galino A, et al. Endoscopic endonasal transclival approach and retrosigmoid approach to the clival and petroclival regions. Neurosurgery 2009;65:42–50 [discussion: 50–2].

16. Kassam A, Snyderman CH, Mintz A, et al. Expanded endonasal approach: the rostrocaudal axis. Part II. Posterior clinoids to the foramen magnum. Neurosurg Focus 2005;19(1):E4.

17. Kassam AB, Gardner P, Snyderman C, et al. Expanded endonasal approach: fully endoscopic, completely transnasal approach to the middle third of the clivus, petrous bone, middle cranial fossa, and infratemporal fossa. Neurosurg Focus 2005; 19(1):E6.

18. Kassam AB, Thomas A, Carrau RL, et al. Endoscopic reconstruction of the cranial base using a pedicled nasoseptal flap. Neurosurgery 2008;63: ONS44–52 [discussion: ONS52–3].

19. Kasemsiri P, Carrau RL, Otto BA, et al. Reconstruction of the pedicled nasoseptal flap donor site with a contralateral reverse rotation flap: technical modifications and outcomes. Laryngoscope 2013; 123(11):2601–4.

20. Prevedello DM, Pinheiro-Neto CD, Fernandez-Miranda JC, et al. Vidian nerve transposition for endoscopic endonasal middle fossa approaches. Neurosurgery 2010;67(2 Suppl Operative):478–84.

21. Osawa S, Rhoton AL Jr, Seker A, et al. Microsurgical and endoscopic anatomy of the vidian canal. Neurosurgery 2009;64:385–411 [discussion: 411–2].

22. Falcon RT, Rivera-Serrano CM, Miranda JF, et al. Endoscopic endonasal dissection of the infratemporal fossa: anatomic relationships and importance of Eustachian tube in the endoscopic skull base surgery. Laryngoscope 2011;121(1):31–41.

23. Kasemsiri P, Solares CA, Carrau RL, et al. Endoscopic endonasal transpterygoid approaches: anatomical landmarks for planning the surgical corridor. Laryngoscope 2013;123(4):811–5.

24. Kassam AB, Prevedello DM, Carrau RL, et al. Endoscopic endonasal skull base surgery: analysis of complications in the authors' initial 800 patients. J Neurosurg 2011;114(6):1544–68.

25. Kono Y, Prevedello DM, Snyderman CH, et al. One thousand endoscopic skull base surgical procedures demystifying the infection potential: incidence and description of postoperative meningitis and brain abscesses. Infect Control Hosp Epidemiol 2011;32(1):77–83.

26. Gardner PA, Tormenti MJ, Pant H, et al. Carotid artery injury during endoscopic endonasal skull base surgery: incidence and outcomes. Neurosurgery 2013;73:ONS261–9 [discussion: ONS269–70].

27. Zanation AM, Snyderman CH, Carrau RL, et al. Endoscopic endonasal surgery for petrous apex lesions. Laryngoscope 2009;119(1):19–25.

28. Ceylan S, Koc K, Anik I. Extended endoscopic approaches for midline skull-base lesions. Neurosurg Rev 2009;32(3):309–19 [discussion: 318–9].

29. Fernandez-Miranda JC, Morera VA, Snyderman CH, et al. Endoscopic endonasal transclival approach to the jugular tubercle. Neurosurgery 2012;71(1 Suppl Operative):146–58 [discussion: 158–9].

30. Chivukula S, Koutourousiou M, Snyderman CH, et al. Endoscopic endonasal skull base surgery in the pediatric population. J Neurosurg Pediatr 2013; 11(3):227–41.

31. Battaglia P, Turri-Zanoni M, Dallan I, et al. Endoscopic endonasal transpterygoid transmaxillary approach to the infratemporal and upper parapharyngeal tumors. Otolaryngol Head Neck Surg 2014; 150(4):696–702.

32. Velutini Ede A, Balsalobre L, Hermann DR, et al. The endoscopic endonasal approach for extradural and intradural clivus lesions. World Neurosurg 2014; 82(Suppl 6):S106–15.

Endoscopic Endonasal Management of Orbital Pathologies

Paolo Castelnuovo, MD[a,b], Mario Turri-Zanoni, MD[a,b],*,
Paolo Battaglia, MD[a,b], Davide Locatelli, MD[b,c],
Iacopo Dallan, MD[b,d]

KEYWORDS

- Endoscopic assisted • Endonasal approach • Skull base • Orbit • Optic nerve • Paranasal sinuses

KEY POINTS

- Endoscopic endonasal techniques are able to reach the medial orbital structures as well as the orbital apex region without skin incision and brain retraction.
- The endoscopic endonasal management of orbital pathologic conditions may include the complete removal of the lesion or only a tissue sampling for diagnostic purposes.
- The lateral limit of the transnasal approach is represented by the course of the optic nerve that must not be crossed.
- Endonasal approaches can be used in combination with superior/inferior eyelid approaches to manage complex lesions involving the orbit, the superior/inferior orbital fissure, and the anterior/middle skull base (multiportal surgery).

INTRODUCTION

External approaches to the orbit are well established, including transconjunctival, transcranial, or lateral orbitotomies, depending on the localization of the lesion. Among these, orbitozygomatic craniotomy is generally used for lesions that extend intracranially and into the orbit and is used for exposure of the optic nerve and canal.[1]

The transnasal endoscopic route, initially developed for treating inflammatory sinuses disease, has emerged in the last decades as a minimally invasive corridor to approach adjacent anatomic areas such as ventral skull base, orbit, and orbital apex regions.[2] What is paramount for the application of endoscopic transnasal approaches to the orbit is the close anatomic relationship between the paranasal sinuses and the orbital content, summarized in the concept of sino-orbito-cranial interface.[3] In this respect, endoscopic visualization from the transnasal route has provided surgeons the possibility of reaching the medial orbital structures as well as the orbital apex region without skin incision, major bony work, or brain retraction.

Given these facts, endoscopic endonasal orbital and optic nerve decompressions have become accepted treatments for thyroid eye disease[4] and traumatic optic neuropathy that is unresponsive to steroids.[5] The endoscopic endonasal technique is widely used as well for ophthalmologic procedures such as drainage of subperiosteal abscesses and dacryocystorhinostomy. Recently, some

All the authors certify that they have no conflict of interest or financial relationship with any entity mentioned in the article. No sponsors or grants are involved in the article.
[a] Unit of Otorhinolaryngology, Department of Biotechnology and Life Sciences (DBSV), Ospedale di Circolo e Fondazione Macchi, University of Insubria, via Guicciardini 9, Varese 21100, Italy; [b] Head and Neck Surgery & Forensic Dissection Research Center (HNS&FDRc), DBSV, University of Insubria, via Guicciardini 9, Varese 21100, Italy; [c] Unit of Neurosurgery, Civic Hospital, via Papa Giovanni Paolo II, Legnano 20025, Italy; [d] First Otorhinolaryngologic Unit, Azienda Ospedaliero-Universitaria Pisana, via Paradisa 2, Pisa 56124, Italy
* Corresponding author. Unit of Otorhinolaryngology, Azienda Ospedaliero-Universitaria Ospedale di Circolo e Fondazione Macchi, University of Insubria, Via Guicciardini 9, Varese 21100, Italy.
E-mail address: tzmario@inwind.it

Neurosurg Clin N Am 26 (2015) 463–472
http://dx.doi.org/10.1016/j.nec.2015.03.001
1042-3680/15/$ – see front matter © 2015 Elsevier Inc. All rights reserved.

studies concerning the endoscopic endonasal biopsy, debulking, or even radical resection of tumors involving the orbit also have been reported, expanding the indications for such endonasal approaches.[6,7] Herein are described the anatomic principles, indications, technical nuances, and limitations of the endoscopic endonasal approaches for the management of selected orbital pathologic conditions.

INDICATIONS AND CONTRAINDICATIONS

Endoscopic endonasal technique allows reaching adequately the medial compartments (**Fig. 1**). The lateral limit of the transnasal approach is represented by the course of the optic nerve that must not be crossed. Thus, tumors that are localized to the superior and lateral compartments of the orbit are contraindicated for a pure endoscopic endonasal approach.[8] When dealing with orbital lesions, the intents of surgery can be not only the radical removal but also the partial removal (to decompress the orbit), the drainage of the mass (in the case of cyst, abscess, or hematoma), or the tissue sampling for diagnostic purposes. The current indications and contraindications for this minimally invasive approach are detailed in **Table 1**.

SURGICAL TECHNIQUE
Preoperative Planning

Nasal endoscopy is useful to explore the sinonasal spaces in close relation with the orbit that will be approached transnasally. Ophthalmologic evaluation (including visual acuity, pupillary reactions, visual fields, ocular motility, and color discrimination) and cranial nerves function examination are important as well to assess the preoperative conditions.

Radiological studies with computed tomographic (CT) scan and contrast-enhanced MRI are mandatory for the evaluation of the sino-orbito-cranial interface. Probably the coronal views are the most important perspective to analyze when dealing with intraorbital lesions. Radiological examinations allow the precise evaluation of the site, size, and extent of the lesions and in some cases can provide preoperative diagnosis. Imaging scans give information on anatomic details (Onodi cell pneumatization, anterior and posterior ethmoidal arteries position, supraorbital cell pneumatization, position of the lesion in respect to extraocular muscles, and optic nerve course) that can influence the surgical procedure. Based on patients' features, evolution of the disease, and its radiological appearance, surgery has to be planned with diagnostic or curative intent.

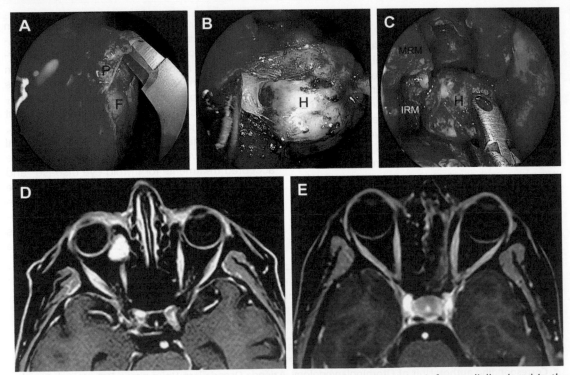

Fig. 1. Endoscopic endonasal resection of an extraconal cavernous hemangioma inferomedially placed in the orbit. (*A*) Periorbit incision; (*B*) hemangioma dissection from intraorbital fat and muscles; (*C*) transnasal removal of the lesion; (*D*) preoperative contrast-enhanced MRI; (*E*) postoperative contrast-enhanced MRI. F, intraorbital fat; H, hemangioma; P, periorbit.

> **Table 1**
> **Indications and contraindications for the endoscopic endonasal management of orbital pathologic abnormalities**
>
> | Indications | Contraindications |
> | --- | --- |
> | Orbital and optic canal decompression (Graves disease, posttraumatic optic neuropathy) | Orbital high-flow vascular malformations (OA aneurysms, arteriovenous malformations) |
> | Medial orbital wall fractures repair | Lateral and superolateral orbital wall fractures repair |
> | Sinonasal benign tumors invading the orbit (medial compartment). In these cases, the surgical corridor to pass through is represented by the tumor itself.[8] | Sinonasal malignancies extending to the orbit (relative contraindication) |
> | Lesions of the medial extraconal orbital spaces (mainly inferomedially located) | Lateral and superolateral extraconal and intraconal lesions |
> | Extraconal medially located orbital apex lesions | Intraconal orbital apex lesions (posteriorly, the annulus of Zinn is difficult to open) |
> | Selected lesions of the medial intraconal space (mainly inferomedially located) | |

Data from Turri-Zanoni M, Dallan I, Terranova P, et al. Frontoethmoidal and intraorbital osteomas: exploring the limits of the endoscopic approach. Arch Otolaryngol Head Neck Surg 2012;138(5):498–504.

Preparation and Patient Positioning

The transnasal approaches to the orbital spaces require adequate instrumentation for a correct procedure. The surgical set should include several dissectors of different sizes, and delicate scissors of different angles (like for cranial base surgery). Delicate bipolar forceps with straight and angled tips can be very useful. Moreover, in all intraorbital procedures, an intraoperative navigation system is strongly advisable.

Patients are placed in the anti-Trendelenburg position and under general anesthesia. A perioperative prophylactic antibiotic regimen is followed, including third-generation cephalosporin. Some minutes before surgery, the nasal cavities are packed with cottonoids soaked in 2% oxymetazoline, 1% oxybuprocaine, and adrenaline (1/100.000) solution to reduce bleeding and improve transnasal operative spaces.

Step-by-Step Surgical Procedure

Different pathologic conditions affecting the orbit and optic nerve can be treated transnasally, requiring a different combination of the following surgical steps, as described.

Transnasal corridor setup and lamina papyracea exposure

To gain adequate operative space, the middle turbinate has to be partially or completely resected, paying attention to preserve the olfactory mucosa. Natural ostium of the maxillary sinus is opened after a partial uncinectomy, to expose

the inferomedial angle of the orbit. A standard spheno-ethmoidectomy and a large medial antrostomy are performed to expose the medial orbital wall (mainly given by the lamina papyracea). The choice to use an anterior septal window depends on the position of the orbital lesion. Once the lamina papyracea is exposed, the sphenoidotomy is enlarged laterally to expose the bony bulging of optic nerve and internal carotid artery. When present, Onodi cell represents a key marker for the optic canal and must be opened with caution.

Optic canal opening (if needed)

The optic canal is opened by a gentle drilling out, under continuous irrigation, from proximal (orbital apex) to distal, obtaining a bony pellicle that is finally removed with a spatula. The orbital apex identification is crucial for starting the procedure to localize the optic nerve course even in the case of low pneumatized (conchal) sphenoid sinus. When a clockwise 180° of freedom of the optic nerve is obtained, the nerve becomes pulsatile. Finally, the dural layer covering the nerve is incised superomedially to reduce the risk of damaging the ophthalmic artery (OA) situated inferomedially.[5]

Lamina papyracea removal and periorbit exposure

Lamina papyracea is gently drilled out and finally removed with a spatula. Entry through the lamina papyracea should occur below the level of the ethmoidal foramina to avoid damage to the ethmoid arteries and to reduce the risk of retrobulbar hemorrhage and vision loss. Once the lamina papyracea is removed, the medial aspect of the periorbit is exposed. Generally, the superomedial angle of the orbit is preserved to keep the patency of the frontal recess (**Fig. 2**).

Extraconal fat exposure

After removal of the periorbit, the extraconal fat is exposed. Posteriorly, the extraconal fat is less evident; therefore, sometimes, medial rectus muscle (MRM) can be found immediately below the periorbit. At the level of the orbital apex, the annulus of Zinn is rapidly exposed below the periorbit and not infrequently an extraconal venous channel is evident connecting the orbital system with the cavernous sinus.[9]

Extraconal fat removal and medial muscular wall exposure

By removing the extraconal fat, the "medial muscular wall" comes into view. It is given mainly by the MRM and inferior rectus muscles (IRMs) and, to a lesser part, by the superior oblique

muscle (SOM). Between the medial and IRM, it is possible to identify intraconal fat (**Fig. 3**). The anterior ethmoidal artery (AEA) passes between the MRM and the SOM, while the posterior ethmoidal artery usually passes above the SOM.

Approach to the intraconal spaces

To manage the medial (mostly inferomedial) intraconal spaces, the best corridor lies between the medial and the IRMs. Sometimes, to increase the size of this surgical window, the medial aspect of the orbital floor can be removed, paying attention to preserve the infraorbital nerve, which allows an increased mobility of the orbital structures. In selected cases, for lesions localized posteriorly in the orbit in a superomedial area, a surgical corridor between the MRM and the SOM is preferred. When this superior corridor is indicated, the AEA is generally identified, cauterized, and cut (**Fig. 4**).

Medial intraconal space dissection

Within the orbit, a complex reticular system of fibrous septa divides the fat into distinct lobules.

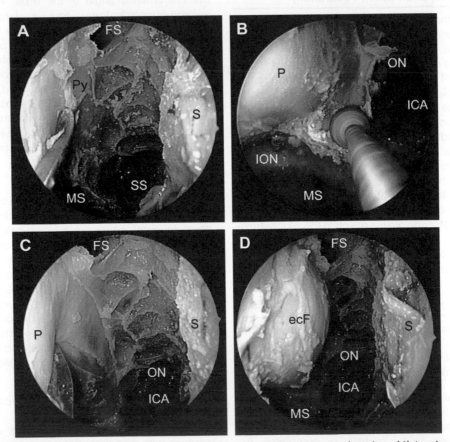

Fig. 2. Endoscopic endonasal step-by-step surgical approach to the extraconal region. (*A*) Lamina papyracea removal; (*B*) drilling out of the inferomedial orbital angle; (*C*) periorbit incision; (*D*) extraconal fat exposure. ecF, extraconal fat; FS, frontal sinus; ICA, internal carotid artery; ION, infraorbital nerve; MS, maxillary sinus; ON, optic nerve; P, periorbit; Py, lamina papyracea; S, nasal septum; SS, sphenoid sinus.

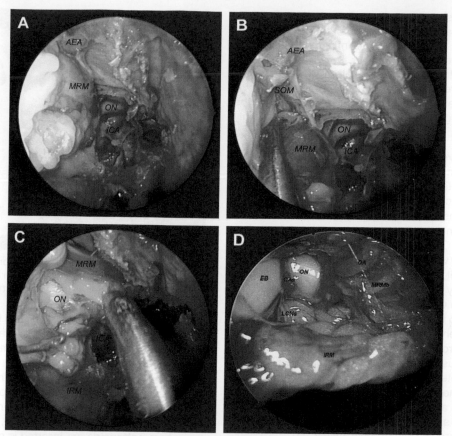

Fig. 3. Endoscopic endonasal step-by-step surgical approach to the intraconal region. (*A*) Medial muscular wall exposure after removing the extraconal fat; (*B*) surgical corridor between MRM and SOM; (*C*) surgical corridor between medial and IRMs; (*D*) intraconal dissection with identification of neurovascular orbital structures. CAs, ciliary arteries; EB, eye ball; ICA, internal carotid artery; LCNs, long ciliary nerves; MRMb, branches of the MRM; ON, optic nerve.

These septa are well evident in the anterior orbit and bridges together extraocular muscles, thus "creating" an intraconal and extraconal space.[10] Posteriorly, this division is less evident. The lateral border of dissection is given by the optic nerve. Obviously, it is critical to avoid crossing the plane of the optic nerve. In the upper part, above an axial plane passing through the optic nerve, the OA, the nasociliary nerve (NCN), and superior ophthalmic vein (SOV) can be seen.[10] In close proximity to OA, the NCN runs branching off the ethmoidal nerves (anterior and posterior) and the infratrochlear nerve. The SOV is the largest and most important vein of the orbit and usually runs close to the OA. It usually originates by the fusion between the continuation of the supraorbital vein and the angular vein. On the internal aspect of the MRM, it is possible to identify the branch of the oculomotor nerve and the muscular arterial branches usually coming from the OA. As a general rule, the muscular branches are nearly all situated in the

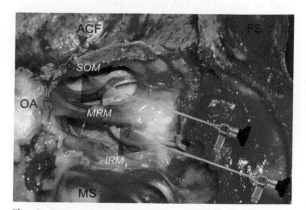

Fig. 4. Anatomic representation of the 2 surgical corridors to approach the intraconal spaces. The surgical window between the MRMs and the IRMs allow approach to the inferomedial intraconal region (especially the anterior portion). The corridor between the MRM and the SOM can be used to address the posterior intraconal region superomedially. ACF, anterior cranial fossa; FS, frontal sinus; MS, maxillary sinus.

intraconal side of the muscles, principally at their posterior part. What is crucial for intraorbital lesion dissection, especially for the intraconal one, is the careful preservation of as much neural and vascular structures as possible, even at the cost of partial resection, since a given procedure will be considered minimally invasive not only for the type of surgical approach adopted but also mainly for the functional outcomes obtained.

Optic nerve exposure

Once the medial intraconal fat is removed, the intra-orbital portion of the optic nerve with its tortuous course becomes evident (see **Fig. 3**). Anteriorly, the optic nerve is closely associated with vascular network, mainly given by ciliary arteries (branches of the OA). Close to these vessels, long ciliary nerves are usually well identifiable.[10] In the posterior aspect of the orbit, posterior ciliary arteries (PCA) can be seen. They arise independently from the proximal part of the OA: the superior PCA is always located superior to the ON. The medial PCA and the central retinal artery (CRA) are usually the first branches of the OA. From an endoscopic transnasal perspective, it is usually possible to identify the CRA that usually enters the optic nerve from its inferior surface. Sometimes it can also reach the nerve from its medial aspect. It should be noted that CRA is one of the smallest branches of the OA and its position is unpredictable preoperatively.[10]

Orbital apex exposure

In the orbital apex region, by splitting the annulus of Zinn between the MRM and IRM, the inferior division of the oculomotor nerve, with its branches, becomes evident.[9] Between them, the proximal part of the orbital OA can be seen.

It is really necessary a medial orbital wall reconstruction?

Contrary to what is reported by some investigators, even in the case of wide removal of the periorbit and extensive intraorbital dissection, medial orbital wall reconstruction is not necessary.[11] In the large majority of cases, where only the periorbital layer is removed, the orbital stability is warranted by the intraorbital connective septal system. However, even in the case of intraconal dissection with interruptions of the connective septa, postoperative scar tissue is enough to restore the orbital continence.

Surgical Tips and Tricks

- Anterior septal window: creation of an anterior septal window allows a 2-nostril technique with a 3- to 4-hands technique and a more favorable angle of attack. A reduced conflict between instruments is also provided (**Fig. 5**).

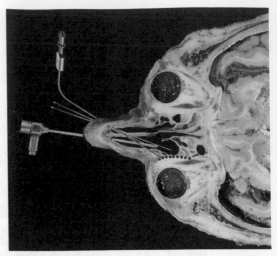

Fig. 5. Anterior septal window illustration. This technique allows approach to the anterior portion of the medial orbital compartment (*red dotted line*).

- Four-hands technique: it is helpful to have one surgeon retracting the mass inferomedially, while the other surgeon uses a bimanual technique to dissect tumor margins.
- Dissection: dissection along the lesion's capsule by inserting cottonoid pledgets, to create space all around the lesion and to increase its mobilization. To note, the space where cottonoids are inserted is given by the increase in volume of the lesion itself that generally has spread out the surrounding neurovascular structures. This surgical trick is particularly useful for superomedially located lesions, approached through a superior corridor (between MRM and SOM).
- Medial retraction of MRM: to increase the working window between the MRMs and IRMs, the MRM can be retracted in the direction of the nasal septum.[6] Usually this is done using a vessel loop or a stitch. This maneuver upturns the ability to dissect and work within the medial intraconal space, reducing at the same time the conflicts between instruments.
- Canine fossa trephination: for introducing a dissector useful to lateralize and lower the IRM. In this way, the surgical corridor lying between the MRM and IRM could be augmented.
- Extraocular muscles anterior stiffening: anterior stiffening of MRMs and IRMs by means of transconjunctival looping represents another help for transnasal orbital dissection, especially for extraconal lesions. By pulling the stitches anteriorly, the muscles become rigid, thus making extraconal dissection easier and safer.

INTRAOPERATIVE COMPLICATIONS
Vascular Damages

- Muscular branches, mainly of the MRM: this vessel can be injured especially in posterior aspect of the orbit. This complication is infrequent especially if a careful blunt perilesional dissection is carried out.
- Central retinal artery: damage of this artery leads to sudden blindness. Unfortunately, the position of the CRA is unpredictable. Most of the time, the artery enters the nerve on its inferior surface, but sometimes it can have a medial entrance.
- Ciliary arteries: this network surrounds the optic nerve and can be seen from a transnasal view. Their damage can be very serious and may lead to severe visual impairment.
- Ophthalmic artery: given the position of the artery, direct damage of the vessel is very rare during transnasal intraorbital procedures

Neural Damages

- Motor nerves (branches of the inferior division of oculomotor nerve): this lesion can lead to a dysfunction of the muscles (MRMs and IRMs). These branches usually enter the muscles on their inner surface, in the posterior orbit. Therefore, their damage during transnasal intraorbital procedures is not common. Notwithstanding, a careful perilesional dissection is strongly advisable because it greatly reduces the risk to damage these branches.
- Long ciliary nerves: these nerves are mainly sensory but can also contain sympathetic fibers for pupillary dilatation. They can be found on the medial aspect of the optic nerve and their damage can lead to some disturbances in sclera's sensation.
- Optic nerve: a direct damage to the optic nerve is infrequent if a careful dissection is performed, but when it occurs, it causes blindness.

Muscular Damages

The extraocular muscle with the highest risk of damage is the MRM. Direct trauma or even surgical maneuvers by themselves can lead to a postoperative impairment of extraocular muscles with consequent diplopia. Usually the dysfunctions disappear within months.

POSTOPERATIVE COMPLICATIONS

- Orbital hematoma: intraorbital blood collection may occur in the case of blood vessel injuries. To avoid increasing of intraorbital pressure, a careful hemostasis (using warm water irrigation, bipolar forceps, hemostatic agents) should be achieved at the end of the procedure. Notwithstanding, given the opening at the level of the periorbital window, rarely a severe intraorbital hematoma develops after this type of procedure.
- Diplopia, especially if related to MRM impairment, is usually transient and should be considered a possible consequence of such an approach. Persistent diplopia is a rare event, generally related to severe injury of extraocular muscles or to medial displacements of the eyeball resulting from connective tissue septae interruptions within the orbital fat.
- Enophthalmos, resulting from orbital fat herniation intranasally, may occur as a late complication of expanded intraconal approaches.
- Nasal obstruction and chronic rhinosinusitis are possible sequelae in the case of paranasal sinuses natural ostia blockage for scar tissue formation or for intranasal orbital fat herniation. For this reason, postoperative endoscopic evaluations and debridements are mandatory to assess the nasal situation after surgery and to ensure patency of nasal cavity and sinuses.

POSTOPERATIVE CARE

Nasal packing, when used, is normally removed under endoscopic visualization on the first postoperative day. Vision and nasal endoscopy are regularly checked for the first few days. During hospitalization, CT or MRI scan is performed only when complications are suspected. During the early postoperative period, the patient is recommended to avoid blowing the nose for some weeks to reduce the risk of pneumo-orbit. Moreover, nasal rinsing with saline solution and sodium hyaluronate is suggested to the patient to optimize the cleaning of the nasal fossae and to accelerate the healing process. Finally, patients should be submitted to adjuvant treatments or to a regular follow-up program, according to the biology of the pathologic condition treated.

OUTCOMES

The efficacy of endoscopic endonasal approaches to decompress the orbit and the optic nerve is well known and proved by several case series describing outcomes of endonasal procedures in the case of Graves ophthalmopathy[4] as well as in posttraumatic optic neuropathy.[5] The management of intraorbital space-occupying lesions still represents a challenge in terms of both radical removal and biopsy for histopathological examination. Excluding single case reports, the outcomes observed in the largest case series are summarized in **Table 2**. Data emerging from these studies underline that the endonasal corridor has some advantages over external approaches for medial lesions. The endonasal approach minimizes external scarring and preserves cosmesis. On the other hand, external approaches require

Table 2
Summary of published case series on endoscopic endonasal approach to orbital lesions

Author, Year	No. of Cases	Biology of the Lesions	Outcomes of Surgery	Complications
Lund & Rose,[12] 2006	12	12, Sph-O meningiomas	12, debulking	None
Sieskiewicz et al,[13] 2008	6	2, pseudotumors 2, inflammatory lesions 1, plasmocytoma 1, carcinoma	6, biopsy	None
McKinney et al,[14] 2010	6	Not specified	4, RR 1, PR 1, biopsy	Not reported
Gavriel et al,[15] 2010	3	3, intraorbital abscesses	3, drainage	None
Murchison et al,[16] 2011	12	44% benign tumors 28% malignant tumors 17% inflammatory lesions 11% infectious diseases	Biopsy debulking RR (numbers not specified)	2, decreased visual acuity 1, transient diplopia 1, CSF leakage
Tomazic et al,[6] 2011	6	2, cavernous hemangioma 1, schwannoma 1, melanoma 1, lymphoma 1, optic glioma	2, RR 1, PR 3, biopsy	None
Castelnuovo et al,[7] 2012	16	6, cavernous hemangioma 2, solitary fibrous tumors 2, optic nerve tumors 2, metastases 2, pseudotumors 1, lymphoma 1, intraorbital abscess	6, biopsy 8, RR 1, PR 1, drainage	5, transient diplopia 1, transient III c.n. palsy 1, periorbital edema
Karaki et al,[17] 2012	4	1, cavernous hemangioma 1, intraorbital hematoma 1, inflammatory lesion 1, metastasis	2, biopsy 1, drainage 1, RR	None
Netuka et al,[18] 2013	3	2, cavernous hemangioma 1, solitary fibrous tumor	3, RR	1, reduced eye abduction
Berhouma et al,[19] 2014	11	4, Sph-O meningiomas 3, optic nerve meningiomas 1, trigeminal neuroma 1, pseudotumor 1, ossifying fibroma	5, debulking 4, biopsy 2, RR	1, epistaxis 1, pneumo-orbit

Abbreviations: c.n., cranic nerve; CSF, cerebrospinal fluid; PR, partial resection; RR, radical resection; Sph-O, spheno-orbital meningiomas.
Data from Refs.[6,7,12–19]

skin incisions, osteotomies, and significant displacement of orbital structures, including the globe. Given the deep, cone-shaped surgical window provided by the external approach, it also has the disadvantage of suboptimal visibility compared with the endonasal approach. In addition, external approaches to intraconal lesions may also require deinsertion of extraocular muscles, with subsequent impact on extraocular mobility. For these reasons, when feasible, the endoscopic endonasal technique can be considered a safe and effective surgical option to manage the optic nerve and orbital compartments (medial side) for various posttraumatic, inflammatory, infective, or tumoral diseases.

FUTURE DIRECTIONS

At present, endoscopic-assisted procedures to the orbit are mainly performed via transnasal routes. However, alternative minimally invasive endoscopic-assisted approaches through superior and inferior eyelid incisions have been recently proposed to treat selected orbital pathologic conditions placed laterally or superolaterally, outside from the orbital regions approachable from the transnasal route. In this way, surgeons nowadays have available different endoscopic-assisted procedures to manage different situations, for a minimally invasive comprehensive approach to the orbit.

Furthermore, pioneering experiences are going to open the door to new surgical corridors for managing not only orbital lesions but also profounder areas. In other words, nowadays the orbit should be considered not only the site of a pathologic condition but also a potential corridor for deeper areas. Clinical experiences seem to demonstrate the feasibility and effectiveness of such "transorbital" procedures. For example, anterior cranial fossa has been approached via the superior eyelid route.[20] More recently, it has been reported as a possibility to address the lateral wall of the cavernous sinus[21] as well as to manage the anterior aspect of the temporal lobe by means of a transorbital approach.[22] The possibility of using different entry windows, each one with its own advantages and limits, will represent the basis for the development of the multiportal surgery concept. Obviously, this new exciting field is only in its beginning and requires multidisciplinary cooperation to increase success rates and decrease risks.

SUMMARY

Endoscopic endonasal procedures are safe and effective to manage orbital pathologic conditions in properly selected cases. They should be considered a valid option for optic nerve or orbital wall decompression in the case of Graves ophthalmopathy and posttraumatic optic neuropathy as well as for addressing extraconal or intraconal lesions placed medially to the optic nerve course. Future evolutions including the development of endoscopic-assisted transorbital surgery and multiportal approaches will contribute to expand the actual indications for such an approach.

REFERENCES

1. McDermott MW, Durity FA, Rootman J, et al. Combined frontotemporal-orbitozygomatic approach for tumors of the sphenoid wing and orbit. Neurosurgery 1990;26(1):107–16.
2. Castelnuovo P, Lepera D, Turri-Zanoni M, et al. Quality of life following endoscopic endonasal resection of anterior skull base cancers. J Neurosurg 2013; 119(6):1401–9.
3. Dallan I, Lenzi R, de Notaris M, et al. Quantitative study on endoscopic endonasal approach to the posterior sino-orbito-cranial interface: implications and clinical considerations. Eur Arch Otorhinolaryngol 2014;271(8):2197–203.
4. Sellari-Franceschini S, Berrettini S, Santoro A, et al. Orbital decompression in graves' ophthalmopathy by medial and lateral wall removal. Otolaryngol Head Neck Surg 2005;133(2):185–9.
5. Emanuelli E, Bignami M, Digilio E, et al. Post-traumatic optic neuropathy: our surgical and medical protocol. Eur Arch Otorhinolaryngol 2014. http://dx.doi.org/10.1007/s00405-014-3408-5.
6. Tomazic PV, Stammberger H, Habermann W, et al. Intraoperative medialization of medial rectus muscle as a new endoscopic technique for approaching intraconal lesions. Am J Rhinol Allergy 2011;25(5):363–7.
7. Castelnuovo P, Dallan I, Locatelli D, et al. Endoscopic endonasal intraorbital surgery: our experience with 16 cases. Eur Arch Otorhinolaryngol 2012;269:1929–35.
8. Turri-Zanoni M, Dallan I, Terranova P, et al. Frontoethmoidal and intraorbital osteomas: exploring the limits of the endoscopic approach. Arch Otolaryngol Head Neck Surg 2012;138(5):498–504.
9. Dallan I, Castelnuovo P, de Notaris M, et al. Endoscopic endonasal anatomy of the superior orbital fissure and orbital apex regions: critical considerations for clinical applications. Eur Arch Otorhinolaryngol 2013;270(5):1643–9.
10. Dallan I, Seccia V, Lenzi R, et al. Transnasal approach to the medial intraconal space: anatomic study and clinical considerations. Minim Invasive Neurosurg 2010;53:164–8.
11. Karligkiotis A, Appiani MC, Verillaud B, et al. How to prevent diplopia in endoscopic transnasal

resection of tumors involving the medial orbital wall. Laryngoscope 2014;124(9):2017–20.

12. Lund VJ, Rose GE. Endoscopic transnasal orbital decompression for visual failure due to sphenoid wing meningioma. Eye (Lond) 2006; 20(10):1213–9.

13. Sieskiewicz A, Lyson T, Mariak Z, et al. Endoscopic trans-nasal approach for biopsy of orbital tumours using image-guided neuro-navigation system. Acta Neurochir (Wien) 2008;150(5):441–5.

14. McKinney KA, Snyderman CH, Carrau RL, et al. Seeing the light: endoscopic endonasal intraconal orbital tumor surgery. Otolaryngol Head Neck Surg 2010;143:699–701.

15. Gavriel H, Kessler A, Eviatar E. Management implications of diagnosing orbital abscess as subperiosteal orbital abscess. Rhinology 2010; 48(1):90–4.

16. Murchison AP, Rosen MR, Evans JJ, et al. Endo-scopic approach to the orbital apex and periorbital skull base. Laryngoscope 2011;121(3):463–7.

17. Karaki M, Akiyama K, Kagawa M, et al. Indications and limitations of endoscopic endonasal orbitotomy for orbital lesion. J Craniofac Surg 2012;23(4):1093–6.

18. Netuka D, Masopust V, Belšán T, et al. Endoscopic endonasal resection of medial orbital lesions with in-traoperative MRI. Acta Neurochir (Wien) 2013; 155(3):455–61.

19. Berhouma M, Jacquesson T, Abouaf L, et al. Endoscopic endonasal optic nerve and orbital apex decompression for nontraumatic optic neurop-athy: surgical nuances and review of the literature. Neurosurg Focus 2014;37(4):E19.

20. Andaluz N, Romano A, Reddy LV, et al. Eyelid approach to the anterior cranial base. J Neurosurg 2008;109(2):341–6.

21. Bly RA, Ramakrishna R, Ferreira M, et al. Lateral transorbital neuroendoscopic approach to the lateral cavernous sinus. J Neurol Surg B Skull Base 2014;75(1):11–7.

22. Chen HI, Bohman LE, Loevner LA, et al. Transorbital endoscopic amygdalohippocampectomy: a feasibility investigation. J Neurosurg 2014;120(6):1428–36.

Endoscopic Endonasal Resection of Trigeminal Schwannomas

Shaan M. Raza, MD[a], Muhamad A. Amine, MD, MS[b],
Vijay Anand, MD[b], Theodore H. Schwartz, MD[b,c,d],*

KEYWORDS

- Trigeminal • Schwannoma • Endoscopic • Skull base • Transpterygoid

KEY POINTS

- Trigeminal schwannomas may appear anywhere along the length of the nerve.
- The endoscopic endonasal transpterygoid approaches provide a direct trajectory with a minimized risk to the trigeminal nerve, abducens nerve, and carotid artery.
- Significant posterior fossa extension or large (>2.5 cm) tumors may be better suited by an alternative or additional approach.
- Complete resection is curative and should be accomplished without causing additional morbidity.

INTRODUCTION: NATURE OF THE PROBLEM

Although only accounting for up to 0.36% of all intracranial neoplasms and often histologically benign lesions, trigeminal schwannomas (TNs) pose significant challenges in their surgical management.[1,2] TNs can occur anywhere along the course of the trigeminal ganglion, root, and nerve branches; consequently, they can exist in the posterior fossa (PPF), middle fossa/Meckel cave, and extend along V1 into the orbit, V2 into the pterygopalatine fossa, and V3 into the infratemporal fossa (ITF). Additionally, they can be intradural, interdural, and extradural. In addition to their involvement of multiple compartments, the surgical resection of TNs can be complicated by an intimate association with surrounding cranial nerves (ie, abducens nerve) and carotid artery depending on their site of origin along the trigeminal nerve system.

Given the benign histology, a gross total resection can be considered curative, providing patients with the best long-term progression-free and overall survival. Hence, the goal of surgery is considered to be a gross total resection as long as this can be done safely with no neurovascular morbidity. However, radiosurgery is also effective in the treatment of TNs and can be included in the treatment algorithm. In some cases, leaving tumor behind for radiosurgery may be acceptable. A spectrum of surgical approaches has been proposed based on the anatomic extent of the tumor.[1,3,4] For the purposes of approach selection, it is best to classify lesions based on their compartmental involvement. For disease involving the Meckel cave and/or the peripheral V2 and V3 trunks, the endoscopic endonasal transpterygoid approaches provide a direct trajectory with a minimized risk to the trigeminal nerve, abducens nerve, and carotid artery. This idea is based on several publications reporting

[a] Department of Neurosurgery, The University of Texas MD Anderson Cancer Center, 1515 Holcombe Boulevard, Houston, TX 77030, USA; [b] Department of Otolaryngology, Weill Cornell Medical College, New York–Presbyterian Hospital, East 68th Street, New York, NY 10065, USA; [c] Department of Neurosurgery, Weill Cornell Medical College, New York–Presbyterian Hospital, East 68th Street, New York, NY 10065, USA; [d] Department of Neuroscience, Weill Cornell Medical College, New York–Presbyterian Hospital, East 68th Street, New York, NY 10065, USA
* Corresponding author. Departments of Neurosurgery, Otolaryngology, and Neuroscience, Weill Cornell Medical College, New York–Presbyterian Hospital, 525 East 68th Street, Box 99, New York, NY 10065.
E-mail address: schwarh@med.cornell.edu

Neurosurg Clin N Am 26 (2015) 473–479
http://dx.doi.org/10.1016/j.nec.2015.03.010
1042-3680/15/$ – see front matter © 2015 Elsevier Inc. All rights reserved.

the use of endonasal approaches to Meckel cave in addition to the authors' own experience with this technique for the resection of TNs.[5–8]

INDICATIONS/CONTRAINDICATIONS

The indications for surgical intervention

- Demonstrated growth of a diagnosed tumor on surveillance imaging
- A newly diagnosed lesion with associated symptoms, which would include trigeminal neuropathy (sensory or motor), diplopia related to an abducens nerve palsy, compressive optic neuropathy
- The lack of medical comorbidities that would prohibit surgery and anesthesia

The indications for an endoscopic transpterygoid resection

- Tumor involving the trigeminal ganglion (Meckel cave), V2 trunk (pterygopalatine fossa), and V3 trunk (infratemporal fossa)
- Limited posterior fossa involvement (note, this is a relative contraindication; see later discussion)

The relative contraindications for an endoscopic transpterygoid resection

- There is significant disease extension into the posterior fossa; the risk of sixth nerve injury is elevated within the posterior fossa via an expanded endoscopic approach (EEA) because of the relationship of the trigeminal trunk to the abducens nerve proximal to the Gruber ligament.[9] However, it is possible to remove limited posterior fossa intradural disease safely based on the skill and experience of the surgeon.
- There is involvement of the peripheral V1 trunk in the orbit. Disease within the orbit will ultimately lie above the optic nerve within the apex and is difficult to reach safely via an EEA.
- The tumor size is larger than 2.5 cm within the Meckel cave and middle cranial fossa.
- It is contraindicated in patients with preexisting V1 neuropathy. The slightly elevated risk of vidian nerve injury with a transpterygoid approach can place patients at risk for a postoperative corneal keratopathy if they have diminished corneal sensation.[6,7]

SURGICAL TECHNIQUE/PROCEDURE
Preoperative Planning

- A detailed preoperative neurologic examination should be performed with attention to the function of the involved trigeminal nerve and its divisions, including evidence of corneal anesthesia (V1 neuropathy), numbness in the V2 or V3 distribution, or masseter weakness/jaw deviation (V3 motor dysfunction).[5,6,10]
- Preoperative imaging should include an MRI scan with thin cuts through the skull base. Imaging is assessed for the tumor site of origin and which anatomic compartments are involved. With regard to the endoscopic approaches, tumor extension into the posterior fossa and into the orbit becomes difficult to manage with this approach. Additionally, on coronal imaging, the size of the tumor should be studied; tumors with large middle cranial fossa components may be more suitable for a transcranial approach.
- Although not obtained on all patients, on a case-by-case basis, the authors obtain CT angiography to determine the caliber of the adjacent segments of the internal carotid artery (ICA) (paraclival and cavernous segments). Additional information regarding the bony anatomy can be ascertained to provide an idea of the extent of drilling necessary for the surgical approach.

Preparation and Patient Positioning

- After anesthesia induction and before lumbar drain placement and fluorescein injection, patients are premedicated with dexamethasone (10 mg) and diphenhydramine (50 mg). Lumbar drains are generally used for patients in whom a high-flow cerebrospinal fluid (CSF) leak is expected (ie, patients with intradural tumors). Patients receive 0.25 mL of 10% intrathecal fluorescein (AK-Fluor). Fluorescein is diluted with 10 mL of CSF and administered over several minutes.
- Cotton patties with 4% cocaine are placed into the nose to allow for mucosal decongestion and topical anesthesia.
- After rigid fixation of the patients' head in Mayfield pins, the head is slightly extended and rotated to the right and surgery is commenced. The patients' face and abdomen are prepped and draped in a sterile fashion in case a fat graft is needed.

Surgical Approach for Disease Within Meckel Cave and/or Restricted to V2

- Starting with a rigid 0° endoscope, the uncinate process, vertical lamella of the ipsilateral middle turbinate, and sphenopalatine foramen are infiltrated with 1% lidocaine with 1:100,000 epinephrine to vasoconstrict the branches of the sphenopalatine artery. Care is made to not infiltrate the vascular pedicle on the side where the nasoseptal flap will be harvested.

- A nasoseptal flap is harvested contralateral to the lesion based on a sphenopalatine artery pedicle. The dimensions of the flap are maximized by extending incisions onto the hard palate toward the inferior turbinate (maximizing width) and anteriorly toward the columella (ensuring adequate length). However, the extent of the anticipated defect should be determined before harvesting the flap in order to avoid reconstructing with a flap that is too bulky for the final defect. This final flap is stored in the nasopharynx for the duration of the approach and resection.

- Focusing attention back to the supravidian transpterygoid exposure (**Fig. 1**), an anterior and posterior ethmoidectomy and sphenoidotomy is performed after which a transmaxillary corridor is developed. This procedure commences with an uncinectomy, middle turbinate resection, and wide maxillary antrostomy. The completeness of the antrostomy is determined once the infraorbital

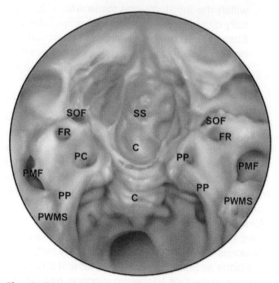

Fig. 1. Bony structures encountered during a transpterygoid approach to Meckel cave. C, clivus; FR, foramen rotundum; PC, pterygoid canal; PMF, pterygomaxillary fissure; PP, pterygoid process; PWMS, posterior wall of maxillary sinus; SOF, superior orbital fissure; SS, sphenoid sinus. (*From* Hofstetter CP, Singh A, Anand VK, et al. The endoscopic, endonasal, transmaxillary transpterygoid approach to the pterygopalatine fossa, infratemporal fossa, petrous apex and the Meckel cave. J Neurosurg 2010;113(5):968; with permission.)

neurovascular bundle can be adequately visualized along the roof of the maxillary sinus.

- The sphenopalatine artery is then cauterized and selectively cut after which the vertical and orbital processes of the palatine bone (posterior maxillary sinus wall) (**Fig. 2**) are removed using a diamond hybrid drill bit, Kerrison punches, and bone curettes. Once the bone is removed, the periosteal layer covering the contents of the pterygopalatine fossa is opened. For resection of V3 disease extending into the infratemporal fossa, PPF dissection is required (*described later*). Otherwise, for the management of disease along V2 or primarily within the middle fossa/Meckel cave, the contents of the PPF are merely retracted laterally to identify the vidian nerve at the junction of the sphenoid sinus floor and medial pterygoid plate.

- A supravidian approach, preserving the vidian nerve, is used for accessing Meckel cave, minimizing the risk of postoperative corneal injury in patients with V1 neuropathy. Using a diamond drill bit, the vidian nerve can be exposed back to the junction of the paraclival and laceral ICA. Once this depth has been determined, the pterygoid wedge (anterior junction of the medial and lateral pterygoid plates) is exposed. When viewed en face, V2/foramen rotundum is identified along the superior aspect of the wedge and is another key landmark. At this point, a tailored pterygoid resection is performed in a superior-to-inferior and medial-to-lateral fashion. This portion of the approach exposes the quadrangular space, which is bound by the carotid artery medially and inferiorly and by the maxillary nerve laterally. The ophthalmic branch of the trigeminal nerve and the abducens nerve traverse along the superior aspect of this anatomic compartment.

- For larger tumors or if access to the posterior fossa is required, then the paraclival and laceral segments of the ICA are fully skeletonized using a combination of endoscopic drills and dissections in order to facilitate safe retraction; otherwise, a full carotid dissection is not required for smaller lesions.

Surgical Approach for Disease Along V3 Extending into the Infratemporal Fossa

- Access into the infratemporal fossa and/or lateral aspect of the middle cranial fossa is required for disease involvement of the mandibular branch (V3) of the trigeminal nerve. This compartment is delineated by

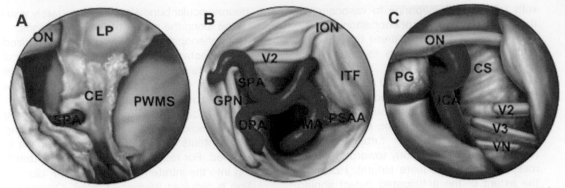

Fig. 2. Key steps in the transpterygoid approach. (*A*) After completion of the ethmoidectomy and sphenoidotomy, the maxillary antrostomy is enlarged to expose the posterior wall of the maxillary sinus. The sphenopalatine artery (SPA) emerges through the crista ethmoidalis (CE). (*B*) The contents of the PPF include the internal maxillary artery (IMA), which gives rise to the SPA and descending palatine artery (DPA) as well as the posterosuperior alveolar artery (PSAA). The pterygopalatine ganglion is found at the intersection of the greater palatine nerve (GPN) and the second division of the trigeminal nerve (V2). The infraorbital nerve (ION) and IFT can be seen laterally. (*C*) Removal of the pterygoid process and CE provides exposure to the medial and posterior to the PPF covered by the lateral wall of the sphenoid sinus. Removal of this bone reveals the medial wall of the cavernous sinus (CS) as well as the second (V2) and third (V3) divisions of the trigeminal nerve and the vidian nerve (VN), often used as a landmark to identify the internal carotid artery (ICA). ITF, infratemporal fossa; LP, lamina papyrcea; ON, optic nerve; PG, pituitary gland; PWMS, posterior wall of maxillary sinus. (*From* Hofstetter CP, Singh A, Anand VK, et al. The endoscopic, endonasal, transmaxillary transpterygoid approach to the pterygopalatine fossa, infratemporal fossa, petrous apex and the Meckel cave. J Neurosurg 2010;113(5):968; with permission.)

the lateral pterygoid plate medially, mandible laterally, styloid diaphragm/stylopharyngeal aponeurosis posteriorly, and the PPF/posterior maxillary sinus wall anteriorly. Anterior to the styloid diaphragm, the ITF contains the medial and lateral pterygoid musculature and the V3 along with its trunks and divisions.

- In order to gain access to the ITF, after completion of the maxillary window, the greater and lesser palatine nerves must be exposed and transposed from their canal within the vertical portion of the palatine bone.
- Once the PPF is exposed as described earlier, the periosteum is opened and branches of the internal maxillary artery are sequentially clipped. Once this has been completed, the vidian nerve is identified and transected. This maneuver allows full inferior and lateral transposition of the PPF in order to gain access to the infratemporal fossa.
- The lateral pterygoid plate is then dissected in a subperiosteal fashion in order to separate the inferior head of the lateral pterygoid muscle to avoid bleeding from the pterygoid venous plexus. Any venous bleeding at this point can be dealt with using standard hemostatic agents.
- Dissecting along the lateral pterygoid plate in an anterior-to-posterior fashion, the foramen ovale will be identified at the skull base along

with V3 and any associated tumor. Disease within the infratemporal fossa with TNs typically displace the pterygoid muscles laterally, Eustachian tube (and associated musculature) posteriorly and the styloid diaphragm posteriorly; these adjacent structures must be identified and can be safely dissected away.

Tumor Resection

Tumor resection proceeds using standard microsurgical techniques (**Fig. 3**). Based on the growth of the tumor, the trigeminal nerve and any associated branches are displaced superiorly and laterally toward the middle cranial fossa. Depending on the coronal plane, the sixth nerve has a variable course. More distally, particular attention should be paid along the superior aspect of the tumor where the abducens nerve is displaced. When in the same coronal plane as Meckel cave, CN VI lies just above the superior aspect of V1; when working toward the posterior fossa, the nerve can lie more along the medial aspect of the tumor and within the posterior fossa, the nerve lies inferomedial.

Closure

- A multilayer closure is used generally for all skull base reconstructions although extradural tumors may require little by way of closure absent a CSF leak.[11,12] Clearly, the

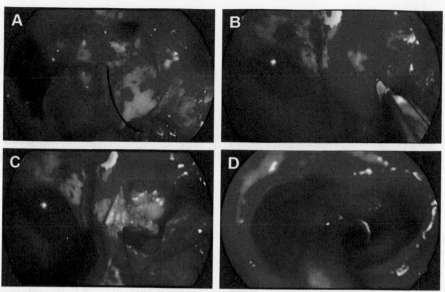

Fig. 3. (*A*) View obtained after sphenoidotomy, maxillary antrostomy, opening, and transposition of the PPF contents were performed. Note the expanded appearance of Meckel cave because of the tumor. Paraclival ICA, solid red line; medial and inferior borders of Meckel cave, solid black line. (*B*) After removing the ventral and medial bone overlying Meckel cave, the authors incised the periosteal dura to gain access to tumor. (*C*) The tumor was internally debulked. (*D*) After resection of the tumor capsule, the gasserian ganglion is visible. (*From* Raza SM, Donaldson AM, Mehta A, et al. Surgical management of trigeminal schwannomas: defining the role for endoscopic endonasal approaches. Neurosurg Focus 2014;37(4):E17; with permission.)

risk of a CSF leak is lower for TNs within the Meckel cave/PPF/ITF; the meningeal dural layer is often not breached during surgery and can serve as a barrier against a high-flow leak. Of course, the risk of a CSF leak is higher with disease extension into the posterior fossa.

- If there is no CSF leak, thrombin-soaked Gelfoam (Baxter International, Inc) or Floseal (Baxter International Inc, Deerfield, IL) can be used for hemostasis and this may be sufficient.
- If there is a CSF leak, typically, a fat graft is placed into the resection cavity and then covered by a nasoseptal flap harvested earlier in the procedure. The flap is then covered with DuraSeal (Covidien, Waltham, MA), at the authors' institution, to keep it in place, although other institutions have described the use of a Foley balloon.
- Particular attention should be paid to any exposed segments of the carotid artery; exposed vasculature should be covered with the reconstruction.
- A limited time period (24–48 hours) of postoperative lumbar drainage is used in situations when a high-flow CSF leak was encountered.

POSTOPERATIVE CARE

The postoperative care of patients who have undergone an endoscopic endonasal resection is no different than from standard EEA care. Perioperative antibiotics (ie, cefazolin) are administered for 24 hours after resection; an MRI scan, to assess the extent of resection, is obtained before discharge. After discharge, patients are seen at predetermined time intervals (ie, 10 days, 3 weeks, and so forth) for debridement of nasal crusting. Of particular concern to those with postoperative trigeminal neuropathy, patients with V1 neuropathy should be carefully assessed for corneal anesthesia or dry eyes if there is iatrogenic vidian nerve sacrifice; natural tears are prescribed in such situations to prevent corneal keratopathy.

OUTCOMES

Because of the limited number of cases performed at any one center, there are limited data published regarding the endoscopic endonasal resection of TNs. A recent study published by Raza and colleagues[6] reported a case series of 4 patients after endoscopic resection (**Fig. 4**). All patients had disease within the Meckel cave, and 1 patient had

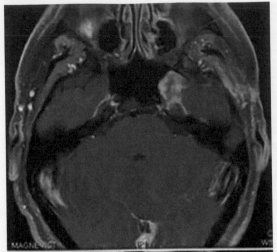

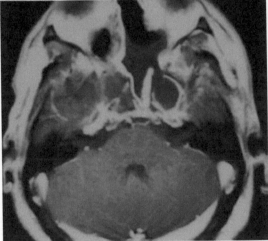

Fig. 4. (*Upper*) Preoperative T1-weighted MRI with contrast demonstrating and enhancing mass restricted to Meckel cave. (*Lower*) Postoperative T1-weighted MRI with contrast confirming gross total resection. (*From* Raza SM, Donaldson AM, Mehta A, et al. Surgical management of trigeminal schwannomas: defining the role for endoscopic endonasal approaches. Neurosurg Focus 2014;37(4):E17; with permission.)

tumor extension into the posterior fossa. In the reported series, volumetric analysis of preoperative and postoperative MRI was performed in order to determine the extent of resection of different anatomic compartments. Additionally, clinical charts were reviewed for postoperative clinical outcomes. The results indicated that gross total resection was achieved in 100% of Meckel cave involvement; in the one patient with posterior fossa extension, gross total resection was achieved with the Meckel cave portion of the tumor, whereas only 52% of the posterior fossa component was resected. Shin and colleagues[7] similarly reported

their experience of nonvestibular schwannomas resected via endoscopic endonasal techniques. In this cohort, there were 11 patients with TNs whereby 4 had primarily middle fossa disease, 2 had combined middle–posterior fossa disease, 3 had combined middle fossa–extracranial disease, and 2 had isolated extracranial disease. Those patients with posterior fossa components to their disease underwent 2 stage resections with a retrosigmoid approach. In this series, the rate of gross total resection was 63% with a postoperative trigeminal neuropathy (sensory and/or motor) rate of 45%.

Adverse cranial nerve events were noted in 2 instances in the Raza and colleagues[6] series, highlighting the limitations of endoscopic endonasal resection versus laterally based cranial base approaches. An iatrogenic sixth nerve injury occurred during an endoscopic transpterygoid suprapetrous approach to the posterior fossa component of a patient's tumor; the rate of such injury was 9% in the report by Shin and colleagues.[7] This injury is thought to have occurred because of the complicated anatomic course of the abducens nerve in relation to the trigeminal nerve. Within the posterior fossa, the abducens nerve lies inferomedial to the trigeminal nerve as it courses up to Dorello canal.[9] At the coronal plane of the petroclinoid ligament, the nerve is directly medial to the gasserian ganglion and within the cavernous sinus and anteriorly; it then lies just medial and superior to V1, the superior most extent of the trigeminal system along the lateral cavernous sinus wall. Given the anatomic trajectory of the sixth cranial nerve, the management of posterior fossa disease represents a limitation of the endoscopic approaches relative to the transpetrosal or retrosigmoid approach.

Another nerve-related adverse event was 1 incident of corneal keratopathy in a patient with a preoperative V1 neuropathy. As a result of an iatrogenic vidian nerve deficit, preexisting corneal anesthesia compounded by diminished lacrimation yielded significant corneal problems requiring a tarsorrhaphy. The rate of postresection dry eye was 54% in the Shin and colleagues[7] series. Given the consequences of postoperative vidian nerve dysfunction from a transpterygoid approach, significant attention is paid to preserving this neurovascular bundle. In situations when vidian nerve preservation is less likely (ie, when infratemporal fossa exposure is required) and there is a presenting V1 neuropathy, a transcranial skull base approach is likely to provide a better outcome with regard to corneal sensation.

With regard to open cranial base approaches in managing all anatomic categories of TNs, the reported outcomes in the larger series demonstrate gross total resection rates between 70% and 83%, new cranial nerve injury rates ranging from 1.4% to 33.0%, and worsened trigeminal neuropathy incidences of 11.6% to 33.0%.[1–4,13–17] Based on the early outcomes from endoscopic endonasal approaches, it is evident that the open and endoscopic skull base approaches provide complementary approaches through which optimal outcomes can be achieved. The laterally based open skull base approaches (ie, orbitozygomatic, transpetrosal, retrosigmoid suprameatal approach) seem to be well suited either for larger tumors with posterior fossa disease, tumors with extension along V1, or in patients with preoperative V1 neuropathy. The endoscopic approaches preliminarily have improved outcomes for smaller tumors restricted to the middle fossa and those lesions with extracranial extension along V2 and V3.

SUMMARY

The surgical management of TNs poses unique challenges because of the anatomic diversity encountered, the varied goals of treatment, and the multiple cranial nerve functions at risk because of the varied relationship along different compartments of the skull base. Although the reported outcomes for expanded endoscopic resections are based on smaller retrospective series, the limited data support a role for endoscopic transpterygoid resection for tumors isolated to the Meckel cave, tumors with middle fossa–extracranial extension, or tumors with pure extracranial involvement along V2 or V3. As with many skull base diagnoses, ideal surgical management does require an understanding of complementary open skull base and radiosurgical techniques.

REFERENCES

1. Samii M, Migliori MM, Tatagiba M, et al. Surgical treatment of trigeminal schwannomas. J Neurosurg 1995;82:711–8.

2. Yoshida K, Kawase T. Trigeminal neurinomas extending into multiple fossae: surgical methods and review of the literature. J Neurosurg 1999;91:202–11.

3. Day JD, Fukushima T. The surgical management of trigeminal neuromas. Neurosurgery 1998;42:233–40 [discussion: 40–1].

4. Wanibuchi M, Fukushima T, Zomordi AR, et al. Trigeminal schwannomas: skull base approaches and operative results in 105 patients. Neurosurgery 2012;70:132–43 [discussion: 43–4].

5. Kassam AB, Prevedello DM, Carrau RL, et al. The front door to Meckel's cave: an anteromedial corridor via expanded endoscopic endonasal approach-technical considerations and clinical series. Neurosurgery 2009;64:ONS71–82 [discussion: ONS3].

6. Raza SM, Donaldson AM, Mehta A, et al. Surgical management of trigeminal schwannomas: defining the role for endoscopic endonasal approaches. Neurosurg Focus 2014;37:E17.

7. Shin SS, Gardner PA, Stefko ST, et al. Endoscopic endonasal approach for nonvestibular schwannomas. Neurosurgery 2011;69:1046–57 [discussion: 57].

8. Van Rompaey J, Suruliraj A, Carrau R, et al. Meckel's cave access: anatomic study comparing the endoscopic transantral and endonasal approaches. Eur Arch Otorhinolaryngol 2014;271:787–94.

9. Barges-Coll J, Fernandez-Miranda JC, Prevedello DM, et al. Avoiding injury to the abducens nerve during expanded endonasal endoscopic surgery: anatomic and clinical case studies. Neurosurgery 2010;67:144–54 [discussion: 54].

10. Hofstetter CP, Singh A, Anand VK, et al. The endoscopic, endonasal, transmaxillary transpterygoid approach to the pterygopalatine fossa, infratemporal fossa, petrous apex, and the Meckel cave. J Neurosurg 2010;113:967–74.

11. McCoul ED, Anand VK, Singh A, et al. Long-term effectiveness of a reconstructive protocol using the nasoseptal flap after endoscopic skull base surgery. World Neurosurg 2014;81:136–43.

12. Patel KS, Komotar RJ, Szentirmai O, et al. Case-specific protocol to reduce cerebrospinal fluid leakage after endonasal endoscopic surgery. J Neurosurg 2013;119:661–8.

13. Goel A, Muzumdar D, Raman C. Trigeminal neuroma: analysis of surgical experience with 73 cases. Neurosurgery 2003;52:783–90 [discussion: 90].

14. Guthikonda B, Theodosopoulos PV, van Loveren H, et al. Evolution in the assessment and management of trigeminal schwannoma. Laryngoscope 2008;118:195–203.

15. Hasegawa T, Kato T, Iizuka H, et al. Long-term results for trigeminal schwannomas treated with gamma knife surgery. Int J Radiat Oncol Biol Phys 2013;87:1115–21.

16. Pollack IF, Sekhar LN, Jannetta PJ, et al. Neurilemomas of the trigeminal nerve. J Neurosurg 1989;70:737–45.

17. Taha JM, Tew JM Jr, van Loveren HR, et al. Comparison of conventional and skull base surgical approaches for the excision of trigeminal neurinomas. J Neurosurg 1995;82:719–25.

Index

Note: Page numbers of article titles are in **boldface** type.

Neurosurg Clin N Am 26 (2015) 481–486
http://dx.doi.org/10.1016/S1042-3680(15)00037-6
1042-3680/15/$ – see front matter © 2015 Elsevier Inc. All rights reserved.

Moving?

Make sure your subscription moves with you!

To notify us of your new address, find your **Clinics Account Number** (located on your mailing label above your name), and contact customer service at:

Email: journalscustomerservice-usa@elsevier.com

800-654-2452 (subscribers in the U.S. & Canada)
314-447-8871 (subscribers outside of the U.S. & Canada)

Fax number: 314-447-8029

Elsevier Health Sciences Division
Subscription Customer Service
3251 Riverport Lane
Maryland Heights, MO 63043

Printed and bound by CPI Group (UK) Ltd, Croydon, CR0 4YY

14/10/2024

01773630-0001